Manual of Simulation in Healthcare

Manual of Simulation in Healthcare

SECOND EDITION

Edited by

Richard H. Riley

School of Medicine and Pharmacology,
University of Western Australia

and

Department of Anaesthesia and Pain Medicine
Royal Perth Hospital, Australia

OXFORD
UNIVERSITY PRESS

OXFORD

UNIVERSITY PRESS

Great Clarendon Street, Oxford, OX2 6DP,
United Kingdom

Oxford University Press is a department of the University of Oxford.
It furthers the University's objective of excellence in research, scholarship,
and education by publishing worldwide. Oxford is a registered trade mark of
Oxford University Press in the UK and in certain other countries

First Edition published in 2008
Second Edition published in 2016

Impression: 1

Published in the United States of America by Oxford University Press
198 Madison Avenue, New York, NY 10016, United States of America

British Library Cataloguing in Publication Data

Data available

Library of Congress Control Number: 2015944564

ISBN 978–0–19–871762–1

Printed in Great Britain by
Clays Ltd, St Ives plc

Foreword to the first edition

There is a long history of using simple devices to simulate the real experience in healthcare education. A simple example would be teaching students to handle needles and sutures using a pig's foot or a piece of simulated skin. A more complex example is the use of the famous Resusci Anne™ to teach a partial task such as chest compressions associated with positive-pressure ventilation. The development of sophisticated, instrumented, mannequins coupled with computerized physiology and pharmacology programmes began a new era in healthcare simulation. These new mannequins had the ability to react to student interventions in a realistic and automatic manner not requiring instructor intervention. The mannequins were originally developed and popularized within the field of anaesthesiology. It was quickly realized that not only could these mannequins be used to simulate an anaesthetist's interaction with a patient but also that they can be used for team-building situations leading to the development of 'crisis resource management'. In the short period of the past two decades, the use of mannequins to create simulated experiences has been adopted by diverse healthcare providers including nursing, various medical subspecialties, and other allied health providers.

Healthcare educational institutions around the world are recognizing the need for providing their students with simulated experiences not only to enhance the educational experience but also to improve on patient safety. When embarking on the development of a simulation centre, some of the questions inevitably asked are:

+ How large should the centre be?
+ What types of rooms do I need in a simulation centre?
+ How will I run the centre?
+ What equipment should I buy?
+ Who will the users be?

Dr Riley has chosen contributors for this book who have the experience necessary to answer these questions. Section one provides simulation centre logistics, section two discusses the various equipment available, and section four addresses the needs of the different subspecialties.

For me, the most important section of this book is section three—Education Components. A machine is simply a machine unless it is integrated into the learning environment using sound educational principles. The question concerning educational integration of the simulation modalities is often left off the initial list when planning a simulation programme. Dr Riley needs to be congratulated for devoting a large section of this book to education; education is the pivotal element in determining a centre's success.

2008
David H Wilks MD
Professor and Chair
Department of Anesthesiology
West Virginia University
School of Medicine

Foreword to the second edition

Confucius made the case for the utility of simulation and debriefing some 2,500 years ago by observing that real experience, however profound in nature, was always tinged with risk or potential harm. He suggested that rehearsing or imitating practice was perhaps a sensible and pragmatic way to mitigate some of this experiential risk. Perhaps even more importantly Confucius also highlighted that without meaningful reflection all activity runs the risk of being meaningless . . . So from across antiquity Confucius offers wisdom as to the potential utility of simulation in professional education.

His analysis of wisdom would appear to support the fundamental importance of experiential learning; he makes a clear case for emulation and rehearsal and highlights the utility of debriefing and reflective practice. All of these concepts are basic tenets of adult and humanistic learning and deeply enshrined in contemporary thinking in simulation-based education.

It would appear, therefore, that the concepts underpinning the value of simulation are nothing new!

In modern times simulation has become established as a major educational modality in healthcare education. Over the last decade simulation has moved from being an emergent and disruptive educational innovation into a mainstream element of most healthcare curricula. This renaissance has been fuelled in part by the enthusiasm, evangelism, and passion of many of the early adopters and advocates of simulation. Organizations have also been keen to demonstrate their innovative credentials by boarding the innovation bandwagon. Many such initiatives or programmes have brought about a stepwise improvement and transformation of healthcare education.

Not all strategies, however, have been so successful.

It is therefore timely and apposite that Richard Riley and colleagues have taken the opportunity afforded by a second edition to bring their original and trusted text up to date. This edition brings current advances in contemporary simulation practice and thinking into one place.

Effective simulation-based education is a complex and challenging field of educational practice. It is a wide family of educational techniques and technologies, contexts, and applications with many distinct forms, opportunities, and challenges. These are explored and considered in detail throughout the new edition.

This second edition offers many hard won insights, experiences, and learning from an international cadre of simulation experts. They share learning from their successes but with a commendable degree of openness and humility; they offer their cautions and mistakes so providing the reader with the unique opportunity to learn from their wisdom and experience.

rous offering of innovative and thoughtful insights from many
on in healthcare. Further this manual reflects that simulation
acteristics of a maturing field of academic practice, the ini-
usiasm replaced by principle and concept, construct, and utility.
criticality, collegiality, and community reflected in this new edition sug-
that simulation has now come of age as an academic discipline.

expect that this book will find a prominent home in the offices and centres of those engaged in high quality, simulation-based education.

Confucius could only wonder at the technology available today but in many ways I suspect he would immediately recognize and approve of the current application and utility of simulation in healthcare.

2015
Ian Curran
Professor of Innovation and Excellence in Healthcare Education
Queen Mary University of London

Preface to the first edition

The idea for this manual came to me during the inaugural Simulation and Skills Training Special Interest Group of the Australian and New Zealand College of Anaesthetists held in Perth, September 2000. At that time the chief references for those of us who had entered the world of medical simulation were David Gaba's book *Crisis Management in Anesthesiology* and his chapter in Miller's textbook of *Anesthesia*. Learning how to use the commercially available medical simulators was achieved through attendance at Dr Gaba's ACRM Instructor's Course at Stanford and old-fashioned on-the-job practice. Subsequent discussions with colleagues in this growing field made it apparent that many of us were struggling with common problems but that there were some very creative solutions. However, the process of mustering these collective talents and experiences was quickly subdued by the pressures of teaching and administration in a new simulation centre.

My association with local and international simulation meetings not only enriched my knowledge of simulation in healthcare but also brought me into contact with many leaders in simulation. I am deeply grateful that many of these simulation leaders have kindly shared their expertise with us. Thanks must also go to hospital and organizational administrators and heads of departments who have supported the simulation community. I thank those who have mentored and inspired me: David Wilks, Myroslav Klain, Peter Winter, and Peter Safar. I also would like to thank Sara Chare, Clare Caruana, Eloise Moir-Ford, Anna Winstanley, Catherine Barnes, Georgia Pinteau, Kelly Hewinson, Kate Wanwimolruk, and the team from Oxford University Press who kept me on track. Finally, I wish to express thanks to my wife Vera who has been my support and strength through the simulation journey.

2008
Richard H Riley
Perth, Western Australia

Preface to the second edition

The response to the publication of the first edition of this manual has been gratifying. It has been more than enough reward to know that many have found it to be helpful as they seek to enhance their healthcare programmes with simulation-based education. For this edition, I had the sad task of replacing some sub-specialty areas with combined chapters and new topics. The advent of web-based storage has allowed us to supplement these paperback and digital editions with additional resources that are in current use at various simulation and skills centres.

Any success that this book achieves is due to these talented authors and I remain very thankful that they have shared their expertise with us. Further, I continue to learn from colleagues, educators, and students in the simulation community. If I have learnt only one thing from simulation, it is that the historic concept of a teacher and students as separate entities is not only wrong but that it can be a barrier to education. I cling to the hope that at some time in the distant future I will achieve some level of expertise in this field. I also would like to thank Caroline Smith, Nicola Wilson, James Cox, Cherline Daniel, Paul Nash and the team from Oxford University Press, who kept me on task; and Ian Curran and Brydon Dunstan. Thanks to David Gaba and Ray Page for being so inspirational. Finally, I thank my wife Vera who has been my support on the simulation journey.

Richard Riley
Perth, Western Australia 2015
Richard@pobox.com

Contents

List of Contributors

Dale C Alverson, MD
Professor Emeritus of Pediatrics and
Regents' Professor
Professor, Health Sciences Center Library
and Informatics Center
Medical Director, Center for
Telehealth and Cybermedicine
Research
University of New Mexico
Albuquerque, NM, US

Andrew Anderson
Chief Executive Officer
Association for Simulated Practice in
Healthcare (ASPiH)
Managing Director
Crawford Medical Limited
London, UK

Fernando Bello, BSc (Hons), PhD
Reader in Surgical Graphics &
Computing
Division of Surgery
Department of Surgery and Cancer
Imperial College London
Paterson Centre
St Marys Hospital
London, UK

Joshua S Botdorf, DO
Department of Medicine
Division of Pulmonary and Critical Care
Medicine
Mayo Clinic
Rochester, MN, US

John R Boulet, BSc, MA, PhD
Vice President, Research & Data Resources
Foundation for Advancement of
International Medical Education and
Research

Educational Commission for Foreign
Medical Graduates
Philadelphia, PA, US

**Col (ret) Mark W Bowyer, MD, FACS,
DMCC**
Ben Eiseman Professor of Surgery
Chief, Division of Trauma and Combat
Surgery
Surgical Director of Simulation
Uniformed Services University
Bethesda, MD, US

Thomas P Caudell, PhD
Professor
Department of Electrical & Computer
Engineering
Department of Computer Science
(secondary)
Department of Psychology (secondary)
University of New Mexico
Albuquerque, NM, US

**Chris Chin MBBS, FRCP, FRCA, MA
Clin Ed**
Staff Anesthesiologist
British Columbia Children's Hospital
Clinical Instructor, University of British
Columbia
Vancouver, BC, Canada

Jeffrey B Cooper, PhD
Professor of Anaesthesia
Harvard Medical School
Massachusetts General Hospital
Founder and Executive Director,
Center for Medical Simulation
Boston, MA, US

Robert Davies, MBBS, FRACS
Australian and New Zealand Surgical
Skills Education and Training Committee

Royal Australasian College of Surgeons
East Melbourne, VIC, Australia

COL Shad H Deering, MD, FACOG
Chair, Department of Obstetrics and
Gynecology
Uniformed Services University of the
Health Sciences
Bethesda, MD, US

Michael DeVita MD, FCCM
Director, Critical Care
Harlem Hospital Center
Assistant Professor, Internal Medicine
Columbia College of Physicians and
Surgeons
New York, NY, US

Mantosh Dewan, MD
Professor
Department of Neurosurgery
SUNY Upstate Medical University
Syracuse, NY, US

Thomas Dongilli, AT
Director of Operations, WISER
University of Pittsburgh
Pittsburgh, PA, US

William F Dunn, MD
Mayo Clinic Multidisciplinary
Simulation Center
Rochester, MN, US

Simon Edgar, MBChB, FRCA, MMed
Consultant Anaesthetist
Director of Medical Education NHS
Lothian, Edinburgh
Education Coordinator, Scottish Centre
for Simulation and Clinical Human
Factors (SCSCHF)
Stirling, UK

Anthony Errichetti, PhD
Chief of Virtual Medicine
Director, MS in Medical/Healthcare
Simulation Program

New York Institute of Technology-College
of Osteopathic Medicine
Old Westbury, NY, US

**Sheena M Ferguson, MSN, RN, CCRN,
CNS**
Chief Nursing Officer & Administrator
University of New Mexico Hospitals
Albuquerque, NM, US

Brendan Flanagan, MBBS, FANZCA
Department of Anaesthesia &
Perioperative Medicine
The Alfred Hospital
Melbourne, VIC, Australia

Rhona Flin, PhD
Chair of Applied Psychology
School of Psychology
University of Aberdeen
King's College
Aberdeen, UK

Janene H Fuerch, MD, FAAP
Fellow in Neonatal-Perinatal
Medicine
Division of Neonatal and Developmental
Medicine
Department of Pediatrics
Stanford University School of Medicine
Center for Advanced Pediatric and
Perinatal Education
Packard Children's Hospital at
Stanford
Palo Alto, CA, US

**Alexander (Sandy) Garden, MBChB,
PhD, FANZCA**
Rotational Supervisor
Department of Anaesthesia
Wellington Hospital
Adjunct Professor
School of Biological Sciences
Victoria University
Wellington, New Zealand

Timothy E Goldsmith, PhD
Associate Professor
Department of Psychology
University of New Mexico
Albuquerque, NM, US

Joseph S Goode Jr, CRNA, MSN
Faculty, University of Pittsburgh
School of Nursing
Department of Nurse Anesthesia
Staff Nurse Anesthetist, Presbyterian
Hospital
University of Pittsburgh Medical
Center
Pittsburgh, PA, US

Louis P Halamek, MD, FAAP
Professor and Associate Chief for Training
and Assessment
Division of Neonatal and Developmental
Medicine
Department of Pediatrics
Stanford University School of Medicine
Director, Center for Advanced Pediatric
and Perinatal Education
Packard Children's Hospital at Stanford
Stanford Children's Health
Palo Alto, CA, US

Jeffrey M Hamdorf, MBBS, PhD, FRACS
Winthrop Professor of Surgical
Education
Director, Clinical Training and Education
Centre
Head, School of Surgery
The University of Western Australia
Nedlands, WA, Australia

Cindy Hein, DipAppSc, BHSc, PhD
Extended Care Paramedic
SA Ambulance Service
Postdoctoral Research Fellow
Flinders University
Bedford Park, SA, Australia

**Chris Holland, MBBS, BAO, MMedEd,
FRCA, FFICM, FAcadMEd**
Consultant in Intensive Care
Director of Clinical Practice
Lecturer in Clinical Education
King's Healthcare Partners
London, UK

Ross Horley, CEng
Adjunct Lecturer, School of Medicine
University of Notre Dame Australia
Director, Medical Synergies Ltd
Stirling, WA, Australia

Yue Ming Huang, EdD, MHS
Education and Operations Director,
UCLA Simulation Center
Associate Adjunct Professor, Department
of Anesthesiology
David Geffen School of Medicine at UCLA
University of California,
Los Angeles, CA, US

**Russell W Jones, BSc, DipEd, BEd
(Hons), PhD**
Professor of Clinical Education, Edith
Cowan University
Professor of Clinical Education, Royal
Flying Doctor Service
Edith Cowan University
Joondalup, WA, Australia

Kianoush Kashani, MD, FASN, FCCP
Assistant Professor in Internal Medicine
Division of Nephrology and
Hypertension
Division of Pulmonary and Critical Care
Program Director—Critical Care Fellowship
Mayo Clinic Multidisciplinary Simulation
Center
Rochester, MN, US

**Roger Kneebone, PhD, FRCS, FRCSEd,
FRCGP**
Professor of Surgical Education

Division of Surgery
Department of Surgery and Cancer
Imperial College London Clinical Skills
Centre
St Marys Hospital
London, UK

Satish Krishnamurthy, MD
Professor
Department of Neurosurgery
SUNY Upstate Medical University
Syracuse, NY, US

Fiona Lake, MD, FRACP
Respiratory Physician, Sir Charles
Gairdner Hospital
Eric Saint Professor of Medicine
School of Medicine and
Pharmacology
The University of Western Australia
Crawley, WA, Australia

**Anthony R Lewis, BSc, PhD, MB BCh,
FRCA, FANZCA**
Consultant Anaesthetist
Department of Anaesthesia
St George Hospital
Director, iSimulate Pty Ltd
Sydney, NSW, Australia

Geoffrey K Lighthall MD, PhD
Associate Professor
Anesthesia and Critical Care
Stanford University School of
Medicine
Stanford, CA, US

Christine C Myo-Bui, MD
Assistant Clinical Professor
Department of Anesthesiology and
Perioperative Medicine
David Geffen School of Medicine at
UCLA
University of California,
Los Angeles, CA, US

Christine L Mai, MD
Instructor in Anaesthesia
Harvard Medical School
Massachusetts General Hospital
Boston, MA, US

Nicola Maran, MBChB, FRCA, FRCSEd
Consultant Anaesthetist
Associate Medical Director for Patient
Safety, NHS Lothian, Edinburgh, Scotland
Educational Coordinator, Scottish Centre
of Simulation and Clinical Human Factors,
NHS Forth Valley, Larbert, UK

Rima Matevosian, MD
Chair, Department of Anesthesiology
Olive View—UCLA Medical Center
Associate Dean
David Geffen School of Medicine at UCLA
University of California,
Los Angeles, CA, US

Al May, MBChB, FRCA, FCARCSI
Educational Coordinator
Scottish Centre for Simulation and
Clinical Human Factors
Larbert, UK

Rebecca D Minehart, MD
Assistant Professor in Anaesthesia
Harvard Medical School
Massachusetts General Hospital
Boston, MA, US

**Nicolette C Mininni, BSN, RN, MEd,
CCRN**
Advanced Clinical Education Specialist,
Critical Care
University of Pittsburgh Medical Center
UPMC Shadyside
Pittsburgh, PA, US

**Jonathan Mould, PhD, MSc, RSCN,
RGN, RMN, Adult Cert Ed**
Lecturer and Researcher, School of
Nursing, Midwifery and Paramedicine

Curtin University
WA, Australia

Robert P O'Brien, EdD, MEd, BA, BTeach
Honorary Senior Fellow
Melbourne Medical School
University of Melbourne
Melbourne, VIC, Australia

John M O'Donnell, CRNA, MSN, DrPH
Professor of Nursing and Chair,
Department of Nurse Anesthesia
Director, Nurse Anesthesia Program
Associate Director, WISER
University of Pittsburgh
Pittsburgh, PA, US

Harry Owen, MBBCh, MD, FANZCA
Professor, School of Medicine
Flinders University
Bedford Park, SA, Australia

Ray Page, Dip Radio Technology, Dip Television, Dip Industrial Electronics
Former Manager
Simulator Services
QANTAS Airways
past Chair, IATA Flight
Simulator Technical Committee
Inaugral Chair
Simulation Industry Association Australia
(SIAA)
Australia

Janice C Palaganas, PhD, RN, NP
Principal Faculty
Director of Educational Innovation and
Development
Center for Medical Simulation
Massachusetts General Hospital
Department of Anesthesia, Critical Care,
& Pain Medicine
Harvard Medical School
Boston, MA, US

Mary D Patterson MD, MEd
Medical Director for Simulation Center
for Safety and Reliability
Akron Children's Hospital
Professor of Pediatrics
Northeast Ohio Medical College
Akron, OH, US

Richard H Riley, MBBS, FANZCA
School of Medicine and Pharmacology
University of Western Australia
Anaesthesia and Pain Medicine
Royal Perth Hospital
Perth, WA, Australia

Brian Robinson, MSc, PhD
Senior Lecturer
Graduate School of Nursing, Midwifery &
Health Te Kura Tapuhi Hauora
Victoria University of Wellington
Wellington, New Zealand

Maria D D Rudolph, MD
Visiting Scholar
UCLA Simulation Center
David Geffen School of Medicine at
UCLA
University of California,
Los Angeles, CA, US

Chris Sadler, BSc, PhD (Physiol), MBBS, FRCA
Consultant Anaesthetist
Training Programme Director,
Barts & The London School
of Anaesthesia
Director of Strategy for Simulation &
Essential Clinical Skills
Barts Health, London, UK

Usha Satish, PhD
Professor
Department of Psychiatry
SUNY Upstate Medical University
Syracuse, NY, US

Julie A Schmidt, MSN, RN
Department of Nursing
Mayo Clinic
Rochester, MN, US

Robert Simon, EdD
Senior Director, Educational
Leadership & International
Programs, Center for Medical Simulation
Department of Anaesthesia, Critical Care,
and Pain Medicine
Massachusetts General Hospital
Harvard Medical School
Boston, MA, US

Cyle Sprick, BSc, PhD
Paramedic, South Australian Ambulance
Service
Director, Clinical Simulation
Unit
Flinders University
Bedford Park, SA, Australia.

Randolph H Steadman, MD, MS
Professor and Vice Chair
Department of Anesthesiology and
Perioperative Medicine
Director, UCLA Simulation Center
David Geffen School of Medicine
at UCLA
Los Angeles, CA, US

Nusrat Usman, MBChB, FRCA
Consultant Anaesthetist
Barts Health NHS Trust
London, UK

Iris Vardi, BAppSc, DipEd, MEd, PhD
Principal Consultant Higher Education
Director, Vardi Consulting
Perth, WA, Australia

John A Vozenilek, MD
Chief Medical Officer for Simulation
Jump Trading Simulation and Education
Center, OSF Healthcare System
Duane and Mary Cullinan Professor in
Simulation Outcomes
Associate Professor, Emergency
Medicine
University of Illinois College of Medicine
at Peoria
Associate Professor of Bioengineering
University of Illinois College of
Engineering Urbana Champaign, Peoria,
IL, US

**Leonie M Watterson, MB BS, FANZCA,
MClinEd**
Clinical Associate Professor, Sydney
Medical School, University of Sydney
Director, Sydney Clinical Skills and
Simulation Centre, Simulation
Division
Royal North Shore Hospital
St Leonards, NSW, Australia

**Jennifer M Weller, MD, MBBS, MClinEd,
FANZCA, FRCA**
Associate Professor and Head of
Centre for Medical and Health Sciences
Education
School of Medicine, University of
Auckland
Specialist Anaesthetist, Auckland City
Hospital
Auckland, New Zealand

Nicole K Yamada, MD, FAAP
Clinical Assistant Professor
Division of Neonatal and Developmental
Medicine
Department of Pediatrics
Stanford University School of Medicine
Associate Program Director, Center
for Advanced Pediatric and Perinatal
Education
Packard Children's Hospital at
Stanford
Palo Alto, CA, US

Part 1

Design, logistics, equipment, and history

Chapter 1

Lessons from aviation simulation

Ray Page

Overview

- Simulation was previously described as having achieved an integral role in the aviation industry. This role can now be described as **essential** for this industry.

- The standards developed by the industry have been maintained and regulation continues to evolve, driven by technological changes, and changes to the training environment brought about by developments in aircraft technology.

- Until relatively recently, aviators were required to manually fly their aircraft within very tight tolerances of just a few knots, and basic airmanship skills learned during initial training were maintained during operational flying. Now, automated control of aircraft flight parameters prevent a pilot from exceeding the flight envelope of the aircraft.

- With progression to fly-by-wire control of modern aircraft, the pilot is even further removed from the rigours of basic aircraft control and handling; unless some unforeseen event arises which suddenly requires skills that are not used in normal operation.

- The extent of computer-controlled operations in normal procedures has highlighted the need for basic skills to be taught and maintained in all conditions. Advanced simulator training is the only practical means available to complete such advanced training.

- The use of fly-by-wire control of commercial aircraft has raised concerns with the Federal Aviation Authority (FAA) that will lead to a 'fundamental rewrite' of flight training rules to require all enhanced training to take place in flight simulators.

- This has arisen from a number of major accidents where pilots failed to recognize and react to some fundamental problems, being totally dependent on the aircraft automatic flight controls and possibly suffering from a lack of skill in manually flying the aircraft for recovery.

Overview *(continued)*

- To provide and maintain pilot skills will require a boost in simulator fidelity to handle the new training scenarios. Costs of implementing new standards, in part due to simulator upgrades, have been estimated to be at least $354 million.

- In Australia, CASA has recently updated regulations to mandate the use of Simulation for certain flight crew training requirements in the air transport and other sectors where this may be considered appropriate. This resulted from a number of accidents and incidents that occurred when dangerous abnormal conditions were being practiced in the aircraft.

1.1 Introduction to lessons from aviation simulation

In the original edition of this manual, there were historical references to the invention and development of simulation devices, as well as training methods used, to illustrate the progress made with the use of flight simulation. This was shown to be based on the advances of technology, especially in the areas of computing science, as well as experience gained with use of the flight simulator as both a training and checking device. Specific areas were highlighted as the basis of the success and acceptance of simulation as a complete and valid form of training and testing.

- Comprehensive training analysis of what was required to be simulated
- Accurate data and performance of what was to be simulated
- Accurate modelling of the simulation
- Simulation device constructed to standards using adequate computational power and speed (fidelity of simulation)
- Full acceptance testing (any area not tested cannot be regarded as correct)
- Testing and compliance to international standards to ensure regulatory control

Since the initial publication there have been advances in all areas, though none more so than the actual method in which modern aircraft are controlled, and this has had, and will continue to have, a significant impact on training.

The world has suffered a financial crisis which has had a dramatic impact on aviation, with airlines experiencing the need for cost reduction resulting in moves to newer, more efficient aircraft. These new aircraft, however, also now feature new piloting techniques.

While the crisis has somewhat abated, the need for cost savings has not and demand for air travel has increased enormously, with the industry now facing major challenges to be able to meet the demands of increasing training throughput while maintaining standards and managing the introduction of new and more complex aircraft.

In this environment, standards play a vital part in ensuring pilots receive and maintain the skills necessary to fly safely every time they take to the air.

1.2 **Flight simulation standards**

Prior to the 1970s there were no standards for flight simulation devices and accreditation was based on individual country regulatory authorities, providing vastly differing performance criteria requirements.

In the early 1970s a small group of flight simulator maintenance engineers from the world's airlines formed an association to be known as IAFSTA (International Airline Flight Simulator Technical Association). This group was formed to discuss the lack of standards, data, and performance problems with flight simulators then in service. The simulator manufacturers did not react kindly to open forum criticisms and legal threats were made.

IAFSTA was disbanded and the membership looked to IATA (International Air Transport Association) to form a committee. In October 1973 the IATA FSTC (Flight Simulator Technical Committee) held its first meeting in Denver, Colorado.

The FSTC set about the task of forming sub-committees and working groups to examine what was needed to develop and publish standards for flight simulation. There was a huge wave of cooperation, though many avionics and airframe manufacturers at that time could not really understand or appreciate the need for the levels of fidelity being sought and many closed, volatile sessions were held along the way.

In 1980 the first edition of the IATA publication 'Flight Simulation Training Device Design and Performance Data Requirements' was published and became an automatic contractual document in the purchase of flight simulators and training devices. This document is now in its seventh edition.

With the standards established, a push was made to offer incentives to the aviation industry to increase flight simulator fidelity, with an objective to eventually move all training and checking from the aircraft to the flight simulator. Discussions were held with the FAA, which agreed to an incentive programme with landing credits as the initial goal. This became the start of a long process of driving technology and improved aircraft data collection and testing to achieve 'zero flight time' (the ability to use the flight simulator as a total replacement for all aircraft training and testing).

This was a total cooperative effort between all parties. As an example, it was a Qantas simulator engineer, endorsed by the FSTC, who actually controlled the Boeing flight test for the data required for the Boeing B747–400.

1.2.1 **Regulation**

The aviation industry remains highly regulated and as a basic element of flight safety aircrew training and simulation are well covered in these regulations.

All nations have to abide by their own regulatory authority and agreement was reached to produce The **ICAO** (International Civil Aviation Organization) **Manual of Criteria for Qualification of Flight Simulators**, which now forms the basis of most nation's regulations.

1.3 **The aviation industry**

Towards the end of the last century, the world economy was slowing and airlines were feeling the effects, resulting in major cost-cutting. Airlines were restructured and, in some cases, national carriers were 'privatized'. This resulted in many cases of stripping of experienced technical personnel to improve the financial bottom line of the airline. Cost-cutting also placed restrictions on technical and training personnel being able to attend conferences and meetings of airline organizations, such as IATA.

In order to ensure that airlines continued to maintain their understanding of technical developments and investigation for solutions to technical problems, alternative approaches and organizations were sought by the flight simulator fraternity.

Fortunately, this happened as the aircraft being operated moved to the 'fly-by-wire' aircraft concept, and the flight simulators used actual aircraft flight control computers, which were simulated, or the now-accepted practice of the aircraft software integrated into the simulator under licence, from the software provider. The acceptance of the flight simulator into the mainstream avionics world was now complete.

The following describes how existing aircraft organizations have incorporated the flight simulator into their existing operations, therefore ensuring the ongoing fidelity of the simulator in parallel to the actual aircraft.

1.3.1 **ARINC (Aeronautical Radio Incorporated)**

This organization was originally incorporated in 1929 and chartered to serve as the airline industry's single licensee and coordinator of radio communications. ARINC was also responsible for all ground base radio stations and transport communications, as well as supporting commercial aviation and the US military.

In 1978, ARINC introduced ACARS (Aircraft Communications Addressing and Reporting System), a data link system that enables ground stations, as well as aircraft maintenance bases, to communicate with an aircraft without voice, but with data, including interfacing to on-board units such as the FMS (Flight Management Systems) to allow updating of flight-planning information.

With the introduction of the B767, the FMS on this aircraft presented tremendous difficulties for flight simulator training, as faults and repositioning introduced for training in the simulator caused the FMS (aircraft unit) to signal a systems failure and remove themselves from controlling the simulated aircraft—as it perceived this as a disaster situation. This presented huge training problems and the obvious solution was to incorporate simulation software in an aircraft-certified on-board unit which could be locked out during regular aircraft use.

The incorporation of any non-aircraft software in airborne avionics was unheard of and initially vehemently opposed by ARINC engineers with a long battle, originally led by the IATA FSTC, and later by a group of airline simulator engineers led by Qantas and British Airways. This was finally agreed when it was revealed that the FMS manufacturers actually used such a feature for their testing of this unit.

This was an historic first for flight simulation, as it recognized the importance of the role played by simulation training and also the safety of coexisting software between aircraft and flight simulator, which would be imperative for the future of fly-by-wire aircraft simulation. The battleground also extended to the aircraft manufacturers, as this problem impacted on the production cycle of the B767.

1.3.2 Aviation committees

Flight simulation was now entering the world of avionics and the advent of fly-by-wire aircraft would dictate a new role of adherence to ARINC standards and participation in associated aviation committees.

1.3.3 AEEC

The Airline Electronics Engineering Committee (AEEC) develops the engineering standards and technical solutions for avionics, networks, and cabin systems that would provide interchange ability with reduction in life-cycle costs.

More than 4,000 engineers and scientists, representing some 250 sponsoring organizations, participated in the development of consumer-based ARINC standards. These standards define the key elements of equipment and systems installed in more than 10,000 aircraft worldwide.

1.3.4 AMC

The Aviation Maintenance Committee (AMC) is concerned with the maintenance and reliability of avionics and the development of technical standards, in compliance with ARINC standards. The annual meeting is attended by more than 750 avionics maintenance experts from around the world and identifies issues with both immediate and long-term maintenance improvements.

1.3.5 FSEMC

The Flight Simulator Engineering Maintenance Committee (FSEMC) provides cost-effective solutions to flight simulator operational and maintenance problems. The annual conference is attended by more than 300 flight simulator experts from around the world to discuss technical solutions to engineering and maintenance issues, with long-term savings as well as increased efficiency for simulator users.

The activities of the FSEMC are led are led by a steering committee with the Terms of Reference approved by the ARINC Board of Directors. The ARINC Standards Development Document specifies the procedures to develop voluntary consumer-based ARINC standards.

1.4 Fly-by-wire aircraft

This is a system which replaces the conventional manual aircraft flight controls with an electronic interface which allows the pilot to input his commands (fly up)—(turn left) through either conventional flight controls, or a side or centre stick (like a computer game controller) which provides a signal to a computer. This computer then performs calculations based on the flight control laws programmed into the flight control computers, which along with inputs from other sensors and the air data internal reference units commands the flight control surfaces to adopt a configuration that will achieve the desired flight path.

1.4.1 Weight saving

Digital fly-by-wire systems are now used in the majority of new commercial aircraft as they provide many advantages over the earlier aircraft by replacing hardware such as cables and linkages with associated pulleys and push rods. Overall, this reduces weight, equipment space areas, and the number of potential failure points that require maintenance and routine service checks.

Electronic systems require less maintenance, as opposed to traditional mechanical and hydraulic systems, which require tension adjustments, lubrication, leak checks, and fluid changes.

Preflight safety checks can now be performed using the Built-in Test Equipment (BITE), which allows a number of control movement steps to be performed automatically and to report any fault or failure automatically.

1.4.2 Safety and redundancy

Aircraft control systems may now be a multiplex to prevent loss of control, in the case of a failure of one or two channels. High-performance fighter-type aircraft are basically unstable to gain performance, and could not be flown manually as they required some 20 to 30 on-board computers to rapidly compute high-speed manoeuvres. The control system will attempt to prevent a stall or can stop the pilot from over-stressing the airframe.

The Space Shuttle, for example, had an all-digital fly-by-wire control system. This system was first exercised (as the only flight control system) during the unpowered flight 'Approach and Landing Tests' carried out on Space Shuttle Enterprise in 1977.

1.4.3 Airbus vs Boeing

The fundamental difference between the two main commercial aircraft suppliers is that, with Airbus aircraft, the computer always retains the ultimate control and will not allow pilots to fly outside performance limits.

With Boeing 777 airliners, the two pilots can completely override the computerized flight-control system to permit the aircraft to be flown beyond its usual flight control envelope during emergencies.

1.4.4 Intelligent Flight Control Systems (IFCS)

This is a later development spearheaded by NASA, which is designed to compensate for any aircraft damage or failures during flight. This system, for example, would automatically use engine thrust and other avionics to compensate for loss or failures of other control surfaces such as rudder or ailerons. These advances are believed to be achieved by software upgrades to existing fully computerized fly-by-wire systems.

1.5 **FAA requires training simulator updates**

In November 2013, the FAA issued a rule that will give airlines and training providers five years to upgrade flight simulators and begin more comprehensive training of pilots for stall and upset incidents, as well as for crosswind and gust events. The agency has stated that implementing the rule, in part due to simulator upgrades, will cost as much as $354 million, while benefits from accidents averted will be $689 million.

This primarily stems from two major aircraft disasters:

1 The crash of a Colgan Air Bombardier near Buffalo, New York, in February 2009. The captain inappropriately responded to a stall warning system alert and the aircraft stalled and crashed killing 49 people on board and one death on the ground.

2 The crash of an Air France Flight 447 Air Bus A330–200 in mid-Atlantic, June 2009. This resulted in the loss of 216 passengers and 12 crew. The official report identified that one of the pilots made a fatal and sustained mistake that was not corrected by his experienced colleagues in not recognizing that he was operating in a manner bound to induce a stall by attempting to climb, despite repeated stall warnings.

In both cases, pilot error was accepted as the cause, which has resulted in the FAA looking closely at pilot training with particular attention to the area of stalls and other areas for which training has lapsed on modern aircraft. It should be noted that although pilot error was identified as the primary cause, accident investigations always examine the whole aviation system, including pilot training, and make findings that address weakness in whatever aspect of the system contributed to the accident. Recommendations to address training weaknesses are often made as the outcome of such investigations.

With earlier model aircraft, such as the B747, the former simulator organization of the Australian carrier Qantas had developed an unusual attitude towards recovery positions for pilot training in the flight simulator, where the aircraft was placed in an unusual config- uration, such as caused by stall, wind gust events, or system failures. The pilot was expected to use his skills to recover from these situations. One specific training exercise was related to the early recognition of wind shear, where the recovery method had been established in the flight simulator by simulator engineering and Flight Training.

This was well proven by an incident, as published in the Qantas News by a First Officer who was in command for the take-off of a Qantas service from South Africa when as de- scribed that immediately after take-off, the aircraft speed started to drop rapidly and he recognized the symptoms from his training and called 'wind shear'. He then proceeded to firewall the engines, reduce his rate of climb, and slowly climbed through the wind shear. The first officer's comment in the news article 'It was just like the simulator'.

It could be that the industry may adopt a similar approach as part of a training upgrade, although the procurement of data to ensure these flight regimes are accurately simulated is difficult.

1.6 **Air traffic control (ATC) training**

Concern has also been raised regarding the number of reports of multiple errors, such as landings and take-offs taking place without clearance, approaches to, or landing on the wrong runway, airport runway incursions, and loss of communications. Radio communications have played a major role in 72% of incidents. This demands that inadequate or even erroneous ATC instructions are reportable.

Given the evidence presented, it is clear that both airlines and the simulator industry are striving to improve radio communication realism for training. Among the most realistic efforts has been United Airlines Interactive Real-time Audio System (IRAS) based on recordings of actual ATC communications. This system is no longer operational due to high production costs. Lufthansa and the German ATC organization are collaborating in a joint programme where up to eight Lufthansa flight simulators can be linked to two DFS ATC simulators, which will result in highly effective recurrent training of both pilots and controllers. Other approaches involve using computer-based voice recognition and text-to-speech programs to simulate ATC operators. Such programs are becoming more accurate, and more varied and realistic in terms of voice reproduction.

Figure 1.1 shows a Qantas Airways Radio Aids Station, which was connected to a number of simulators in training, with the recorders in the background providing weather and traffic simulation, including voice-altering technology to give the illusion of foreign accents. The use of Off Board Radio Communications was used by Qantas from its very first flight simulator in 1958 up to the 1990s, when this aspect of training was removed.

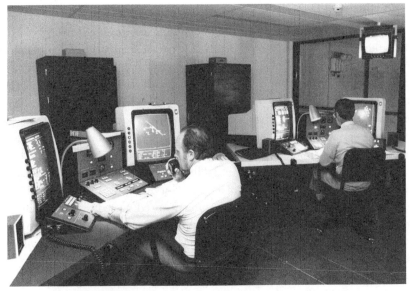

Fig. 1.1 Qantas Airways Radio Aids Station.
Reproduced by kind permission of Ray Page. Copyright © 2015 Ray Page.

1.7 **Advances in simulation**

There have been continuing advances in many areas of aviation simulation, such as flight simulator motion systems and visual presentation to pilots. In general, many of the actual technical advances have come from outside the simulation industry.

1.7.1 **Computer science**

Ongoing improvements in computer-systems performance now allow development in many new applications. In the case of flight simulators, these advances have led to widespread use of PC technology and distributed processing to provide the majority of computing platforms, where previously specialized and dedicated high-performance computers were used. This has reduced the cost of the basic computing elements of flight simulators, and allowed the use of part task trainers and other lower-level training devices. Specialized computer equipment is still, however, required to run the software that is provided by the avionics equipment manufacturers.

Since the first digital computer was used for flight simulation in the 1960s, up until the turn of the century the capacity, operational speed, and architecture of the computing systems used has been a major factor in flight simulator performance.

Many problems were identified in training where, for example, deficiencies in resolution and computer computational throughput delays resulted in pilot-induced oscillation and motion sickness. While these problems were a great distraction at the time, the investigation and studies undertaken have resulted in a greater understanding of 'man-in-the-loop training' using simulation devices.

1.7.2 **Visual systems**

Nowhere is this constant ratcheting up of performance more than in the area of visual imagery. Although general purpose CPU performance has increased exponentially, graphics chips are now used to draw the scenery simulating the out-the-window view and these are processed by a GPU (graphics processing unit), and the programs that run on the GPU and generate the visual output seen on the screen are called Shaders. The term Shader is a little misleading as they also define a 2D or 3D scene as well as vertices, colours, texture, and lights.

In fact, the raw computing power of high-end GPUs exceeds that of the general purpose CPU in a computer, especially when operating on large sets of data in parallel, as is the case when drawing a scene. The level of scene complexity and detail in the imagery that can be drawn by these GPUs is now very realistic.

This huge increase in performance has not been driven by the simulation industry, but the games and entertainment industry. There are tens or hundreds of millions of dollars invested in new game titles, with gamers looking for ever more realistic and complex effects generated in real time as the game unfolds.

Not only has the technology in computers used to generate the imagery moved ahead, but also in the last few years a range of technologies has superseded the once ubiquitous cathode ray tube-based (CRT) projector. Liquid crystal display (LCD) digital matrix projectors have been followed by liquid crystal on silicon (L Cos), and lately digital light processing (DLP). The DLP projector utilizes an array of tiny mirrors, the orientation of each of which is flipped many times a second, each mirror being oriented to either reflect light onto a screen or away from it, depending on the image being drawn.

This new technology does not offer improvements in all aspects of the operation, however, as the CRT projector, when operated in calligraphic mode, can provide a better depiction of runway lights than the current digital matrix projector. This disadvantage will be overcome and for the present does not detract significantly for training.

Until recently, all new technology digital projectors have relied on high-brightness lamps for the light source. Now, light-emitting diodes (LEDs) have reached a level of brightness that is sufficient to achieve the display illumination levels required by the regulations. Unlike lamps, and CRT projectors before them, LED illumination sources are stable for tens of thousands of hours.

The combination of LED illumination and DLP matrix, along with relatively simple auto-calibration systems, has resulted in a projector system that is so stable it requires almost no maintenance action for extended periods of time, possibly even years. In the future, laser-based illumination sources will offer ever-greater brightness and contrast and richer colour imagery. Once again, this technology has not arisen from the simulator industry, but in this case, from the advent of digital cinema. In both these areas relating to visualization, simulators are reaping the benefits of significant investments made in other industries.

The combination of high-performance PC-based image generators and LED- or laser-based DLP projectors has brought the simulation industry to a point where it is now possible to realize the 'holy grail' of visualization—so-called eye-limiting resolution displays. The displays provide imagery for the trainee where it is not possible to distinguish individual lines or pixels, and the scene is as sharp as the real world. Some military aircraft simulators, particularly for fast jet air superiority fighters, have already implemented technology at this level, although it is still very expensive. The need for such high-performance displays in training commercial pilots, whose aircraft spend most of their time at high altitudes, is questionable, but highly detailed imagery is important for civil helicopters, particularly public safety helicopter operations, which frequently fly close to terrain and buildings.

In the area of visual displays, the regulatory standards have been slow to keep pace, and, in general, improvements in visualization have been integrated into simulators more in order to meet increasing expectations, rather than meeting regulatory requirements.

1.7.3 **Motion systems**

In contrast to computing systems, the improvements in the generation of motion and vibration cues have been developed by or for established simulation companies. The original motion-cueing systems for commercial flight simulators (known as a synergistic six degree of freedom, or six axis motion system, due to its ability to move a cockpit in the six axes) have been powered by hydraulics. They utilized a large hydraulic power unit, and involved bulky hydraulic hoses and accumulators, with the risk of a high-pressure leak of hydraulic fluid, which can be extremely dangerous.

In recent times, however, hybrid electro-hydraulic and, more recently, fully electric motion-cueing systems have come on to the market. This change has been driven more in an effort to reduce simulator costs, including both the cost of the motion system itself and the cost of the facility required to house it, as well as reducing through life costs. Fully electric motion systems are much simpler to maintain, consume significantly less power, and are much quieter than the hydraulic equivalent.

In addition to cost benefits, some of the new fully electric motion systems offer improved performance, particularly in terms of smoothness of operation and increased frequency response.

An example of a fully electric motion system is the Hexaline EML, recently developed by Thales (see Figure 1.2). In place of six hydraulic or electric actuators, each driving linearly though an extending and retracting leg, this system utilizes electric motors to move the payload via a belt drive. This consumes approximately a quarter of the power required by a conventionally powered motion system, as well as smoother operation and enhanced frequency response, which are essential for motion-cue fidelity.

1.7.4 New flight simulator profiles

With the advances in both visual projection and motion systems, the flight simulator available today and in the future certainly has a vastly reduced external and weight profile. This has enormous cost-factor reduction implication for installation requirements. The new

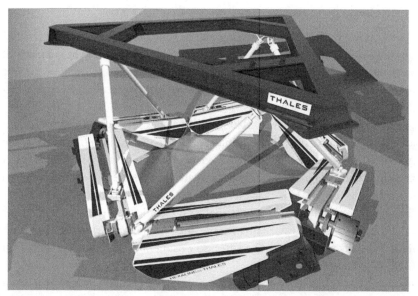

Fig. 1.2 Thales Hexaline EML Motion System.
Reproduced by kind permission of Thales Group. Copyright © 2015 N Durand/THALES.

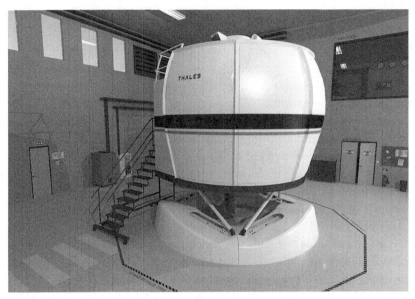

Fig. 1.3 Thales Reality Helicopter Simulator.
Reproduced by kind permission of Thales Group. Copyright © 2015 N Durand/THALES.

Hexaline motion system can be fitted to the Thales Reality H helicopter simulator (Figure 1.3) and is an example of the new generation of flight simulators.

1.8 **Conclusion**

The standards for the development, testing, and accreditation of flight simulators, as developed by the world's airlines and agreed as ICAO standards continue to be maintained. Due to changed technology in modern aircraft, the organizations and committees that support the ARINC standards for the actual aircraft now include full recognition and representation from the flight simulation industry.

The FAA continues to monitor safety of flight issues for the world's airlines and has identified problems with pilot training and checking in the recovery from stalls in the new generation fly-by-wire aircraft, which have led to a number of tragic airframe losses. A new multimillion-dollar programme has been legislated to upgrade flight simulators for these aircraft, as well as training to ensure these aspects can be fully covered.

Flight simulators continue to include the latest technical developments in all technological areas with vast improvements now in the areas of their motion and visual out-of-window display systems, with the latter now using high-tech developments from the multibillion-dollar gaming industry.

Finally, the lessons learned from all the above should be heeded in respect to all areas that use automated devices to accomplish difficult and complex tasks, that basic operator skills must be maintained to provide safe recovery from failure and unforeseen circumstances.

References

1 ARINC History: Activities and Services arinc.com (<http://www.arinc.com>)

2 ARINC 2012 Reports on activities of Committees AEEC, AMC, and FSEMC.

3 *Aviation Week* (5 November 2013), FAA Requires Training Simulator Upgrades.

4 AV web: Air France Flight, 447 Final Report (5 July 2012).

5 FAA Flight Simulator Training Device Qualification Guidance Bulletins (2007–2014).

6 FAA National Simulator Program FSTD Guidelines for Full Stall Training Manoeuvres FSTD Bulletin 14–01. Effective 22/1/2014.

7 NASA History of Fly-By-Wire Project (Tomayko JE 2000).

8 NASA Arnstrong Fact Sheet: F-8 Digital Fly-By-Wire Aircraft (28 February 2014).

9 Proceedings of the 11th International Symposium on Aviation Psychology (March 2001).

10 Swadling P, Flight Simulation Advances 2014, Australian Technical & Engineering Manager, Avionics, Training & Simulation, Thales-Australia.

11 *Wall Street Journal*. February 2009: <http://online.wsj.com/articles/SB124200193256505099>

Chapter 2

Simulation centre design

Ross Horley

Overview

- Key elements in the design of a simulation centre are building form, room usage (function), and technology.
- Important design criteria are space planning for traffic flow, adequate breakout spaces, storage, and entrance and exit design.
- Room usage includes mock operating theatre, control room, procedure rooms, debriefing rooms, wards, communications/standardized patients rooms, lecture theatres, external areas, breakout spaces, and catering areas.
- Technical aspects include a high level of lighting with flexible control, air-handling system with fresh-air cycle, access control security system, high level of sound insulation, digital high-definition audiovisual system permeating all training areas.
- The simulation centre needs to have sizable broadband connectivity to enable tele-education, video streaming, and videoconference applications.

2.1 Introduction to simulation centre design

Simulation centre design can be broken into a number of key components, building form, room usage (function), and technology.

Building form references how the building or space appears. Room usage is the actual function of the room or space referencing to the types of training or activity that will be carried out in those rooms. The technology component focuses on the application of technology to best enhance the learning process. A simulation centre is an educational facility in a clinical setting; the technology, the physical location, the relationship of the rooms, the relationship of nearby clinical areas, the intended training activities, and the current and future training trends should all be taken into account during the design process.

However the design process starts with the following questions:

- What type of training will we do in the first year and subsequent years (define the target market)?

- How many people will we train and where will they come from (define the size of the market)?
- How much space do we have now and will we be able to expand?
- How much money can we spend?
- Do we have courses that we can deploy now or do we need to write courses?
- How do we fund the ongoing operation?
- How do we achieve sustainability?

Answers to these questions will determine the building components and layout but also lay the foundation for developing the business plan.

2.2 **Building form**

The internal building form or visual architecture of a simulation centre, while often varied, needs to be complementary to the educational activities. The facility should be designed to enhance the learning process.

Important elements to be considered in the design and space planning are traffic flow, storage and breakout capacity, entrance and exit statements, and goods and technical movements.

Further factors such as colour, brightness, energy efficiency, and building finishes are also important to create the clinical and educational ambience. However, a simulation centre doesn't need to represent the total clinical aspects of a hospital, but it does need to emulate a medical facility.

2.2.1 **Space planning and traffic flow**

Once the types of intended training and training numbers have been established and, therefore, the required training rooms and areas have been identified, then it's a matter of determining the best location within the building.

One design criteria that is critical in space planning is ensuring traffic flow does not impede or adversely affect the diverse activities that are carried out in the simulation centre. In the past, many simulation centres were single service (catering for a single clinical discipline) and traffic flow was less of a critical consideration. Today, a more sustainable and increasingly deployed model is a multidisciplinary simulation centre which can deliver a diverse number of training activities to a diverse market. The target market for a multifunctional simulation centre can include medical and nursing students, surgeons, nurses, anaesthetists, paediatricians, physicians, allied health workers, paramedics, multiple agency teams; efficient traffic flow and very effective space utilization become important elements in the management of the training activities for these different groups. Basic design principles apply in keeping noisy training areas separate from quiet areas, training groups separate from other training groups where possible, wet activities (wet laboratories) separate from dry activities (bench-top tasks, immersive simulation, etc.), and avoiding bottlenecks.

2.2.2 **Breakout spaces**

Breakout spaces are important and should be included in the design of all simulation centres. There is numerous research that highlights the importance of breakout spaces not only for refreshment breaks, but also more importantly for casual discussion about participants' experiences on the course. The process of peer discussion relating to the course experience is proven to be beneficial when it comes to retention of educational content. However, there requires to be significant thought on the location of these spaces and on the management of traffic flow during breaks to and from the training event without disruption to the other users of the centre.

The following situation could easily occur: surgical training is taking place in one section of the simulation centre, anaesthesia training in another, and nurse training in a third area, but all 'breaking' at the same time. There needs to be logical areas for these groups to congregate separately without interfering with the other groups.

Therefore, a number of breakout areas within the centre may be required. Each breakout space should be associated to specific training areas if possible. Mixing the different disciplines at this point, between participants who have just finished one course with participants who have just finished a separate course, could hinder the flow of communication, discussion, and reflection.

Thus, the location of breakout spaces need to be well planned. Ideally, the breakout spaces are separate or a common area is large enough to accommodate pockets of groups. A centralized cafeteria can be a solution, which also solves a catering issue. Effective breakout spaces are very beneficial, but many times in the planning phase their significance is underestimated.

2.2.3 **Technical traffic flow**

The flow of traffic for technical staff and the course participants through the centre is important and can have a positive or negative impact on the efficiency of the simulation centre. The ideal situation is to have dedicated technical circulation space separate from course participant circulation space. This is not dissimilar to what happens in a hotel, for example, where there is a back-of-house area for maintenance and general staff transfer, thus avoiding the public space. This is sometimes difficult to achieve in simulation centres due to space limitations. An example of a common problem is when there are a number of concurrent training courses, all of different durations, and the setting up of one course interferes with the running of another. The desired situation is for training rooms to be able to be set up and cleared away without ingress into the course participants' circulation space or affecting adjacent training areas. Efficient technical traffic flow will considerably add to the efficient running of the simulation centre.

2.2.4 **Storage**

Storage is one of those elements within a simulation centre that is never adequately considered. In a multifunctional simulation centre, the training rooms are usually generic and the equipment that is used for one course will need to be removed from that room and stored, as different types of equipment may be used for the next course. A minimum of 20% of the entire floor area should be allocated for storage. Storage should always be in close proximity to the training area and can consist of high- and low-perimeter cupboards in the training area, under bench storage, compactus storage, as well as store rooms for larger equipment. Off-site storage can be advantageous for equipment that is used infrequently.

2.2.5 Building entrances and exits

First impressions of a simulation centre are important and can influence the attitude of the course participant. The German physiologist Hermann Ebbinghaus (1850–1909) coined the phrase 'serial position effect' where we recall best the first and last items in a series and the middle items the worst. Therefore, if the entrance to a simulation centre can capture the 'wow' factor then that will leave a long-lasting positive effect on the course participant. The course participant's journey from the moment they enter into the simulation centre to the moment they leave should be an extremely positive and rewarding experience.

There needs to be a designated point of entry and exit for course participants, goods and equipment, and staff. Even when simulation centres are located within a teaching hospital or university campus, there is still a need for a controlled point of entry and exit. Such a control has two critical roles:

1 To meet and greet course participants, and to guide them to the appropriate area, answer questions, facilitate storage of personal items (coats, laptops, bags, etc.).

2 To create a point of security, as equipment theft is a considerable problem in many simulation centres.

The controlled entrance could be in the form of a reception foyer, which can also be used to display interesting medical technology, advertise upcoming courses, be linked to a cafeteria or coffee shop, and provide a dynamic and themed environment representing advanced simulation training.

2.3 Room usage

Depending on the simulation centre's focus and business model, the layout of the rooms and the number or type of rooms will vary. However, the following are identified as fairly typical in a multifunction simulation centre. These rooms include:

+ mock operating theatre with associated control room
+ mock procedure room/intensive care or emergency room with associated control room
+ debriefing rooms
+ communication and standard patient training rooms
+ lecture rooms
+ mock ward with associated control room
+ task-training laboratory

- external areas for external training activities
- breakout spaces
- catering area, coffee, tea-making facilities

2.3.1 Mock operating theatre

Many simulation centres have been established around the mock operating theatre concept. This type of training is generally associated with mannequin-based activities and includes both single discipline procedural training and multidisciplinary team-based training. In a multifunctional simulation centre the mock operating theatre is a recommended inclusion.

The mock operating theatre needs to be a similar size to an actual operating theatre, approximately 40–50 m². The theatre does not always need medical gases, a specialized air-handling system, equipotential earthing system, or any of the specific hospital-based services that exist in an actual operating theatre. However, some anaesthesia and respiratory equipment may require the use of medical-grade gases to avoid loss of warranty or to operate correctly during a simulation. A mock theatre recreates the environment whereas training activities are centred on a simulated patient—usually a full-body mannequin. The room can be constructed in a more conventional manner rather than medical-grade. For example, the ceiling system can consist of lay-in tiles rather than flush plaster. The light in the centre of the mock operating theatre is there as a working prop and in many training centres this light has not been installed, as it limits the flexibility of the space. The same applies when it comes to surgical and anaesthetic pendants.

One important exception is when certain high-fidelity mannequins are used as the patient. These mannequins do require gas such as nitrogen, oxygen, carbon dioxide, nitrous oxide, and compressed air. In this case the gases can be installed in a mock anaesthetic pendant, brought through floor ducting to the location of the mannequin or located on the wall adjacent to the mannequin. Further design issues relating to reticulating medical gases is covered under the heading 'Medical gases'.

In the design of the mock operating theatre, it is also important that there is sufficient access to allow for future pipework and cable, and although many mannequins are now wireless it is good for future-proofing to include additional access. Raised computer flooring has been used as a solution as has floor ducting. Floor ducts are more cost effective than raised floor; however, in each case, access for future cable and piping will need to continue from the floor to the ceiling space and to the control room. This access can be hidden within walls and behind removable panels.

It is important that the training space is as flexible as possible. If floor ducts are specified then they are preferably installed in a cross configuration (north/south/east/west) through the centre points of the room.

Other equipment necessary in the mock operating theatre are multiple pan-tilt-zoom (PTZ) cameras and microphones (wired and wireless) to record the training scenarios for playback in a debriefing session, monitor screens to show X-ray/scan images or even a remote viewing audience, a significant number of power outlets, data outlets, ceiling speakers, telephone (connected to the control room to simulate calling hospital services, e.g. pathology, during a scenario), nurse call, and ceiling speakers (connected to the control room).

2.3.2 Control room

A control room is required immediately adjacent to the scenario-based simulation areas such as the mock operating theatre, ward, procedure room, etc. This usually means that there is more than one control room. Common control rooms are not efficient or effective when there are concurrent training activities as the audible activities from one training session will interfere with the other.

The control room shall be fitted with one-way glass so that the people in the control room can view the simulation training area but the participants within that area cannot view into the control room. It is preferable that the top of the glass is angled slightly towards the simulation room to assist in minimizing reflective glare. Special mirror glass can be used; however, this can be expensive. Reflective film is a low-cost and effective solution.

A desk top shall be installed within the control room along the full length of the viewing window. The lighting system in the control room should consist of work lights along the centre line of the room and low brightness fully recessed down lights as task lights directly over the desk top. The work lights shall be on a separate dimmable switch to the task lights. The work lights are used as general lighting in the control room where as the task lights are used during training sessions.

The control room is where the scenario and simulated environment is controlled from. Operators will control the mannequin, audiovisual (AV) devices and lighting in the simulation training area including being the voice of the patient and providing instruction via ceiling mounted speakers.

The control room can also be the logical location for communication racks and AV equipment; however, consideration will need to be made for the increased heat load and equipment indicator lights will need to be shielded so that they cannot be seen through the glass from the simulation room. The control room will need to be relatively soundproofed to eliminate sound transfer into the training areas. Audible activity within both the control room and the simulation training area can become quite loud due to the intensity of the scenario that is being simulated.

2.3.3 Debriefing rooms

A simulation centre requires a number of debriefing/discussion rooms. The debriefing rooms should generally be able to accommodate not less than ten people, but there may be the need to increase the capacity when necessary. Operable walls can provide this increased capacity in opening up two rooms to make one.

The debriefing rooms serve a number of functions. One is for the debriefing of activities that have concluded in a training scenario. The participants return to the debriefing room where the facilitator can walk them through the appropriateness, or otherwise, of their actions; and review what they did well and what they might do differently next time and apply to clinical practice. The scenario is played back via the AV system with multiple camera views as well as patient vital signs.

Debriefing rooms can also be used as small meeting rooms or locations for videoconferencing. Debriefing rooms can fulfil the role of an observation room so that people who are associated with the skills training course, but are not actually located within the simulation training area, can view what's happening. Where the debriefing room is alongside the training room then one-way glass may be installed to view into the training area; however, where the debriefing rooms are remote, the training activities can be viewed via the AV system. It is recommended that multiple video links are provided into a debriefing room in all cases—at least three cameras viewed simultaneously plus patient vital signs. Debriefing rooms should be in close proximity to the training areas so that the debriefing process can happen as soon as possible after the training scenario.

2.3.4 Communication/standardized patient (SP)/human-factor rooms

An emerging activity deployed in simulation centres is communication training, standardized patient and human-factor analysis. Training focuses on the communication within teams, or communicating adequately to patients. Effective communication is a very important skill but has not previously been adequately addressed in medical training. Poor communication has been identified as a significant contributor to medical error and now increased emphasis is placed on improving communication skills within and between teams and to the patient.

The simulation centre will need space designed to support communication training. The space includes small surgical communication suites with a control room to visually view and record the communication activities. The suites can be set up as a doctor's office, a day surgery facility, a consultation room, or any variation on this theme including for Objective Structured Clinical Examination (OSCE). Actors play the part of patients or as part of a team and the trainee or participant is immersed into the scenario and their actions are video recorded and/or viewed in real time for analysis and assessment.

A good layout for a series of communication rooms is a hub and spoke arrangement: the control room is at the hub and the communication rooms are the spokes. There have been numerous other configurations, such as a corridor design, where the control room is a service corridor behind the communication rooms. The participants enter the communication rooms through the opposite side to the service corridor. The layout is very much dependent on how much space can be allocated within the simulation centre.

2.3.5 Lecture theatre

It is important that at least one lecture theatre be provided within the simulation centre that can cater for a significant number of people, preferably greater than 50. The lecture theatre can be level or tiered. It is preferable to have lecture theatres flat because this style enables reconfiguration in keeping with the multifunctional concept; however, there are viewing and line-of-sight benefits for tiered lecture theatres. The style of lecture theatre needs to be assessed at the time of design.

The lecture theatre should be equipped with appropriate AV and communication equipment to not only view multimedia content but also to participate in videoconferencing and to record activities that are happening within that lecture theatre.

2.3.6 External training areas

Where possible, it is beneficial to incorporate an external training area as a component of the simulation centre. External training areas may be fitted out with props, such as wrecked motor vehicles, building rubble, or ambulance facility, and aim to provide a realistic training environment in an outdoor area. AV devices can link this external space back into the simulation centre so that the activities are captured on video and audio and then viewed in the debriefing rooms or lecture theatre.

2.3.7 Breakout spaces

The importance of breakout spaces has been covered previously; however, breakout spaces need to be designed as a relaxing environment to facilitate freedom of communication and encourage discussion by participants. There may need to be some e-learning facility or Internet access in close proximity to the breakout space so that further information can be accessed during this time.

Beverage facilities should also be nearby. Breakout spaces have the potential to be noisy and, therefore, acoustic consideration is required.

2.3.8 Catering capacity

Many training courses will be greater than a half day so catering also needs consideration. Whether food is brought in or catered on site, refreshments need to be provided. It is better for session continuity that the participants do not leave the simulation centre to purchase lunch or for any tea breaks. Areas will need to be allocated for food handling, serving, and removal.

2.3.9 Change rooms and lockers

In many training activities the course participants are required to change into scrubs or wear laboratory coats. Change rooms are required and shall preferably be located near the training areas such as the mock operating theatre, as well as laboratories. Change rooms also shall be equipped with lockers for the secure storage of participants' belongings, as well as shelving for storing scrubs, etc.

2.3.10 Standard patient lounge and moulage room

Consideration should be made for the inclusion of a *moulage* room, which can double as a standard patient or actor lounge. It is recommended that this room be as close as possible to the training areas so that made-up actors do not need to travel down public areas. The *moulage* room requires make-up mirrors, a change area, and a sink, as well as lockers for personal belongings.

2.3.11 **Loading dock**

In many situations, large-size equipment and materials will need to be bought into and removed from the simulation centre. It is recommended that a loading dock or a designated goods area be allocated for this purpose. The loading dock or goods area should be away from public areas and secured when not in use. Vehicle access is required directly to the loading dock and goods area.

2.4 **Technical aspects of a simulation centre**

2.4.1 **Lighting**

Apart from providing good lighting levels, lighting is very important to generate the appropriate ambience and to create the feel of the environment. Lighting needs to be variable, low glare, and energy-efficient. Lighting levels need to be at least 1,000 lux within the surgical training areas and laboratories, greater than 800 lux within the mock training areas, and standard lighting levels for lecture and debriefing areas to match local building standards and codes. The lighting should be controllable within each space served and the ability to vary the intensity of the light is recommended either by dimming or individually switching banks of lamps. Colour-rendered lighting is important in surgical training areas and laboratories and additional task lighting should be used where appropriate.

In laboratories and surgical training areas where training tasks may be computer/video screen-based, such as minimally invasive surgical procedures, then a further system of green lighting may be considered. The green lighting system consists of green lamps either installed within the normal light fittings or within separate light fittings but separately switched from the main lighting. The eye is very efficient in processing green colour at 560–490 nm. This is at the highest point in the visible spectrum, therefore maximizing stimulation to the retina with the lowest possible light level. Where there needs to be high levels of contrast between the computer/video screens and the surrounding area in order to optimize the image on the screen, green lighting will create a very efficient visual environment which does not appear dark and enhances the screen image. In many new operating theatres, green and sometimes blue (490–450 nm) lighting systems are now being installed.

2.4.2 **Air-handling systems**

Air-handling systems should be designed for the maximum occupancy of the building. For laboratories, the system should be fresh air-based with the number of air changes per hour to suit local building by-laws and requirements. Air-handling systems in surgical training areas need to be fully compliant with environmental and occupational health and safety laws pertaining to the activities being carried out within those spaces, especially if there is cadaveric or animal material, or any other material that is chemically preserved or emits gases. Specific air handling for mock operating theatres is not required, as generally the type of activities within those spaces has no requirement for any further air treatment apart from what is expected in an educational facility. The exception is when medical gases are installed and, therefore, the air-handling system will need to comply with the specific local building standards and codes relating to exhausting those gases.

2.4.3 Security

The simulation centre should be provided with an access control and security system. If the simulation centre is a part of a hospital or educational campus, it would be expected that the access control and security system would be extended from the hospital's or campus' existing system. If the simulation centre were stand-alone, it would require a stand-alone access control and security system. Access control systems serve a number of purposes: to secure the space and safeguard against equipment theft; enable authorized after-hours access to training spaces, equipment, and simulators; and monitor and control access to specific areas. The security components would include movement detectors, break-glass alarms, and perimeter monitoring. Access control and security systems connected to a CCTV video and audio system recording after-hours activities provide an enhanced level of security.

2.4.4 Acoustic treatments and sound transmission

In the case of a multifunctional simulation centre, each of the training spaces should be acoustically isolated from each other so that the transmission of sound from one training environment to another is minimized. There is a considerable reduction in the effectiveness of a training session when there are activities that can be heard from an adjoining room. A further important element is the confidentiality and respect of participants that are undergoing the training or assessment, and some, who in a scenario may not be performing well.

Sound insulation should be provided within all walls of the training, debriefing, and lecture areas.

2.4.5 AV system

The AV system is an important component within a simulation centre, as much of the activity that occurs within the centre is recorded and replayed during debriefing or for subsequent analysis or assessment. Therefore, good video imagery and audio clarity is critical. The ability to record multiple AV feeds, to take multiple camera views from each of the training spaces, to route that video and audio signal to a remote destination and to receive multiple inputs from external locations such as actual operating theatres or other simulation centres, and then display those feeds in a lecture environment within the simulation centre is essential.

There is a significant number of AV solutions available ranging from proprietary stand-alone systems, primarily designed for scenario-based training, to large centralized whole-of-building systems.

With all systems, a minimum technical specification should be as follows:

+ digital high-definition system (preferably 1080p)
+ capacity for a minimum of four video feeds from each scenario-based training areas (three cameras; one simulated patient vital signs)

- all cameras to be PTZ
- ability to event stamp (bookmark) video streams and replay by selection of events at random
- ability to connect to videoconference equipment
- integrated echo cancelling
- ability to catalogue and store content
- local control of recording/routing/AV levels/cameras/event stamping/playback, etc.
- cable shall be generic data-grade
- ability to connect to multiple sources, including VGA, DVI, HDMI, S-Video, and Composite Video

Further recommended features include:

- touchscreen control and tablet integration
- integral video streaming and videoconference capability
- cloud-database archiving

The AV system should permeate all training areas. AV systems shall be designed so that all areas can interlink, enabling live and stored content to be displayed in any area anywhere across the AV system. Individual devices, however, should be controllable from within those spaces.

The AV system should have significant broadband connectivity to enable high-quality videoconferencing and streaming to support tele-education to and from external locations. These external locations could be other simulation centres, actual operating theatres and clinical treatment areas, educational facilities, conference venues, and telehealth networks. This enables greater collaboration with other parties, to not only participate in remote training activities but also to extend the geographical reach of training activities.

Choosing correct AV equipment is still challenging as the choice nowadays is considerable and new products are launched daily. The most important element to get right is the AV infrastructure and to ensure that it can adapt to new AV technologies as they evolve. Monitors, projectors, and cameras can be upgraded relatively easily but unless the AV infrastructure can support the new devices the whole system will quickly become obsolete.

Most new AV systems are now fully digital and able to accept numerous modes of input such as VGA, DVI, Composite, Display Port, and HDMI. The backbone cable used for these systems is data cable—the same as used for data networks and commonly referred to as Cat 5 or Cat 6. This reference pertains to the ANSI/TIA/EIA-568-A/B classification of the cable where Cat 5 is an eight-core cable (with cores twisted in pairs) providing performance of up to 100 MHz and Cat 6, also eight-core twisted pair cable, provides performance of up to 250 MHz. Cat 5 is now superseded, so all new installations should use Cat 6 as a minimum.

Fibre-optic cable for cable runs of more than 80 m is also used. The advantage of these types of AV systems is that the installation is much more streamlined and the amount of cabling required is significantly reduced. Upgradeability, however, varies between AV vendors and it is important that any limitation in migration to new technology is fully understood.

Decisions will also need to be made on the use of various types of equipment such as large LCD/LED screens vs video projection, and wireless microphones vs wired microphones. The answers will be based on the specific application.

With regards to microphones, high-quality voice capture is necessary in all areas but can be challenging in scenario-based training. There is ongoing debate whether course participants should wear wireless microphones or rely on ceiling-mounted microphones. Wireless microphones will provide clearer audio but could be distracting to the wearer and interfere with the immersive experience. Key scenario participants will also need to wear microphones. Ceiling microphones over the training location won't be intrusive but will pick up all audible sound, not just voices. Each system has its positives and negatives; therefore, both systems should be deployed as it becomes a user preference and can change depending on the scenario. Ceiling microphones should not be placed near air-conditioning registers or loud equipment to minimize the effect of unwanted noise.

Portable AV systems specifically designed for capturing scenario-based training are available, which apart from external or mobile use may also suit single simulation areas where an inbuilt system is not possible. An example is where an actual operating theatre is used for simulation-based training. These systems include cameras, tripods, microphones, and the event recording system.

2.4.6 Medical gases

In certain situations, reticulated medical gas is required. This may be due to the operational requirement for a high-fidelity mannequin or necessary in a task-training laboratory. In either case, planning is required for the location of gas bottles, air compressor, and vacuum pump. Gas bottle stores need to be well ventilated and easily accessible to change out the used bottles. Gas bottles shall be connected to a manifold which allows a number of bottles to be connected, ensuring that there is always backup capacity available. A low gas alarm shall be provided and shall indicate in a nominated area in the simulation centre, in many cases a control room.

Compressor and vacuum pump rooms also need to be well ventilated and in locations where machinery noise will not disturb the activities in the building.

In certain situations, it may be possible to connect into existing services.

A laboratory will usually be supplied with tool air and suction to each work bench, although portable vacuum pumps can be an alternative. A high-fidelity mannequin will require nitrogen, oxygen, carbon dioxide, nitrous oxide, and compressed air. Nitrogen, carbon dioxide, and nitrous oxide gas will necessitate the inclusion of a gas-scavenging system and specific ventilation requirements in the simulated training area that uses the gases.

In the situation where the demand for medical gas is not yet required but will be in the future, it is recommended that the pipework is installed initially and sealed. This will save the cost of retrofitting pipework through an existing building.

2.5 **Conclusion**

The key elements in the design of a simulation centre relate to building form, room usage (function), and technology. The building should be designed to cater for various modalities of healthcare training, future-proof as best as possible, and inspire and enhance learning. To achieve a good design there are numerous factors to consider, which include storage, traffic flow, interrelationships of the rooms, the ambience, and the technical components. Understanding these concepts will assist greatly in the design of an efficient and effective simulation centre. Above all, the training space needs to be flexible to cater for a multitude of training activities and future training technologies. Consideration for flexibility and the seamless incorporation of new technologies is fundamental to good design practice. The success of a simulation centre starts with a clear understanding of the issues associated with the training activities at the design stage and the ability to provide design solutions to overcome these issues.

Chapter 3

Simulation centre operations

Yue Ming Huang and Thomas Dongilli

Overview

- This chapter presents a practical and disciplined approach to simulation centre operations, with ideas from two simulation centres that have been in operation for 18–20 years and have a combined 35-year personal working experience in simulation.

- Begin with people: at the core of operations is the personnel team with defined roles and responsibilities and a professional development and succession-training programme for organizational growth.

- Develop lean processes: build standard operating procedures and follow lean methods with transparent policies, create organized systems for programme development, course creation, scheduling, equipment maintenance, and data documentation, storage, and reporting.

- Use checklists: pay careful consideration to integrate educational goals, space, equipment, and staffing needs in order to balance daily operations with time for creative innovations.

- Practise continuous monitoring: conduct routine briefing and debriefing to review quality of processes and to improve communication and teamwork.

- Stay connected and prepared: borrow and share best practices within the simulation community, and always have contingency plans for unexpected events.

3.1 Introduction to simulation centre operations

Simulation centres are businesses with educational programmes. High-quality training is every centre's goal and we all seek to deliver great programmes. Greatness, however, comes with hard work, discipline, and innovation. As Jim Collins states, 'A culture of discipline is not a principle of business; it is a principle of greatness.'[1] At the core of simulation centres are their people, processes, and products. A successful simulation programme relies on a disciplined team to support the administration and operations in order to produce valuable outcomes. As simulation-based education relies on people and technology, both very dynamic entities, it is crucial to have an organizational infrastructure that is dependable and flexible to evolve with changing needs. In this chapter, we share our experience and ideas on how to establish and maintain a disciplined and sustainable approach to managing your daily operations.

3.2 Administration

3.2.1 First people, then processes

Over the last 18–20 years, we have experienced the growth and expansion of our centres from a small single-suite facility where the director did everything from setting up and operating the simulator to debriefing the learners, to our current full-functioning multiple room interprofessional training facility with a team of staff responsible for a variety of administrative, programme, and technical roles. People are the key drivers of a successful programme; thus, it is critical that we wisely select the operations team members. For start-up programmes, the organizational chart may be as simple as a two-person team with a director (typically a clinician or educator) and a combined simulation technologist who also coordinates and provides administrative support. Larger programmes call for specialized positions, including addition of departmental liaisons or champions and division of labour into programme/curricular development, technical, operations, and administrative work (see Figure 3.1).

Regardless of the maturity level or size of a simulation centre, clearly defined responsibilities and roles are needed. The growth of simulation has created a demand for specialized skills.[2] To attract and retain good people, adequate compensation and professional development opportunities are desired. Such opportunities may include: attendance or presentation at national conferences, special skills training workshops, project leadership roles, programme coordination responsibilities, staff incentive awards, and social gatherings to build network and teamwork. People want to invest time and energy when they feel that they are part of the team and can contribute meaningfully to an organization's vision and mission. A professional development programme could be used to evaluate performance, as well as promote creativity, learning, and career advancement and satisfaction. Performance reviews and progress reports should occur routinely.

With job descriptions defined and the right people hired, the simulation centre team needs training according to clear, established operational processes. Standard operating procedures (SOPs) are written policies and processes that are followed to ensure standard work and consistent quality, and every business has them. All personnel should agree with and understand the SOPs, as well as consistently reinforce and demonstrate such policies and behaviours. The Society for Simulation in Healthcare provides its members with access to sample job descriptions and a SOP template.

3.2.2 Business planning and pricing

A solid business model is needed to sustain operations along with a strategic vision for innovation and expansion. Annual discussions of the centre's business strategies, service/

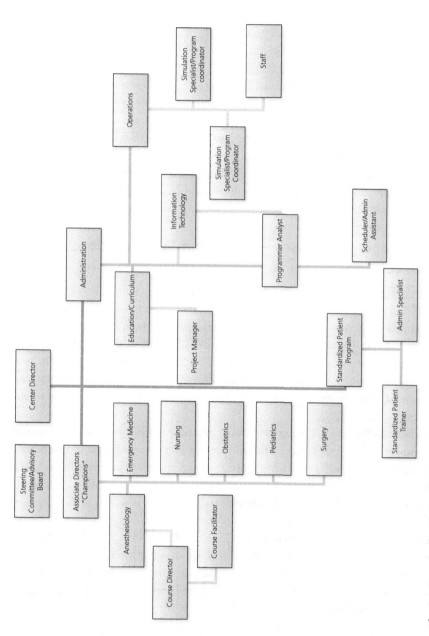

Fig. 3.1 Organizational chart example.

educational goals, and resources help bring all team members to the same vision and mission. Many simulation centres receive funding for operational support from schools of medicine or nursing, or hospital systems. Some are also expected to generate income and maintain a self-sustaining budget. There are many ways to generate revenue, including: charging users for instructional time; renting out facility and equipment; providing continuing education to paying community professionals; partnering with industry for training programmes; and applying for grants.[3–5] Fee structures reflect the high cost of operations, with different rates for internal and external users. Examples of pricing schedules can be found on various simulation centre websites.

To get an accurate accounting of true financial costs, use 'Lean' or 'Six Sigma' methods to conduct real-time observations of front-line work to determine what it actually takes in terms of resources (personnel time, equipment, and space) to run a course.[6–8] This not only helps in creating a reasonable budget and reporting of finances and usage to funding sources, but also enables identification of opportunities to be creative in eliminating waste, cutting costs, generating revenue, improving processes, and minimizing staff burnout.

3.3 Developing processes—organizing the operations of your centre

There are many moving parts in the daily operations of your centre. Daily operations of a centre include: course creation, calendar management, class set-up, class turnover, scenario programming, preventive maintenance, equipment repair, ordering supplies, and curricular support. Creating documentation to assist with management of these tasks is critical to the success of your programme. If you are not organized, things can be missed or done poorly. Educational objectives as well as instructor and learner satisfaction can be compromised. Many of these issues can be eliminated or reduced with clear documented processes.

In addition to the staff following established procedures, processes should be very clear to everyone utilizing your centre. Ground rules for all participants should be made apparent. Instructors should know what they can expect from staff and vice versa. Learners should be aware of expectations and given proper orientation materials. A safe learning environment can be set to optimize learning and teamwork when all parties engaged in simulation follow established professional codes of conduct.

In creating processes, we can practice the 'Lean' method of Plan, Do, Check, Act.[6–8] The planning phase should always take up the biggest part of your time, illustrating the importance of careful preparations, which typically take place months before the actual training sessions. Another way of organizing operations is to break work into three categories or time frames: 'Pre – During – Post'.

3.3.1 Plan: pre-course

The majority of time should be spent in the design or planning phase of the course. The better planned, the better implemented. Think of the pre-course phase as everything you need to do prior to running the first class. Key considerations are: course creation, scheduling and coordination, scenario programming, equipment preparation, supply purchasing, and instructor training. The instructor must work closely with the operations team to identify equipment needs, room configurations, and staff support needs. Details such as who should run the simulator, set up the equipment, play roles, and train the instructors should all be identified.

Consider utilizing forms and checklists to assist you with your efforts (see Figures A3.1; A3.2; A3.3; A3.4, and Tables A3.1; A3.2; A3.3 in Appendix 3.1). Forms provide information and documentation of the process and allow sharing and transmission of ideas with new instructors and staff. For example, a course creation form should explain the step-by-step process of course development and what the instructor and the simulation centre are responsible for and can expect at the end of the process. Checklists provide reminders of task and set-up requirements. An equipment list and room-configuration options should be discussed in the process of course development and incorporated as part of the forms and checklists. Prior to testing or piloting the simulation session, set up the room with the instructor and take a photograph of the room configuration as reference. When programming or running scenarios, a scenario creation form or scenario template can be utilized for the instructor to document scenario flow and key interventions and reactions. The scenario form should capture all the information needed to start and end a scenario. It also serves as a guide for the operator running the simulator.

A scheduling process is critical to ensure coordination and accommodation of your programmes. Most facilities utilize a schedule request form that includes all the information needed for the scheduling manager to approve or deny the request. We will discuss this in more detail in the calendar and booking portion of this chapter.

Before a class is scheduled, verify availability of equipment, supplies, and simulators needed for the scheduled events. One person should maintain the supply inventory for the centre with the inventory list accessible to the entire team. An inventory sheet with minimal stock levels should be created for standard supplies offered or maintained at the centre. This person and/or list should be part of the calendar review process as well to assist with forecasting of supply utilization and purchases. We recommend a weekly review of the calendar (looking one month ahead) as part of your operations plan. This will allow you to foresee upcoming courses, and to review inventory and staffing to ensure you are prepared.

3.3.2 Instructor and staff training

Long before the course, we need to make sure that instructors and staff are properly trained in: learning how to run the simulator; developing a scenario or course; programming scenarios; understanding the resources, equipment, policies, and procedures; and leading a debriefing session. Industry in-services can help provide training and updates on clinical equipment and new simulation products. Learning directly with the simulator is an important aspect of the hands-on training. As part of our faculty development process, we require that all core instructors take a formal debriefing or instructor course prior to leading a session on their own. Co-teaching, peer evaluation, and formative feedback are provided and encouraged. Instructors and staff are evaluated regularly. We set aside regular times each week for training and development via meetings and workshops to improve our simulation programmes.

3.3.3 Scenario development and programming

Designing curricular material takes considerable time and effort. Thus, case contribution by your instructors is critical to the development of a simulation curriculum. The operational and administrative team should enforce systematic standards for scenario development. We have already discussed the importance of using a form to aid instructors in scenario design and to make the programming process easier. Following is a recommended process for scenario development:

1 Instructors speak with a simulation team member to discuss feasibility of scenario with current resources.

2 Instructors complete the scenario form and return to simulation centre team for review.

3 Staff programmes the scenario and pilots scenario with instructor, considering the following:

   a Does it run the way programmed and expected?

   b Clinically, does it make sense?

   c Logistically, is it feasible to set up and run within time constraints?

4 Maintain a log of changes to the scenario and clearly label a printout of the latest version of the programming code or scenario frames.

5 Create checklists for each scenario (list equipment and educational material needed as well as steps for setting up the simulation, room configuration/photo, instructor notes, and simulation programming codes).

6 Create a summary page for each case listing all related files and locations. This is important especially when imaging studies are linked to be displayed during a simulation.

7 Store everything electronically and physically, clearly labelled, in a common location accessible to the entire team.

8 Hold regular instructor meetings to review existing scenarios and develop new ones.

3.3.4 Do: day of and during the course

In the do- or during-course phase of operations, we put all our plans to action: room set-up (including equipment list and room configuration); pre-class equipment check; briefing with instructors; direct support for the class (running the simulator); learner flow through multiple stations; room transition/turnover plan for sessions with multiple scenarios; and contingency plans for unexpected events such as faulty equipment. Checklists should be utilized to ensure that rooms are prepared per instructions and last-minute troubleshooting is accounted for. Ideally, everything should have been checked the day before, but if time constraints do not permit advance preparations, allow a minimum of one hour to set up. A 'Pre-Course Equipment Check' form can be used to test the equipment and simulators prior to the class. To save some time, only test the features of the equipment being used for the course. If your checklist is sufficiently comprehensive, any staff or student worker should be able to set up by following the instructions. Plan for administrative support and staff to greet and direct learners and other participants, provide orientation and logistic information, and play roles as needed during a simulation.

Once the class is up and running, courses may or may not need direct support. For task training sessions, a set-up is sufficient, but for high-technical/fidelity scenario-based simulations, some centres require that simulation technology specialists operate the simulators and audiovisual controls while others have trained instructors running equipment and teaching while the simulation specialists are available for support. Utilizing small two-way radios is a great way to stay in communication with an instructor, especially if staff is not planning on staying in or near the room where the session is held.

For classes running multiple scenarios or the same scenario multiple times, a transition plan is advised. A 'Room Reset' form can be useful in resetting the room to the state you want, and may include reminders such as: empty the Foley bag, fill the IV fluids, return the crash cart to the hallway, etc. If you are running a variety of scenarios in one class, then you can rely on your room configuration and equipment list for each to assist with set-up.

Develop a mechanism for taking notes on what worked well, what did not go smoothly, and what needs improvement so feedback can be provided to both instructors and staff. In addition, note what and how the equipment was utilized, need for supply replenishment, and any observations on instructor/staff and participant interactions as well. This should be a regular part of quality assurance for your simulation centre.

3.3.5 Check: post-course

The post-course phase (after the classes end) includes room turnover, equipment checks, restocking supplies, staff debriefing, and quality review. You may need to collect forms completed by participants, save scenario data, and transition the rooms to the next class. After the room and equipment have been cleaned, perform a preventive maintenance on the simulation equipment. This should be a detailed check of all the features on the simulator or equipment to ensure the equipment is fully functional and ready for the next class. If a class utilizes equipment or supplies from your inventory, restock the room as well as order replacement supplies. An equipment list of basic room supplies is helpful for this purpose.

You may also want to check in with the instructor(s) of the class. After each teaching session, we recommend a quick debrief with instructors and staff, and allotting time to update simulation logs and enter critical notes for later discussions. Follow up with action plans so changes are made for the next course.

3.4 Calendar and booking system

The operational infrastructure of a simulation centre depends on an established process for scheduling training sessions, reserving rooms and equipment, and arranging staff support. However, managing your simulation centre calendar can be a logistical nightmare. Who gets priority? Can anyone add something to the calendar? What if you need to deny a request? This is why we need to explicitly document our scheduling process and identify an owner or designated scheduler. One person should manage the calendar for your centre, with input from the rest of the team. This person should be the key contact for all schedule requests, know the logistics and facility, and have an understanding of the resources (people, rooms, equipment) available to conduct these courses. The owner of the calendar should control all schedule request approvals, denials, and rescheduling functions. Linking equipment with room use could prevent scheduling conflicts. For example, you would not be able to schedule the use of a particular simulator that requires gas use without also scheduling for a room with gas outlets. If a simulator requires a staff to operate the entire time, there should be a note to ensure that staff is available during the entire session.

Your scheduling process should be transparent and shared with instructors and users. In creating your process for scheduling requests, consider the requirement that instructors fill out a form (online or on paper). What should be included in this form? We suggest the following information as standard on your schedule request forms:

1 name of course
2 instructor/requestor name and contact information
3 date of request
4 frequency of activity—how many times per (week, month, year) will this occur?
5 date(s) of the course or educational activity
6 number of learners
7 number of rooms or different stations needed
8 names of instructors for different rooms/stations
9 equipment and supplies needed

Details such as educational objectives and other curricular content can be added, though we have found that oftentimes it is best to speak directly with the requestor to get these data. The simulation centre team can determine how many staff members, what equipment, and which rooms to assign. Once the basic request form is complete and received, consider the approval process and time frame: how long does it take? Who in your centre can approve these schedule requests? As an example, all schedule requests are sent to Jim, the operations manager. He reviews all resources with the team and either denies or approves the request. Jim notifies the instructor within two business days. Once the request is approved, it will be placed on the simulation centre calendar.

The following policies should be considered when creating your scheduling process:

1 schedule request form utilization:
   a all must complete the form
   b the form must be sent to the 'schedule manager' or 'scheduler'

2 request review:

   a review of the request will occur within '#' of business days

   b all schedule requests are reviewed by 'schedule manager'

3 notification:

   a the instructor will be notified by email within '#' business days

   b if the course is denied, an explanation of the denial will be included in the documentation

3.4.1 Scheduling tips

Scheduling conflicts will occur. It is inevitable that you will be looking at two schedule requests for the same day, room, and equipment. How could you manage this? One option is the 'first come, first serve' policy, which if used should be clear to everyone. This method allows you to manage requests based on when you receive them. It is probably the easiest way to manage requests and avoids many conflicts. When you receive a request, if you have the resources, approve it. Some centres also utilize the 'block time' method. This method allocates specific times to specific users. As an example: every Wednesday and Friday emergency medicine uses the centre from 12.00–4.00 p.m. Since these are recurring sessions, we block the centre calendar for the year for these courses.

Another way to avoid scheduling conflicts and to reduce the amount of conflicting requests is to make your centre's calendar public. This allows anyone to see what is happening at your centre. This also allows instructors to see what is occurring on the potential dates they may be interested in requesting as well.

3.4.2 Scheduling 'down time'

There will be times that rooms and resources are available but you do not want to schedule an event in them. Scheduling 'down time' for things like preventive maintenance of equipment, scenario programming, instructor training, and course development is critical to the long-term success of your programme. While we would like to tell others that we use our simulators every hour of the day, it is not possible logistically. Placing dedicated time on the calendar for operational reviews is as important as scheduling actual learner sessions. Take advantage of this down time to also check inventories, order supplies, and accomplish other related duties. Operations staff should allow 1–2 hours per week per room for these activities.

3.4.3 Back-to-back and concurrent courses

When scheduling courses back to back, allow time for room turnover, equipment set-up, and instructor and participant orientation. Simulator preparation inevitably takes time, particularly if the sessions require an elaborate set-up. Consider that trainees will need to leave, equipment will need to be moved and cleaned, and new equipment will need to be set up and tested. You should allow at least 15 minutes between courses, although most have a standard 30-minute turnover. Even without any need for a room turnover, the simulation centre staff would appreciate a restroom or coffee break.

If a course will be utilizing more than one room, schedule those courses next to each other for easier access. Ideally, control rooms should be designed to facilitate operation of a simulator from any room. This would allow multiple, highly scripted scenarios to run from a single control room. However, more than one simulator operator will be needed to run simultaneous sessions, and soundproofing may be a concern if both are in the same room.

3.5 Simulator repair and maintenance

Repair and maintenance of the equipment in your centre is critical. When a simulator is not displaying signs properly or the ultrasound machine is not scanning during a session when they are supposed to, the learning objectives are compromised, and the course integrity and misuse of instructor and learner time are at stake. To proactively anticipate and reduce mishaps, we recommend establishing two systems: routine maintenance and course-related maintenance, both considered as preventive maintenance. Along with an inventory list, we suggest creating a routine maintenance checklist for each piece of equipment in your centre. Simulator equipment should be treated like regular patient care equipment that requires scheduled inspections. Regularly scheduled routine maintenance days should be placed on your simulation calendar and recorded in the routine maintenance log. Custodial work such as dusting electrical devices and cleaning the simulator with alcohol and recommended solvents should be included in the routine maintenance.

The routine preventive maintenance should occur on a weekly, monthly, or quarterly basis depending on how busy your centre is. Typically, this is done at the 'room' level and all equipment in the room is reviewed for functionality and reliability. Equipment in the storage room is also accounted for and tested. The course-related preventive maintenance is done and the functionality of the equipment being utilized for the course is tested prior to the start of the course. Not all equipment in the room needs to be tested. The tests apply to the audio and video equipment, the simulator(s), and clinical equipment that may be used for the session.

All routine checks and repairs should be documented in a master Excel spreadsheet. We suggest including date out of service, equipment name and identification number, description of problem, description of work, date back in service, name of service contact person, and name of responsible simulation staff.

3.6 Data storage and data organization

A simulation centre generates a significant amount of data. Data can include usage and progress-tracking reports, test scores, simulation videos, research information, and records of completion and attendance. Having a systematic way of organizing data is invaluable to a centre's success. Besides allocating physical space and cyberspace for data storage, some general tips on establishing a 'Lean' system of organization[6-8] within your centre include clear documentation and data tracking on Excel files, using a standard file labelling system (e.g. save electronic files using the same format, and include the file name/path and revision date as a footnote for reference), and use of colour labelling and photographs. Not all data need to be saved or stored. To prevent data overload, identify what needs to be saved, how it needs to be saved, and for how long. If there are research studies involved, follow your Institutional Review Board (IRB) policies pertaining to data storage and confidentiality. By keeping track of data, year-end financial and usage reports can be quickly generated.

We recommend the following items to be included in your database:

1 course name
2 category (e.g. medical student education, resident education, continuing medical education, nursing education)
3 interprofessional (yes/no)
4 primary, secondary, and tertiary departments
5 learner type (medical student, nursing student, resident, fellow, nurse, attending physician, non-clinical staff, etc.)
6 start/end date
7 start/end time
8 set-up/tear-down time
9 learner contact hours
10 number of learners
11 video release signed
12 confidentiality agreement signed
13 first, second, and third instructor names
14 activity type (training, research, tour, meeting)
15 number of rooms used and which rooms
16 number of full-body simulators, task trainers, virtual reality simulators used
17 number of staff required
18 notes about cancellation or special accommodations

Data storage can occur in various methods. Most centres opt for local and remote storage plans. One option is to go paperless to accommodate the vast data collected. Consider a learning management system/data collection system that can store your data electronically. Another option is to scan the original documents.

Video storage seems to be the most complicated when it comes to storage issues. Most simulation centres have video recording systems that are local. The memory/storage capacity of these systems can fill quickly. Additional storage (extra server space) is typically the answer. This extra storage space can be local (within your centre) or remote (outside your centre). We suggest consulting with your local IT department on what option(s) work best for your centre. Accessibility to remote data should be verified.

Management of data can be made easier and safer if you automate some of the processes. As an example, videos stored locally on simulation room computers can consume a substantial amount of memory. An IT team can create an automated process where every night, at a specified time, videos are removed locally and sent to a remote server for storage, where they will remain for a specified number of years and then destroyed unless needed for research purposes.

3.7 **Publicity, outreach, and website development**

A website for your simulation centre is not only a useful marketing tool for your learners and the public, but could also be a valuable online resource for staff and instructors. The challenge is having dedicated simulation centre computer support personnel or a webmaster to do the time-consuming task of designing, programming, and updating the web pages. If you do have the resources to host a website, determine what content is needed or desired (static vs dynamic pages) to populate the pages. Some items to consider are: key personnel contact information, directions, interactive facility map, policies and procedures, scheduling request forms, course/scenario creation forms, course descriptions, research publications and news highlights, donor/volunteer site, user portfolios, instructor forum with scenario library repository and teaching resources, and a public calendar.

Other than a website, consider other avenues for marketing and disseminating information, as well as controlling access to the simulation centre. Public media are often handled through your media relations office according to institutional policies. Media requests should also align with your centre's mission and focus. Outreach programmes and interested parties may contact the simulation centre for various reasons, such as for course information, tours and demonstrations, or meetings to discuss potential training contracts. Some may even show up at your door unannounced. It is important to develop policies such as procedures for visitors, standards for sharing cases, dealing with requests for on-site observations, signing media release forms, and responding to tour requests. Placing clear processes and procedures on your website could help answer many questions.

3.8 **When things really go bad: real-life emergencies**

In simulation, we prepare for the worst and have contingency plans to our back-up plans. Occasionally, real, not simulated, emergencies occur in a simulation centre. These could be medical-, natural-, or weather-related. Any type of emergency can have an impact on the operations and the centre needs to be prepared for both.

First, start by ensuring you have policies and procedures in place to manage emergency events. Share these with your staff and instructors. Real medical emergencies are rare, but do occur. As an example, we have had medical students fainting and falling. Most centres have 'simulated' equipment, so management and treatment of these events can be tricky. The following steps should be considered when preparing your centre for a real medical emergency:

- ◆ Make sure you have real medical equipment to manage a medical emergency:
  - Find a central location for the equipment and train all staff on the location and operation of it.
  - Clearly mark the equipment for real medical use so no one uses it for your simulated events, or if it is used for training, that it is regularly serviced and stocked.
- ◆ Consider the following equipment:
  - automatic external defibrillator (AED)/defibrillator—with pads and an extra battery
  - oxygen tank—full E cylinder size with flowmeter and adapters
  - oxygen face mask
  - pulse oximeter
  - bag valve mask
  - blood pressure cuff
  - wheelchair or gurney/trolley
  - torch
  - IV kit and Epipens (epinephrine autoinjector, or adrenaline) may also be stocked accordingly

Ensure that all staff can demonstrate what to do when a medical crisis occurs. Run a simulation of real emergencies. Identify who should bring the real medical equipment to the patient, and who should call for help. Remember that the emergency medical system may not know your centre, so someone will need to meet them at your entrance and take them to the patient. Certify all your staff in basic life support (cardiopulmonary resuscitation) and ensure they are familiar with medical equipment, including demonstrating how to use the AED.

Severe weather or natural emergencies may be a more frequent occurrence depending on your location. Decisions will need to be made pertaining to centre closure, class cancellation, or delays. In preparation for these events, start by creating a notification system for instructors, staff, and learners. This means that you must maintain accurate contact information for all participants. Establish a time period when they would hear from you or a location where they could check on the status of the centre. If you can anticipate severe weather, then notify your instructors and learners of the possibility of delays or cancellations 24 hours prior to the course. Include specific instructions on how you plan to communicate this. An example of such an e-mail to learners might be: 'With the possibility of severe weather tomorrow, courses may be delayed or cancelled. Please check the simulation centre website by 6.00 a.m. for any delays or cancellation of your programmes.'

A notification mechanism should be clearly established, whether these messages are sent via e-mail, text, or by phone, or listed on a website. As an example, internal learners are asked to check the website for updates while external learners, staff, and instructors are notified by text or direct phone conversation. In general, simulation centres should follow routine protocol to practise disaster drills for fires, earthquakes, and other regional disasters, even active shooter procedures. Everyone should know escape routes and the location of fire extinguishers and emergency kits.

3.9 Concluding remarks

The simulation centre operations team plays a vital role in the delivery of experiential learning and healthcare training. Lessons learned from experience are: (1) create a strong foundational infrastructure with people at its core; (2) document best practices and processes; (3) follow established standards; and (4) continuously review and check the system to improve. Learning is optimized when good teachers, role models, and a support team are aligned with innovative instructional tools to provide high-quality immersive experiences. We hope our tips can help you manage your simulation centre operations even more efficiently. We wish you and your team all the best in developing and advancing your simulation centre.

References

1 **Collins** J. Good to great: why some companies make the leap . . . and others don't. New York, NY: Harper Business; 2001.

2 **Alinier G, Pozzo R, Shields** CH. The simulation professional: gets things done and attracts opportunities. In: Kyle RR, Murray WB, editors. Clinical simulation. Operations, engineering and management. Massachusetts: Elsevier; 2008, 505–511.

3 **Allinier** G. Prosperous simulation under an institution's threadbare financial blanket. In: Kyle RR, Murray WB, editors. Clinical simulation. Operations, engineering and management. Massachusetts: Elsevier; 2008, 491–493.

4 **Doyle TJ, Carovano RG, Anton** J. Successful simulation center operations: an industry perspective. In: Kyle RR, Murray WB, editors. Clinical simulation. Operations, engineering and management. Massachusetts: Elsevier; 2008, 479–488.

5 **Gillespie** J. Creative procurement for your simulation program. In: Kyle RR, Murray WB, editors. Clinical simulation. Operations, engineering and management. Massachusetts: Elsevier; 2008, 495–504.

6 **Kimsey DB**. Lean methodology in health care. AORN J 2010;**92**(1):53–60.

7 **Simon RW, Canacari** EG. A practical guide to applying lean tools and management principles to health care improvement projects. AORN J 2012;**95**(1):85–100.

8 Lean Enterprise Institute, <http://www.lean.org>, accessed 01 Sep. 2014.

Appendix 3.1

Table A3.1 Sample airway course equipment list

Quantity	Description
	Standard Airway Equipment:
1 of each	Oral Airway
1	Nasal Airway
1	Yankauer Suction and Tubing
1	Ambu Bag
	Laryngoscopy:
1	Laryngoscope Handle
1	Miller 3 Blade
1	Mac 3 Blade
1	Mac 4 Blade
	Disposables:
1 of each	5.0, 6.0, 7.0, 8.0 Endotracheal Tube with a Stylet and Syringe
1	Tongue Blade
1	Cotton Tip Applicator
1	Blenderm Tape
1 tube	Surgilube
2	14 Ga. Needle
1	SimMan Cric Repair Tape
6	Gauze 4 × 4 inches (10 × 10 cm)
1	TTJV Needle
1 bottle	Manikin Lube
1	Extra Neck Skin
1 box	Gloves
1	NG/OG Suction Tube
	Alternative Airway Adjuncts/Devices:
1	#4 LMA
1	#4 Fastrach LMA with ETT and Obturator
1	Combitube
1	Lighted Stylet

continued

Table A3.1 (continued) Sample airway course equipment list

Quantity	Description
1	Airway Exchange Catheter
1	COOK Cuffed Emergency Cric Catheter Set
1	Poorman Cric Kit (#11 Scalpel, Curved Hemostat, 5.0 ETT)
1	Hand Jet Ventilator
1	Gum Bougie
1	Trach Light
	Other Equipment:
1	McGill Forceps
1	Foam Head Ring
1	Guide Wire (1 Short, 1 Long J Wire)

Table A3.2 Sample course creation form

Please sign and send this completed form (with any questions) to WISER's Production Manager of Curriculum Development		
Please fill in the blanks below with information about yourself		
* Name:		
* Department:		
* Billable Cost Centre:		
Please fill in the blanks below with information about your course		
* Course Name:		
* Course Description:		
* Course Director(s) Names:		
Course Author(s) Names:		
* Target Audience:		
* # of Participants per Class:		
# of Rooms needed for Class:		
* Total # of Classes per Academic Year:		
* # of Days per Class:		
Approximate Time per Class:		
Class Site:	☐ WISER ☐ Children's Hospital ☐ Passavant Hospital ☐ McKeesport Hospital	☐ East Hospital ☐ Shadyside ☐ Virtual course ☐ Other: _____
Is this a CME/CE course?	☐ Yes ☐ No	
Will you have online material?	☐ Pre-course ☐ During ☐ Post-course	
Do you plan to use a simulator?	☐ Yes ☐ No	
Do you plan to use/or have an IRB?	☐ Yes ☐ No	
Additional Comments:		
Signed:		

MONTHS BEFORE COURSE

- ☐ Select course dates, add to simulation centre and staff calendars
- ☐ Reserve rooms, equipment, and staff
- ☐ Confirm instructor availability and request clinical time off to teach
- ☐ Train instructors/staff if needed
- ☐ Set up registration process
- ☐ E-mail confirmation/welcome/orientation package
- ☐ Prepare agenda, course materials
- ☐ Programme and test out scenarios
- ☐ Purchase/arrange for special equipment and supplies

1–2 WEEKS BEFORE COURSE

- ☐ Inventory/order simulation and office supplies
- ☐ Order food, snacks, drinks, kitchen supplies
- ☐ Confirm registration list
- ☐ Send welcome letter/reminder e-mail to participants/learners, check dietary restrictions, parking information, cancellations, etc.
- ☐ Review course at weekly sim ops meeting
- ☐ Confirm staff assignments and roles
- ☐ Team huddle to create To-Do list for MOCA
- ☐ Send agenda and course materials, scenarios to instructors and staff
- ☐ Make final changes to agenda, scenarios

1–2 DAYS BEFORE COURSE

- ☐ Confirm catering order and arrival time
- ☐ Send instructor(s) reminder
- ☐ Upload final slides and course materials
- ☐ Assign groups if needed
- ☐ Print/assemble nametags, group assignments, room signs, table tents, folders
- ☐ Ensure AV system is working (slide advancer, laser pointer, speakers, video, audio, presentation computer, adapters, etc.)
- ☐ Prepare/check sim equipment, supplies, scenario props
- ☐ Set up rooms: rearrange tables, place materials in room, check AV equipment is working
- ☐ Post signs to direct people

DAY OF COURSE

- ☐ Prepare table for food and snacks including:
  - Water dispenser/bottled waters
  - Tea variety pack
  - Creamers, sugars, sugar substitutes, honey
  - Napkins, small plates, utensils
  - Coffee/tea cups, lids, stir sticks
  - Snack container
  - Trash bins
- ☐ Power on simulators and AV system
- ☐ Set up rooms if not already done day before with proper seating, course materials, pens, paper
- ☐ Put up signs if not already done
- ☐ Assigned staff check/replenish supplies (coffee, hot water, creamer) throughout day
- ☐ Assigned staff will clean up rooms after each session
- ☐ Assigned staff will prepare rooms for next session/repair equipment as needed

AFTER THE COURSE

Immediately/ASAP:
- ☐ Collect participant data (signed confidentiality forms, surveys, course evaluations, CE/CME forms)
- ☐ Debrief with instructors and staff
- ☐ Update usage and troubleshooting database

Within a week:
- ☐ Respond to participant requests for materials/info
- ☐ Complete attendance roster, turn in CE/CME forms
- ☐ Send course report to instructors/staff
- ☐ Take care of any issues needing repair/follow-up

PRINTING LIST

For Instructors and Staff:
- ☐ Course roster/group assignments
- ☐ Instructor agenda
- ☐ Staff checklist/agenda
- ☐ Signage: Check-In/Room Signs, Restrooms, Kitchen
- ☐ Course materials w/ instructions

For Participants:
- ☐ Sign-in sheet (if not done electronically), name tags, table tents, blank paper
- ☐ Participant materials: agenda, basic Information (sim centre rules, housekeeping, orientation, Internet), course handouts/worksheets
- ☐ Course evaluation forms (if not available electronically)
- ☐ Surveys/questionnaires (if not available electronically)

Fig. A3.1 Sample simulation course checklist.

FOR INSTRUCTORS & SIM OPERATORS ONLY

Scenario Synopsis	
Title: Title on B-Line (For Sim Operator use): Diagnosis: Target audience: Prerequisite knowledge and skills:	Set-up time: Scenario time: Debrief time:

Case Stem & Background Information for Learner

Patient Demographics

Name:	MRN:	Gender:
Age:	DOB:	Race:
Height:	Weight:	Religion:
Chief complaint:		

Scenario Events Summary

Sequence of events:
  1.
  2.
  3.

Educational Objectives

  1.
  2.
  3.

Observable Actions Checklist

Debriefing Questions

Take Home Points

Fig. A3.2 Sample scenario creation form.

Table A3.3 Sample Scenario Events Table

FOR INSTRUCTORS & SIM OPERATORS ONLY			
Event State	**Patient Vitals**	**Learner Actions/Triggers**	**Operator Notes**
Baseline or Initial Presentation	ECG: HR: BP: T: SpO2: RR etCO2: CVP: PAP: CO: Others (ICP, gases, TOF): PE findings: Labs, imaging studies:		
	ECG: HR: BP: T: SpO2: RR: etCO2: CVP: PAP: CO: Others (ICP, gases, TOF): PE findings: Labs, imaging studies:		
	ECG: HR: BP: T: SpO2: RR: etCO2: CVP: PAP: CO: Others (ICP, gases, TOF): PE findings: Labs, imaging studies:		

TO BE GIVEN TO LEARNER AT START OF CASE (Optional)		
Patient Chart Information		
Name:	MRN:	Gender:
Age:	DOB:	Race:
Height:	Weight:	Religion:

Chief Complaint:

History of Present Illness:

Past Medical History:

Past Surgical History:

Medications:

Allergies:

Family/Social History:

Review of Systems:

Physical Examination:

Labs:

Fig. A3.3 Sample scenario patient chart information form.

FOR INSTRUCTORS & SIM OPERATORS ONLY
Scenario Variations
Actor Roles/Scripts
Props and Set-up
Simulator (model, position, appearance): Monitors and machines: Clinical supplies: Other props: Room/monitor set-up: What's available if asked:
Curricular Integration
Evaluation Methods & Tools
Additional Notes
References
Author Information
Name: Title: Dept: E-mail: Phone: Pager:

Fig. A3.4 Sample scenario background information form.

Chapter 4

Simulators, equipment, and props

Chris Chin

Overview

+ Effective clinical simulation requires learners to suspend disbelief and interact with the human patient simulator and the simulation environment as if they were real.

+ The simulator manikin is often considered the mainstay of simulation training and an increasing range from low- to high-fidelity manikins are available.

+ Task trainers for procedural and surgical skill training play an equally important role in simulator training.

+ The presence of medical equipment is also essential for providing a sense of realism and a vast array from the less expensive (stethoscopes, intravenous and airway equipment) to the more costly (endoscopes, ventilators, anaesthetic machines) may be required.

+ The use of props can be invaluable if they help or enhance the perception of reality of the scenario being created.

+ Local health and safety policies should be followed in regards to equipment used in the simulation environment.

+ Video playback can be a powerful teaching tool and audiovisual equipment plays and important role in enhancing simulation training.

4.1 Introduction to simulators, equipment, and props

Clinical simulation training and assessment encompasses a range of tools such as task trainers, virtual reality simulators, standardized patients, virtual patients, and computerized full-body manikins (human patient simulators).[1-5] As with any tool, the effectiveness of simulation technology depends on how it is used. During clinical simulation training, learners are often asked to 'suspend disbelief' and interact with the simulator and the simulation environment as if they were real.[6] A simulation centre may, therefore, aim to provide the sights, sounds, and other sensations associated with a real clinical environment by using props to help recreate characteristics of the real world. Setting up a clinical simulation scenario can be likened to a good theatrical production. The simulator and simulation room, the actors/trainers, the equipment, and the props all aim to support the illusion of reality and enable the trainee to become fully immersed in the experience. Audiovisual equipment may also be required to improve remote observation of the scenario by the trainers and observers. Video playback is also commonly used during simulation debriefing with the aim of improving feedback to the participants.[7–9]

Designing, developing, and maintaining a simulation centre that reproduces the patient-care environment is a costly, challenging task which includes the provision of appropriate equipment and the development and use of props to create an appropriately setting and realistic scenarios. Within the simulator environment the terms 'equipment' and 'prop' can sometimes be interchangeable. An item of equipment could be any fully functioning machine, tool, or object that is functional and could be used in the real clinical world. The presence of such medical equipment in the simulator environment helps to provide a sense of realism whether it is being used in a scenario or is background apparatus. When functioning equipment is used purely to create a sense of realism it might, therefore, be considered to be a prop. A prop would normally be considered as anything which has the aim of mimicking the real world but which itself is non-functional. In a safety-conscious training environment, some training devices, e.g. a deactivated defibrillator, can be purchased for use in the simulator or training setting.[10] While they may appear to function in the same way as the real equipment, they are not active and cannot be used in the real clinical setting.

4.2 **Simulators**

Human patient simulators (HPSs), often considered to be the mainstay of training provided by a simulation facility, are computerized full-body manikins that aim to represent patients and reliably present clinical signs and symptoms.[11] The more sophisticated HPSs have a controlling computer workstation which generates a range of realistic physiological signals (ECG, pulse oximetry, blood pressure, $EtCO_2$, and invasive pressure parameters). These waveforms can be selectively displayed on a standard patient monitor. Many of the physical parameters of the HPS can be changed, such as ease of intubation, breath sounds and respiratory movements, heart sounds, and pulses. In addition, whole-body manikin HPSs can be instrumented (venous cannulation, intubation and ventilation, cricothyroidotomy, chest tube insertion). A range of HPS systems from neonate to adult are available allowing a full clinical spectrum of patients to be simulated as real entities.

Simulation training can be effectively accomplished with a range of simulator modalities that extend beyond the HPS manikins. Cumin and Merry have previously identified 83 commercially produced simulators including task trainers that could be used for anaesthesia training.[12] With so many simulators now available for medical education and research, deciding what to purchase can be challenging. When other healthcare specialties are taken into account the range of simulators is huge, continuously changing, and expanding making it impossible to comprehensively detail every simulator available for clinical training. A spectrum of simulators including a few of historical significance will be described in the next section.

4.2.1 Human patient simulators

Many HPSs combine a screen-based computer control system, a patient monitor to display physiological, and a manikin. In some of the early low-fidelity systems there was no direct link between the computer and the manikin. The Anaesthesia Computer Controlled Emergency Situation Simulator (ACCESS) (hardware; script; psychomotor and cognitive) developed at the University of Wales in 1994 to provide simulation training in anaesthesia scenarios is one example.[13]

Other 'home built' low-fidelity and higher-fidelity simulators have been created but these have generally been for local use.[14] For potential purchasers of an HPS system, CAE Healthcare (now incorporating METI), Laerdal, and Gaumard are the three principal manufacturers.[15-17] They all offer a range of HPS models from adult to neonate designed to accommodate specific training needs within the healthcare industry. As an example, the METI HPS® was designed to meet the requirements of anaesthesia trainers and trainees and is able to realistically accommodate the use of anaesthesia machines. In addition, the simulator design is physiologically modelled and is capable of independently replicating an actual respiratory gas exchange system that will respond to the administration of drugs, fluids, and inhaled gases. This allows the METI HPS® to automatically sample gases and agents being delivered. It also allows for the calculation of the most suitable or predictable reactions before responding with the exhalation of proper concentrations of gases such as nitrogen, carbon dioxide, and oxygen. Independent anaesthetic gas machines can be used to monitor these gases. Servo-control mechanisms within the METI HPS® mean that action or inaction of participants will lead to automatic changes in the vital signs of the manikin brought about through the physiological and pharmacological modelling. The METI Emergency Care Simulator® is a simpler and less expensive HPS but also has pharmacological and physiological modelling built into the software.

Gaumard 3201Hal® and Laerdal SimMan® do not have inbuilt physiological modelling. Instead, the computer operator or pre-programmed vital signs adjust physiological variables in response to clinical events.

4.2.2 Task trainers

Despite continual technological advancements in the field of medical simulation, low-tech task trainers remain at the heart of clinical skills and procedural instruction. Resusci Annie (Laerdal), produced in 1960, was initially designed for the practice of mouth-to-mouth breathing. The manikin's face was based on the death mask of the Girl from the River Seine, a famous French drowning victim.[18] Resusci Annie evolved to incorporate a spring in her chest for the practice of cardiopulmonary resuscitation (CPR) and more advanced versions remain the mainstay of CPR training today. The cardiology patient simulator, Harvey, debuted at the University of Miami in 1968, was designed to help learners recognize common auscultatory cardiac findings.[19] Several cardiac conditions can also be demonstrated by varying blood pressure, breathing, pulse, and heart sounds. It is the longest-running continuous university-based simulation project in medical education.

4.2.3 Procedural task trainers

Low-tech task trainers remain at the heart of clinical and procedural skills education. These models are meant to represent only a part of the real thing and will often comprise a limb or body part or structure allowing the learner to focus on isolated tasks. They can be excellent for teaching anatomic landmarks and enabling learners to safely acquire, develop, and maintain the motor skills required to perform specific tasks, such as venipuncture, ophthalmoscopy and catheterization. Several companies produce a variety of manikin- and model-based task trainers and these include Simulution, Simulab Corporation, Limbs & Things, IngMar Medical, and Laerdal, among others.[16, 20–23] These companies offer realistic trainers in plastic or other forms. A few examples among the dozens available include IV arms, airway management heads, urinary catheter, and pelvic exam trainers. Although not part of their original purpose, task trainers have also been imaginatively used along with simulated patients (SPs) to provide learners with realistic clinical scenarios in which both technical and communication skills are combined.[24]

4.2.4 Surgical task trainers

Minimally invasive procedures have transformed surgical care but require complex technical skills. Acquiring these skills can have an extended learning curve and laparoscopic trainers have been shown to be an effective and safe training method. Realism of the early surgical simulations was poor but have improved rapidly in parallel with advances in technical elements and computing power. This form of simulation aims to improve medical education by providing realistic multisensory learning platforms for acquiring psychomotor skills training. Haptic feedback (intended to mimic the feeling of living tissue felt through the instruments) helps to increase realism and fidelity. CAE Healthcare, Mentice, Simbionix, Surgical Science, and Simulated Surgical Systems are a few of the principal manufacturers in the virtual procedure station market, with each offering a selection of unique stations designed for learning specialty procedures including endoscopic- (bronchoscopy and colonoscopy), laparoscopic- (general surgery, urological, gynaecological), arthroscopic-, and endovascular-related (including angio and vascular access) techniques.[25–29]

4.3 Creating a realistic environment

Mobile simulation training outside of a simulation centre is now common practice as many HPS systems are compact and portable enabling their easy transport around and between hospitals. *In situ* simulation training occurs at point of care environments and has many advantages, one of which is that training can take place where the environment and equipment is familiar to the learners. This mobility also allows other non-clinical environments to be used for healthcare training. As with the simulator centre, creating a realistic clinical environment in these non-clinical areas can enhance the learning experience.

Portable walls, virtual wallpapers, and curtain scenes are options that help visually turn any training environment into the realistic scenario of your choice by presenting high-quality images of environments such as the operating room, emergency room, intensive care, etc.[30, 31] Out-of-hospital scenery (e.g. a trauma scene) can also be created on a portable wall or screen. For mobile simulation these visual images have the advantage of creating an instant 'clinical' environment with a simple backdrop instead of having to move several pieces of equipment to provide the same effect. It is also possible to use a portable two-way mirror as a space divider to separate the instructor from the student during *in situ* simulation.[32]

The use of a patient voice is a common technique but additional background sounds can also help create a realistic environment. For example, playing the appropriate background noise into the simulation environment can increase the feeling of entering the Emergency Room or being in an ambulance with its siren sounding. Adding such background noise to simulations can be very easy to do. There are numerous online sites to get free sound files and the quickest way is to download some background noise of the scene you are interested in creating.[33-35] Alternatively, if you have access to a real clinical space you can also record your own sounds.

4.3.1 Medical equipment

Hospitals use a vast array of medical equipment that can range from less expensive items, such as stethoscopes, intravenous and airway equipment, to more costly medical equipment such as ventilators. In order to provide an appropriate and realistic environment, a typical anaesthetic course might include the following: anaesthetic machine with all the peripherals including breathing circuits and vaporizers, patient monitor including electrocardiogram (ECG) leads, non-invasive blood pressure cuff, pulse oximetry probe, intubation equipment, patient trolley, operating table, and syringe drivers. For anaesthesia scenarios based around surgical operations the relevant equipment and props might also include appropriate surgical instruments, a diathermy machine, suction bottles, endoscopic or arthroscopic instruments with television monitors and appropriate videotapes, surgical drapes, sutures, swabs, and dressings. For other specialist courses the list would likely become extensive; for instance, obstetric courses would have to include items related to the care of the expectant mother and the newborn child: babytherm; CTG machine; epidural and spinal equipment; and patient bed.

4.3.2 Props

While real equipment can often be used during simulation training, in many situations it will be necessary to employ the use of props. Props have a place in simulation only if they enhance or help the perception of the reality of the scenario being created and give the outward appearance of being real and useful. Such use of props may include the modification of the manikins or the use of *moulage* to improve the realism of the scenario.[36, 37, 38] The use of poor, unconvincing props, which might handicap the realism of the scenario, should be avoided if this could diminish the impact of the training. A prop should be considered successful if it convinces the participant that it is real and or persuades the participant to perform as they would in real life. The way in which a prop is used can also influence the success of that item. For example, using surgical instruments in a convincing manner, although they may not be intended for that purpose, may be sufficient to convince the participant that a surgical procedure is occurring.

4.3.3 **Intravenous fluids and blood products**

Cost and storage space may be a concern when using several bags of intravenous (IV) fluids during simulation courses. This cost can be reduced by refilling used IV bags with water between courses or between scenarios, but some centres have found that the savings are small compared with the time and effort required and using fresh unopened bags of IV fluids can also add another layer of realism to a scenario to the learners. Some simulation centres may also need fresh bags of IV fluids if they provide task training of medical students and nurses in how to set up IV infusions safely. During such training, students learn the importance of checking the label for name, concentration, and expiration date, and the contents for cloudiness, crystallization, etc. These spiked bags can then be kept for use in future scenarios.

Blood, blood products, and body fluids are props that can be created, simulated, or bought.[37] They provide an interesting challenge for simulation training and there are countless variations of recipes in use. Many of the recipes can be found on the Internet, either through the many acting and theatrical sites, and an increasing number of companies are also targeting their products for healthcare simulation use.

One problem with making blood-like products is that they can involve the use of sugar-based thickening agents (such as corn syrup). These products can be difficult or time-consuming to clean up. As an alternative, blood concentrate can also be purchased from theatrical or joke shops and diluted to requirements. Platelets, fresh frozen plasma, and cryoprecipitate are more straightforward and can be easily reproduced using pineapple or pear juice at various dilutions.

4.3.4 **Body fluids**

Recipes and methods for creating or obtaining fake blood and blood products have already been described. In addition, simulation centres may wish to create other body fluids for added realism during scenarios. These body fluids include **urine** (apple juice with added water to lessen concentrate) and **melaena** (Weetabix®, coffee granules, orange flavour Fybogel®, and black food colouring). The latter should be made fresh before use for a distinctive smell. Another distinctive smell is **ketotic breath** that can be created by the use of nail varnish remover. **Vomit** can also be created quite easily as almost anything can be used; chunky vegetable soup is a good option. Finally, hair gel is very good for simulating **sputum** while glycerine is great for simulating **sweat**.

4.3.5 **Drugs and medications**

Use of drugs plays a large part in clinical scenarios. In many places, regulations may prohibit the use of expired drugs and realistic alternatives are required. Water can often be used to refill empty rubber-capped, labelled drug ampoules for many IV medications.

Donation of empty expired or used drug bottles from operating theatres, wards, hospital departments, as well as the hospital pharmacy is a useful source. When colouring is required for added realism, appropriate food dyes or water-based paints can usually be used as a colourant; e.g. white water-based paint can be diluted as appropriate for lipid emulsion drugs and fluids such as propofol and intralipid. Drugs that take a powder form can be replaced with baking soda and/or flour. Pills and tablets, if required, can be replicated with sweets that come in all sizes and colours.

Where necessary it may be possible to purchase simulated medication training aids. These are commercially provided realistic simulation 'medications' that can be provided in vials, pre-loaded syringes, pills, and sprays and labelled similarly to real medications, including concentrations and expiration dates.[39]

When using simulation medications it is important to clearly mark the containers as training aids and take all precautions to keep these props separate from actual medication. All participants must be made aware at the beginning of the training that no controlled substances are on the premises and that no medications in the simulation are intended for human use.

4.4 **Acquiring equipment and props**

The scope and diversity in medical simulation is continually widening, which also increases the need for equipment and resources. As with simulators, a complete list of equipment is unfeasible within the scope of this chapter and will also vary depending on the training undertaken by the simulation centre. While purchase of new equipment may be necessary, it is generally not the cheapest way, and as there will usually be a limit to the equipment and props budget available, various sources should be considered for the acquisition of the required equipment.

Acquiring equipment and props requires a degree of resourcefulness, imagination, and help. As might be expected, hospitals can be a very useful source of equipment and/or props. Many healthcare simulation training centres will be affiliated to a hospital, or through training staff will have links to hospitals. As hospitals often purchase equipment in bulk for a discounted rate, it might be cost effective to purchase a piece of equipment at the same time as the hospital. In addition, hospital equipment that is no longer being used or that is being replaced, and broken equipment that is unsuitable for clinical use, might be donated to the centre or purchased at a much cheaper price than a new piece of equipment. Operating departments are a good hunting ground for surgical and anaesthetic sundries. There are too many to mention all but items range from IV catheters, epidural needles, swabs, breathing filters, and suction catheters, all of which can still be used safely in simulation after the expiry date has passed.

Equipment loans and donations from health-related companies are a potential source of equipment and are a useful means of providing new and up-to-date products as well as any training required. In addition to the obvious benefits for the simulator centre, such arrangements can also be useful for companies as it provides an opportunity for any participants attending a simulator course to become familiar with equipment they might not otherwise have encountered.

Eventually, after exhausting all other channels, the department may have to purchase equipment, which could be used or obtained at a discount from a company offering exposure for said brand. In addition to the purchase cost, some equipment will also require substantial ongoing revenue fees that will need to be factored into the appropriate budget.

4.5 **Health and safety**

The simulation centre has the potential to be a dangerous environment. Local health and safety policies must be followed with regards to equipment used. This includes anything from the storage and disposal of sharp objects (needles, scalpel blades, glass ampoules) to the use and storage of medical gases. All equipment received from any clinical area will also need to be decontaminated before use and any electrical equipment should be subject to an annual audit. Regular safety checks should be carried out by the medical or clinical engineering department at which time the equipment can be certified safe for use. In some cases, adjustments to equipment may be needed. This might include alarms and monitoring on the anaesthetic machine or decommissioning a defibrillator for safe use.

Simulation sessions can often involve critical situation scenarios with multiple personnel and learners. There has been little reported in the literature of the occupational hazards associated with simulation training but personal experience has shown that learners may respond to a scenario with unexpected and potentially unsafe behaviours. All attendees should be familiarized with the simulator setting and the equipment before commencing a training session. This time can also be used to highlight any issues and adjustments made to equipment that may affect candidate safety.

4.6 **Audiovisual equipment**

+ For more information on audiovisual equipment, see Chapter 2, 'Simulation centre design'.

Reviewing video of high-stakes situations is associated with improved clinical performance, and video capture and playback is widely used during high-fidelity patient simulation.[40] It can also be applied to low-fidelity simulation or part-task training.[41] When designing a simulation programme, consideration is usually given to the provision of audiovisual (AV) equipment.

AV recording and playback has several distinct purposes:

+ To allow anyone not in the simulation room (e.g. the simulation operator, observers in the console room or participants observing from the seminar room) to clearly see the patient monitor and simulation room.

+ To provide the participants with a video feedback of the simulation during the debriefing.

+ Education research methodology often involves video-recording simulation events that may then be analysed.

The main HPS providers (CAE, Laerdal, Gaumard) have their own AV products for sale, but there are also several independent AV companies (e.g. B-line Medical, SMOTS, Sz-Reach) which market packages for use in healthcare simulation.[42-44] Most AV packages include the ability for users to add predefined and free text annotations to the timeline, which can be a useful aid when reviewing the video at a later stage for debriefing or research purposes. Additional software products such as Studiocode are designed specifically to enable users to assign workflows and tags to any video content.[45] Once categorized, video clips can be easily searched, reviewed, and compared.

Many factors will affect the choice of an AV solution for medical simulation activities. A fixed location (such as a simulation centre) may allow a system that is a static, hard-wired solution integrated into the infrastructure. Wall- or ceiling-mounted cameras may be used and camera angles and zoom may be controlled. The equipment design and the camera and monitor placements should maximize the amount of information gathered. This can include the vital signs monitor, in addition to audio and video from single or multiple camera feeds. Such a set-up cannot be used beyond the confines of the premises at which it is installed. For *in situ* simulation, outside the confines of the simulation facility, a mobile solution will be required and portability is paramount while complex functionality might be sacrificed. Placement of cameras must be versatile and adjustable. The use of wireless technology may help with this as well as reduce clutter.

In addition, when considering what AV system to install, it is important to remember that unless dedicated staff is continuously available to operate it, the AV equipment is better kept simple and straightforward to use. Many simulator centres will rely on visiting instructor staff to run training courses and the majority of these will not be expert with AV equipment. These instructors will often choose not to use complicated AV equipment.

Systems may be as basic as single camera set-ups or may become more complex. At its simplest there is the potential to use a simple video camera connected to a laptop for the AV recording of a simulation scenario. Other entry-level equipment is available which can allow basic recording and mixing of signals (e.g. overlaying the patient monitor output with that of the video action) for eventual playback. AV products are constantly evolving and beyond these more basic options, simulation centre designers have a wide range of options to choose from. Many HPS companies also market their own AV systems but an increasing number of independent AV companies also provide effective AV solutions. The budget and scope of the project will be significant dictating factors with increasingly sophisticated professional equipment easily available. The potential of using IP video technology, for example, may have cost saving implications if an IP network already exists. Wiring for media transport is not needed and in some cases cabling for electrical power may not be required as many cameras can be function using power over ethernet (PoE). While power to some camera deployments continue to be a requirement (Pan-Tilt-Zoom housings, wireless cameras, and cameras that require fibre connectivity due to distance), PoE can provide substantial cost savings. IP video cameras, once connected to the network, may be remotely configured and managed from a central command centre. This can have a beneficial impact on service costs as well as improving service provision since following the initial installation, camera and software configurations may be completed by a technician from a remote service centre.

Recording and storage of audio and video presents special challenges for any centre. Digital media has largely replaced other systems. The advantages include improved AV quality, and playback of digital video during debriefings or at a later date perhaps for research purposes is also easier and quicker. Additional benefits include ease of storage with a reduction in space required for storage, and increased life span of media. When using digital media, it is important to choose digital storage formats that are well-established standards and are widely accepted. Using standardized formats will increase the likelihood of forward portability of the media. While a variety of options are also available for storing the large amount of compressed data, it is likely that the most popular option now will be the recording AV material direct to a computer/hard drive or disc array. With IP systems this can provide the ability to access the video, by way of the networked digital video recorder, through the IP network at any time, from any place.

Recorded material (and discussion) in simulation training must remain confidential and should be protected to assure the full participation of the participant. The establishment of this trust-bond with the participant is important. While there are circumstances where the use of recorded material outside the centre is permitted, specific permission must be granted by all members of the simulation (including actors).

Additional AV accessories that may be of use are radio headsets. These may be worn by trainers and confederates within the simulation room and allows them to be in contact with the simulator operator. This is useful for allowing the simulator operator to confirm actions by the participant(s) that were not seen on camera. It also allows the simulator operator to feed appropriate prompts (via the confederates) to the participants. These might include physical signs that cannot be portrayed on the manikin such as cyanosis, peripheral perfusion, etc.

4.6 **Conclusion**

The range and availability of simulators, equipment, and props can seem dizzying. Purchasers of simulation equipment should have a clear idea of the range of learning needs of the attendees, the ability of teaching and technical staff, and the technical aspects of the simulation centre or training environment when deciding on what to purchase. As with any tool, the effectiveness of simulation technology depends on how it is used. The appropriate choice of simulator training devices along with the judicious use of appropriate props and *moulage* will elevate the quality of simulation-based training. Simulation centre staff will usually become expert hoarders of healthcare equipment, skilled *moulage* artists and accomplished simulator and AV operators. They are an equally important part of the production process that makes up simulation training.

References

1 **Alinier G.** A typology of educationally focused medical simulation tools. Med Teach 2007;29: e243–250.

2 **Doyle DJ.** Simulation in medical education: Focus on Anesthesiology. Medical Education Online; 2002. Available from URL: <http://www.med-ed-online.org/f0000053.htm> (accessed September 2014).

3 **Issenberg SB, Scalese RJ.** Simulation in health care education. Perspect Biol Med 2008;51:31–46.

4 **Rall M, Dieckmann P.** Simulation and patient safety: the use of simulation to enhance patient safety on a systems level. Curr Anaesth Crit Care 2005;16:273–281.

5 **Rosen KR.** The history of medical simulation. J Crit Care 2008;23:157–166.

6 **Steadman RH, Coates WC, Huang YM, Matevosian R, Larmon, Baxter R, et al.** Simulation-based training is superior to problem-based learning for the acquisition of critical assessment and management skills. Crit Care Med 2006;34(1):151–157.

7 **Birnbach DJ, Santos AC, Bourlier RA, Meadows WE, Datta S, Stein J, et al.** The effectiveness of video technology as an adjunct to teach and evaluate epidural anesthesia performance skills. Anesthesiology 2002;96(1):5–9.

8 **Gaba DM, Howard SK, Flanagan B, Smith B, Fish KJ, Botney R.** Assessment of clinical performance during simulated crises using both technical and behavioral ratings. Anesthesiology 1998;89(1):8–18.

9 **Savoldelli GL, Naik VN, Park J, Joo HS, Chow R, Hamstra SJ.** Value of debriefing during simulated crisis management: oral versus video-assisted oral feedback. Anesthesiology 2006;105(2):279–285.

10 *AED Superstore*, <http://aedsuperstore.com>, accessed 01 Sep. 2014.

11 **Maran NJ, Glavin RJ.** Low- to high-fidelity simulation—A continuum of medical education? Med Educ (Suppl) 2003;37(1):22–28.

12 **Cumin D, Merry AF.** Simulators for use in anaesthesia. Anaesthesia 2007;62:151–162.

13 **Byrne AJ, Hilton PJ, Lunn JN.** Basic simulations for anaesthetists. A pilot study of the ACCESS system. Anaesthesia 1994;49:376–381.

14 **Smith BE, Gaba DM.** Simulators. In: Lake CL, Blitt CD, Hines RL, eds. Clinical monitoring: practical application, New York, NY: W.B. Saunders Company, 2001.

15 CAE Healthcare, <http://www.meti.com/eng/patient-simulators>, accessed 01 Sep. 2014.

16 Laerdal, <http://www.laerdal.com>, accessed 01 Sep. 2014.

17 Gaumard, <http://www.gaumard.com>, accessed 01 Sep. 2014.

18 The Girl from the River Seine: Laerdal website. Available at <http://www.laerdal.com/about/default.htm> (accessed September 2014).

19 **Gordon MS, Ewy GA, Felner JM, et al.** Teaching bedside cardiologic examination skills using _Harvey_, the cardiology patient simulator. Med Clin North Am 1980;64(2):305–313.

20 Simulution, <https://www.simulution.com>, accessed 01 Sep. 2014.

21 Simulab Corporation, <http://www.simulab.com>, accessed 01 Sep. 2014.

22 Limbs & Things, <http://www.limbsandthings.com>, accessed 01 Sep. 2014.

23 IngMar Medical, <http://www.ingmarmed.com/>, accessed 01 Sep. 2014.

24 **Kneebone R, Kidd J, Nestel D, Asvall S, Paraskeva P, Darzi A.** An innovative model for teaching and learning clinical procedures. Med Educ 2002;36(7):628–634.

25 CAE Healthcare, <http://www.meti.com/eng/interventional-simulators>, accessed 01 Sep. 2014.

26 Mentice, <http://www.mentice.com>, accessed 01 Sep. 2014.

27 Simbionix, <http://simbionix.com>, accessed 01 Sep. 2014.

28 Surgical Science, <http://www.surgical-science.com>, accessed 01 Sep. 2014.

29 Simulated Surgical Systems, <http://www.simulatedsurgicals.com>, accessed 01 Sep. 2014.

30 Kb Port,<http://www.kbport.com/products.php#backdrops>, accessed 01 Sep. 2014.

31 SimSpaces, <http://www.simspaces.com>, accessed 01 Sep. 2014.

32 SimScreen, <http://simscreen.com>, accessed 01 Sep. 2014.

33 TheSimtech, <http://thesimtech.com/audio>, accessed 01 Sep. 2014.

34 Freesound, <http://www.freesound.org>, accessed 01 Sep. 2014.

35 Soundbible.com, <http://soundbible.com/tags-hospital.html>, accessed 01 Sep. 2014.

36 Patient Simulation, <http://www.patientsimulation.co.uk/4734.html>, accessed 01 Sep. 2014.

37 TheSimtech, <http://thesimtech.com/moulage>, accessed 01 Sep. 2014.

38 **Merica B**. Medical moulage: how to make your simulations come alive. F.A. Davis Company, 2011.

39 PharmProps, <http://www.pharmprops.com>, accessed 01 Sep. 2014.

40 **Scherer LA, Chang MC, Meredith JW, Battistella FD**. Videotape review leads to rapid and sustained learning. Am J Surg 2003;185:516–520.

41 **Jabbour N, Sidman J**. Assessing instrument handling and operative consequences simultaneously: a simple method for creating synced multicamera videos for endosurgical or microsurgical skills assessments. Simul Healthc 2011;6:299–303.

42 B-Line Medical, < http://www.blinemedical.com>, accessed 01 Sep. 2014.

43 Scotia Medical Observation and Training System, <http://www.scotiauk.com/smots>, accessed 01 Sep. 2014.

44 SZ Reach, <http://en.szreach.com>, accessed 01 Sep. 2014.

45 Studiocode Group, <http://www.studiocodegroup.com>, accessed 01 Sep. 2014.

Part 2

Education

Chapter 5

Developing the skills and attributes of a simulation-based healthcare educator

Al May and Simon Edgar

Overview

- ◆ An effective simulation-based educator requires a specific set of skills and attributes.
- ◆ Some skills are generic but some are specific to simulation.
- ◆ The required skills and behaviours are best learned and developed within an organized programme of faculty development.

5.1 Introduction to developing the skills and attributes of a simulation-based healthcare educator

The core component of education has been described as the arrangement of environments within which the student can interact.[1] This core component is actually a lot more complex than first appears and requires that the educator fulfil a variety of different roles. Each of these roles, in turn, requires the possession or development of a specific set of skills. This description applies of course to nearly all forms of education. However, simulation-based education carries many of its own specific challenges principally related to the psychological risks to the learner being significantly greater than with more conventional forms of education: effective learning will not occur when psychological safety disappears.

To effectively perform an educator role, you will be drawing upon and utilizing many of the generic skills of a medical educator. Throughout this chapter we will attempt to position these generic skills and attributes into the context of a simulation-based education event, but we will also highlight some of the very specific skills required for the unique educational vehicle that is healthcare simulation. To achieve a useful narrative, the chapter is structured as 'A day in the life of a simulation-based educator' (see Box 5.1) and you will, therefore, see some of the skills and behavioural attributes in multiple sections; however, the context will be slightly different each time and this will help to develop our thinking and shared understanding of the descriptors.

Box 5.1 A day in the life of a simulation-based educator

◆ Promoting your simulation event

◆ Setting up the event for success

◆ Running the event

◆ Debriefing and creating the learning

◆ Closing up, reflection, and review

For clarity, all of the attributes mentioned are listed in Box 5.2 (see Box 5.2).

Of note, a textbook chapter can help make explicit some of the theory that underpins practice and can elaborate on the skills that are required for each of the roles described, but there are limits as to how far reading about such skills can develop an individual. Practising under the guidance of an experienced simulation-based educator is vital. We will close out the chapter with some thoughts on considering how to develop a faculty for simulation-based healthcare education. In constructing this chapter we have borrowed heavily from the original work by Dr Ronnie Glavin (*Manual of Simulation in Healthcare*, 1st edition) and are grateful to him for his support in our repurposing of this material.

5.1.1 Teaching, learning, and education

In our descriptions from this point onward, please consider the term educator to be synonymous with any of the following: teacher, simulation-based facilitator, faculty, instructor, or any other similar term. There are clearly some conceptual and some semantic differences between these terms, which are beyond the scope of this chapter. However, we hope that the reader will become aware of the specific attributes required for delivering effective simulation-based healthcare education that sit most comfortably under the title educator.

As referred to earlier, the core of the process of teaching was described by the American educator and philosopher John Dewey as 'the arrangements of environments within which the student can interact'.[1] A model of education is simply a description of that arrangement and interaction between these learning environments. Simulation provides excellent opportunities for controlling and arranging these environments and encouraging interaction with the student. However, the interaction can only be considered educational if it is intended to lead to a set of desirable outcomes on the part of the learner.

The active role of the educator that is being promoted in this chapter may give the impression of the learner as a somewhat passive contributor to this process. We all know from our own experience that this is not the case. Learners come with their own needs and agendas, and a lot of the work on adult learners that appears in the educational literature reflects the importance of taking into account those needs (see Box 5.1 for a list of key features of adult learners[2]).

Box 5.2 Skills and behavioural attributes of a simulation-based medical educator

Engaging

- Establishes rapport
- Manages expectations
- Sincere: genuinely interested in the development of learners

Credible

- Has a proven track record
- Educational literacy: knowledge and ability to apply educational theory
- Knowledge of clinical content (or involvement of a subject matter expert)
- Broad working knowledge of simulation modalities and equipment
- Knowledge and integration of curriculum into activity

Collaborative

Non-threatening

- Sets a safe learning environment
- Flattens the educator-learner hierarchy
- Highlights and respects confidentiality

Situationally aware

- Perception, comprehension, projection
- Active listener
- Emotionally intelligent
- Time aware

Facilitator

- Honest, fair, compassionate
- Inquisitive and shows a desire to understand
- Supportive and challenging
- Accepts learner actions as best intentions
- Displays confluent body language
- Debriefs with 'good judgement'

Reflective

- Uses metadebriefing
- Has a 'critical friend'
- Uses structured debriefing feedback tools
- Maintains a portfolio

Box 5.3 List of features of adult learners[2]

- In children, readiness to learn is a function of biological development and academic pressure. In adults, in contrast, readiness to learn is a function of the need to perform social roles.
- Children have subject-centred orientation to learning, whereas adults have a problem-centred orientation to learning.
- Adults need to know why they need to learn something before commencing their learning.
- Adults have a psychological need to be treated by others as capable of self-direction.
- Adults have accumulated experiences and these can be a rich resource for learning.
- For adults the more potent motivators are internal.

Fish and Coles describe the interaction with the environment as one that affects both educator and learner, each gaining something from the other,[3] in a process that is much more organic than the original description may have implied. We cannot emphasize enough that it is vitally important to get simulation right the first time. As a methodology it is seen as challenging, exposing, and will disengage learners very quickly if attention to learners and their learning needs is not given high priority. It is to this aspect of **engaging** the learner that we will now turn our attention and highlight the first of the key attributes in our framework.

5.2 A day in the life of a healthcare educator: promoting your simulation event

There will be a range of reasons why people will attend your simulation-based learning events and taking a moment to consider this is useful. Is it out of choice, is it a mandatory part of their work or training, are they being forced to attend, and also are they paying themselves or being funded by someone else? The reasons why your participants are attending will alter the dynamic of the day and, to a certain extent, your approach to the individuals or team. As adult learners, intrinsic motivation—for example, being motivated simply by the desire to improve and perform to the best of one's ability—is most powerful. Extrinsic motivation, coming from the need to acquire something—for example, a certificate of mandatory training—or to avoid penalty—for example, disciplinary action—is much less motivating for an adult. You will need to work a lot harder to gain real engagement with the second group, so always bear this in mind (see Box 5.3). Regardless of the motivation for attending, you should strive for a reputation where people really do want to come along to your events, and not just because you're 'nice' to them. One of the keys is to have a **proven track record** of providing developmental and valuable learning so that word of mouth 'sells' the event.

5.2.1 **So how can you do it?**

Primarily, you need to establish and maintain **credibility**. This starts with being able to apply relevant **educational theory** into your activity so that your end product (the learning of the participants) is relevant and important to the learners, but more importantly has been achieved in an efficient and effective way. You also need to have credibility with regard to the **clinical contents** of your events. This does not mean that you need to be a clinical expert in the field that you are teaching, although that is the simplest way. If you are not that clinical expert, you may need to make use of **subject matter experts** with regard to clinical content to ensure the event is appropriate to the learners, and perhaps to be with you on the day (depending on the learner group) to give your event that credibility. The participants need to know that the content has been put together in **collaboration** with an expert in that clinical field. Furthermore, you should be aware of the **curriculum** to which your participants are working. Once participants realize that your whole event has been built around what they need to learn in relation to their everyday practice, and in terms of their curricula they are automatically 'bought in' to your **credibility**. Of note, this links to another fundamental principle often overlooked: being an expert in a clinical field does not automatically correlate to being an expert in delivering simulation-based education in that same field.

5.2.2 **Identify learner needs and create learning objectives**

The old adage 'teachers teach and learners learn' is not necessarily true of adult learners in simulation, where in fact constructivism is more relevant; i.e. an adult learner will construct meaning from the learning activity they participate in. Let us also reference again Box 5.3, which highlights that adults want to learn what they perceive as being relevant to them.

The traits of **educational literacy** and a **collaborative** approach play a role here. Understanding the design and utility of curricula or knowledge and skills frameworks as a source of learning need is important. Awareness of previous learning and experience of the learner group can be fundamental and discussion with experts in the professional group or clinical context will add to understanding and development of learning events. Rather than asking 'What am I going to teach?', consider the question 'What does the learner want or need to learn?' instead. As some examples of this approach we can ask different groups.

We can ask the learners:

'Which clinical scenarios do you feel underprepared for?'

We can ask those people who supervise the learners in their clinical areas:

'Which aspects of practice does your team have problems managing?'

We can interrogate incident reporting systems:

'What are the recurrent themes that underlie problems in this area?'

Not all of these areas may be best suited to simulation-based education and a decision on which aspects are best suited to simulation-based education. Further reading on conducting a needs-assessment exercise is provided by Hesketh and Laidlaw.[4]

5.2.3 **Aligning learning objectives to simulation event**

The same key skill of **educational literacy** will be needed to identify and tease apart the knowledge components, technical skills, and behavioural aspects of the clinical performance that we wish to promote with the learners.

Let us again take a clinical example: suppose that a clinical colleague had approached us and asked if we could develop a simulation-based event on 'the management of major haemorrhage in pregnant women around the time of delivery', then we have to break that down into domains of knowledge, technical skills, and behaviours. What does that involve? We may begin by discussing a range of possible clinical competences such as the ability to recognize major haemorrhage, follow a protocol, and perform certain practical skills, such as intravenous cannulation or setting up and using rapid intravenous infusion devices. We would also want to know whether this was for a particular group of healthcare professionals—obstetricians alone—or for a multidisciplinary group.

The key question we are beginning to formulate is what do you want these learners to be able to do by the end of the educational event that they cannot already do? We may only wish to confirm that they can do these actions, in which case we are moving into the realm of assessment rather than learning. There will be a lot of possible learning objectives even in a fairly specific topic such as major obstetric haemorrhage and this is where the organizational skills of the educator will come into play as they refine **collaboratively** with the subject matter expert, which of these many competences should be converted into learning objectives. For example, the curriculum in which 'major obstetric haemorrhage' is embedded may include 'an understanding of the coagulation cascade pathways'. This, clearly, is not an area that plays to manikin-based simulation's strengths. Whereas 'the ability to interpret coagulation screen results and use that information to manage a patient' would be much more suited to simulation-based education.

It is important to help subject matter experts and commissioners of learning events to understand the effectiveness of simulation stems not solely from the theatrical recreation of clinical reality. Educational impact flourishes from the efficient and organized focus on key learning objectives and the design and running of simulation events specifically to meet those needs.

5.3 **A day in the life of a healthcare educator: setting up the event for success**

Never underestimate how important your first face-to-face contact with your participants can be. This encounter is what will set the atmosphere for the whole of the day ahead and you must take control of it. First of all, you need to be **engaging**; this does involve being able to rapidly build a **rapport** and demonstrate **sincerity**, most easily done in a social context. Put yourself metaphorically close to the participants straightaway by relating to them with a common experience (e.g. travelling to the event). You also want the participants to engage with each other, as this will be the key to having post scenario 'on table' developmental discussions among the participants, guided and facilitated by you. In order to help this process, you may consider using an icebreaker exercise of which there are examples in Chapter 17. Think carefully about this one, as you may be able to get more than interpersonal rapport out of the exercise in terms of information that will help you run the day.

5.3.1 Creating an effective learning environment

We want to create an environment that will stretch and challenge the learners but do so in a supportive manner; an environment conducive to learning. This requires a set of skills that many educators will not have previously had to develop. We introduced this chapter with reference to Dewey and the theory that teaching is all about creating environments that promote interaction with the learner. We want those interactions to be a positive experience in relation to individual or team learning. Simulation-based education can appear very threatening to learners. Learners may worry that they will expose their shortcomings to themselves and their peers. In the context of professional practice this is a serious consideration. A professional's sense of identity is tied up with his or her professional role. If we diminish that role by inappropriate experiences then we may diminish that person's self-esteem and even sense of self.

The participants in your simulation event should quickly form the opinion that you are **sincere**. You can achieve this by describing the day in terms of your **interest being only in their learning** and development. In the previous section we considered building the event on learners' needs. At the outset, the effective educator should acknowledge any other specific needs brought by the learner group on the day. **Managing these expectations** is key, particularly when they do not align directly with the intended learning objectives. Either building these leaner-generated objectives in to the event or simply signposting leaners to alternative materials or activities easily achieves this. Remember: it's your event but it's their learning.

5.3.2 Creating a safe learning environment

As educators we regularly prepare an environment but usually those preparations address the physical and intellectual needs of the learners. Simulation is slightly different and educators must really present themselves as **non-threatening**. A 'bad' experience in simulation will turn participants off very quickly, and you are unlikely to get those individuals to readily reengage (also see Box 5.3).

Attempting to **level the hierarchy** from educator to learner will help to create safety. Highlight that your role is purely to help the participants discuss some of the things that are going to happen during the day so that everyone can learn together. We can also make it very explicit that we do not expect perfection but want to use the interaction with the environment as an opportunity for further reflection. This will demonstrate to participants that you are **non-threatening** and, more importantly, help to set up a non-threatening learning environment and, therefore, a **safe learning environment**. Many of you will have been involved with small-group teaching and will be familiar with the concept of introducing rules to allow smooth functioning of the group. Many of these skills can be used and developed in simulation-based education. Learners must be reassured that they will not be humiliated or held up to ridicule by the faculty or peers if they do not perform well.

The final vital part of this safe environment is **confidentiality**. If the event is formative then we can begin by insisting on confidentiality. Helping everyone agree that the point of the day is learning and, therefore, no performances will be discussed out with the day and any video recordings will be erased at the end of the day (unless you plan to export video for other uses, in which case the participants need to be told about this at the start of the day, and then sign specific and limited consent for this at the end of the day).

Our advice would be to make establishing safety a primary goal of the start of any simulation event—it certainly will impact directly on your ability to manage the learner group and create learning from the interactions during event-running and debrief.

5.4 A day in the life of a healthcare educator: running the event

5.4.1 Engagement with activity

The first aspect to consider here is how to set up the simulated environment and experience to optimally **engage** the learner to encourage and promote the desired learning. For example, in learning the technical skill of peripheral venous cannula insertion, the part-task trainer used must replicate the anatomical and physical properties of the limb and its vasculature. The environment in which the part-task trainer sits is irrelevant. On the other hand, if the learning is focused on more complex learning such as teamworking, the physical space in which the activity takes place must closely replicate the important aspects of the real clinical workspace and there must be a team present that also resembles the learners' usual team in terms of set-up, capability, and action (although, of course, this does not need to be the learners' actual usual team). For immersive simulation, the educator must aim to provide enough stimuli to help promote a constructive interaction that will lead to the attainment of the learning objectives.

In order to get this engagement for learning, a **broad working knowledge of simulation modalities** and equipment and also the specific knowledge of the usual working environment are required. The first point about simulation modalities may be even broader than initial impressions, especially when we take David Gaba's definition of simulation as merely '. . . a technique—not a technology—to replace or amplify real experiences with guided experiences that evoke or replicate substantial aspects of the real world in a fully interactive manner'.[5] This means we must consider things like table-top exercises, tactical decision games, abstract team tasks, and a whole range of activity as simulation, and therefore apply the same methodologies for success. For the second point about the usual working environment, if this is outside the educator's sphere of clinical practice a subject matter expert should be consulted, as mentioned earlier with regard to credibility.

To conclude this discussion about engagement with the activity itself, consider **honesty** and **fairness**. The learners need to understand what is expected of them when they start the simulated activity, what can be effectively simulated, and what aspects cannot. This is easily taken care of with a short orientation and briefing before the activity. Remember that if you don't appear to believe in simulation as an effective learning tool, then they won't either.

5.4.2 Situation awareness

Multitasking in the control room is a learned skill for the educator. The control room can be hectic: driving the manikin, dynamically driving the activity itself, observing behaviours, bookmarking clips of video for debriefing, and planning the debriefing based on observed activity to be centred on the learning objectives. First, consider the description of situation awareness from Endsley as a three-step model: 'the *perception* of elements in the environment within a volume of time and space, the *comprehension* of their meaning, and the *projection* of their status in the near future'.[6] This is a useful framework for analysing the role of the educator in terms of actually running simulation activity.

For example, in the control room of an immersive simulation there are many elements to perceive, which may include: data on current manikin physiology, actions being carried out by learners in relation to the manikin (drugs given, etc.), behaviours of the learners, actions of the faculty confederate, and even simply the amount of time that is passing. There then must be comprehension of those elements: does the current manikin physiology match with the actions being carried out by the learners and, indeed, with the planned course of the scenario, how do the behaviours of the learners translate into the learning objectives to be covered in debriefing, is the faculty confederate feeding the correct information into the activity as required, and is the time spent in the activity encroaching on time for debriefing. To take this to the final step of projection to the future and, therefore, shaping of subsequent actions: will this current manikin physiology flow realistically into the next stage of the scenario, at this stage is there any risk of miscuing the learners causing the activity to deviate from the planned course (and, therefore, the planned learning), is the faculty confederate going to need to intervene with information to get the learners back on track, are any of the next actions of the learners going to damage the equipment, is there any additional value in terms of material for learning in debriefing in continuing the activity further, and what are the opening questions going to be during debriefing.

To conclude this consideration of situation awareness, it is clear that either activity- or scenario-running is not a passive event for the educator. The educator must remain constantly **vigilant** over all aspects of the activity with respect to what's happening, what does it mean for the learning, what could happen next, and, therefore, what actions could be required to guide the experience.

5.5 **A day in the life of a healthcare educator: debriefing and creating the learning**

If there has been constructive alignment[7] throughout the design and active running of the simulation event to this point, then the debriefing conversation should naturally focus on the intended learning. However, in part due to the exposing nature and emotional components of simulation-based learning, the educator must have a specific and solid skill set for debriefing that relies heavily on **facilitation**. To create meaning, the learner will need to make some sort of sense of the simulated experience they have engaged with. The term cognitive dissonance describes a powerful reaction that occurs when an individual's outlook and ideas are confronted with new information that may modify thinking or directly conflict with beliefs. This is almost certainly going to occur with simulation-based learning and, when managed well, it becomes a powerful tool for education. To promote this learning, the educator should be **inquisitive** about the performance they have observed, aligned both to **support** the participant alongside **challenge** of their learning and development. Debriefing is covered in detail in Chapter 15.

5.5.1 **General approach**

The opening comments made by the educator at the very start of debriefing can colour the conversation dramatically. There should already be some **rapport** based on the work done before this moment, but simple things like sitting down with the learners initially will strengthen that bond. Opening questions about how the learners feel are also a powerful acknowledgement of what has happened, but more importantly gives an insight into the level of engagement and the current emotional state. The educator must approach this initial interaction with **honesty, fairness**, and **compassion**. For example, if the scenario has not gone well in the eyes of the learner, opening with 'great job, well done in there' will lose credibility for the educator immediately. A rather more **honest** and, yet, supportive opening would be something like 'from the outside looking in, it looked like quite a tough scenario to manage'.

The educator should take the overall stance that everything that the learner did or said during the simulation activity was done with the **best intentions**, with the aim of showing a gold standard of performance (especially considering that the performance was always going to be reviewed and discussed among the group). Understanding this and tempering all further conversation with this in mind will help in the running of a smooth and yet challenging debrief. Furthermore, the educator must have **confluent body language** so that what is being said or asked is perceived to be absolutely genuine. Even when the educator has made the all-too-easy human assumptions about the performance they have seen, this cannot show through. To expand on this concept, consider for a moment the following two questions: 'How much blood had the patient lost at that point?' and 'How much blood do you think that patient had lost at that point?' Think not about the slight change in words between the two but more about what is behind each question. The first one suggests there is an answer that the educator knows and the learner must guess. The second is entirely different because the initial answer that is given is the correct one; this then opens the door to a conversation about why the learner has come to that conclusion and ultimately to richer and more relevant learning. Debriefing with **good judgement**[8] combines a **genuine desire to understand the performance** with questions based on observation through an advocacy and inquiry model. This approach will put learners at ease and let developmental conversation flourish without attaching any perceived underlying motivation as to why the learner did what they did.

5.5.2 Situation awareness

If we use the same model of situation awareness referred to in the previous section, we can really dissect what makes an effective educator in the simulation debrief. In terms of **perception** of information in the debrief, the educator must be continually alert to hear everything that is said, notice the way it is being said, and sense the things that are not being said (**active listening**). Learner body language can be one of the tell-tale signs to the unsaid items. If you have the facility to record video and audio of debriefing, you will almost certainly be amazed by the amount of things that were missed in the moment. It may sound simple, but without a clock in sight, the educator stands next to no chance of **staying to time**. Picking up all this vital information is far easier when the educator has a structure or model for debriefing and the learning objectives (and thus the direction of conversation) are clear in their mind as this allows concentration on the learners. In terms of **comprehension**, everything that is said should be interpreted with mental reference to the intended learning. By doing this it becomes easier to naturally direct the conversation in a seemingly fluid way. More importantly, because of the revealing and emotive nature of simulation, this is where the educator must be **emotionally intelligent** to interpret those insights and gauge the 'temperature of the room'. Who's talking, who's not talking, and why could that be—is it a problem or are they just thinking?

For the **projection or anticipation**, the educator needs to be watchful for the signs of potential conflict, to be aware of the learners' frames, and when cognitive dissonance will be maximal. For example, where a learner is under the impression that their performance was immaculate, playing a video showing it to be lacking would be a high-risk strategy and likely to result in conflict. Depending on time, momentum, and direction of conversation, the educator may need to move along the spectrum of facilitation[9] from supportively using silence, open questions, and clarification to persuasive or more directive guidance.

5.6 A day in the life of a healthcare educator: closing up, reflection, and review

We encourage learners to reflect on their performance and simulation-based education offers plenty of opportunities for doing that. It would seem contradictory and even illogical if we did not carry out such an exercise ourselves. We may use both **reflection**-on-action and once expertise builds, **reflection**-in-action as described by Donald Schön.[10] **Reflection** is as much a part of being an educator as being a healthcare professional. We can also think of this phase as resembling a quality-improvement cycle for the way in which we have delivered education. Where do we want our participants to be? How close or how far are they from that place? If there is a gap then what are we going to do to minimize that gap? We need to be able to find out where the learners are (end of event evaluation, post-event follow-up, etc.) and then we need to use that information to modify subsequent events.

The process of reflection-on-action is markedly facilitated by the use of video, and, in fact, from our experience, simulation-based educators develop and improve exponentially using this technique either for self-reflection or by after-event facilitated reflection (which we term **metadebriefing**). There are some readily available tools to evaluate debriefing—specifically, the Objective Structured Assessment of Debriefing (OSAD) from Imperial College London[11] and the Debriefing Assessment for Simulation in Healthcare (DASH)[12] from Harvard, to name two accessible via the Internet. The authors would encourage use of one or more of these tools to inform the **metadebriefing** process.

5.7 **Developing the skill set**

All of the skills and attributes that we have highlighted and discussed are best learned and developed through deliberate practice; i.e. repetition with **reflection** or feedback each time for improvement towards expertise.[13] Ideally, this is organized into a programme of educator faculty development with individual components that include: a degree of supervised practice with a **critical friend**,[14] **structured feedback** on performance (as mentioned earlier), maintenance of a **portfolio** of objectives activity and development, guidance via mentorship, and quality assurance via expert review of performance against an agreed set of outcomes, an example of which is provided by the Clinical Skills Managed Educational Network in Scotland.[15]

5.8 **Conclusion**

We have attempted to provide an outline of a set of skills and attributes that define an expert in delivering simulation-based education. We have endeavoured to give varying examples of how and why this is the skill set to work towards. It is not exhaustive. Individual educators will have to use their journey of development in simulation to decide for themselves which skills are most important for them to work to improve.

References

1 **Dewey J.** Democracy in education. New York, NY: Macmillan Inc, 1916.

2 **Knowles M.** The adult learner: a neglected species. Houston, TX: Gulf Publishing Company, 1990.

3 **Fish D, Coles C.** Med Educ: developing a curriculum for practice. Maidenhead: Open University Press, 2005.

4 **Hesketh EA, Laidlaw JM.** Developing the teaching instinct, 4: Needs assessment. Med Teach 2002;**24**:594–598.

5 **Gaba D.** The future vision of simulation in healthcare. Simul Healthc 2007;**2**:126–135.

6 **Endsley MR**. Toward a theory of situation awareness in dynamic systems. Human Factors 1995b;**37**(1):32–64.

7 **Biggs J, Tang C**. Teaching for quality learning at university, Fourth Edition. Open University Press, 2011.

8 **Rudolph JW, et al**. There's no such thing as a 'nonjudgmental' debriefing: a theory and method for debriefing with good judgment. Simul Healthc 2006;**1**(1):49–55.

9 **Bentley TJ**. Facilitation, 2nd Edition. St Weonards: The Space Between, 2000.

10 **Schön DA**. Educating the reflective practitioner. San Francisco, CA: Jossey-Bass Publishers, 1987.

11 **Arora S, et al**. Objective Structured Assessment of Debriefing (OSAD): bringing science to the art of debriefing in surgery. Ann Surg 2012;**256**(6):982–988. Manuals available via <http://www1.imperial.ac.uk/cpssq/cpssq_publications/resources_tools/osad> (accessed 12 October 2014).

12 **Simon R, Raemcr DB, Rudolph JW**. Debriefing assessment for simulation in healthcare—Rater version. Boston, MA: Center for Medical Simulation, 2009. Manuals available via <https://www.harvardmedsim.org/debriefing-assesment-simulation-healthcare.php> (accessed 12 October 2014).

13 **Ericsson KA, Krampe Th.R, Tesch-Romer C**. The role of deliberate practice in the acquisition of expert performance. Psychol Rev 1993;**100**(3):363–406.

14 **Dahlgren LO, et al**. To be and have a critical friend in medical teaching. Med Educ 2006;**40**(1):72–78.

15 **Simulation Based Education**, *Clinical Skills: Managed Education Network, NHS Education for Scotland*, <http://www.csmen.scot.nhs.uk/resources/simulation-based-education.aspx>, accessed 12 Oct. 2014.

Chapter 6

Teaching a clinical skill

Jeffrey M Hamdorf and Robert Davies

Overview

- Successful adult learning requires the identification of clear goals, relevance to clinical practice, and the opportunity for reflection.
- Many senior clinicians will recall their learning was very much an apprenticeship model; today's doctors are expecting a structured learning programme.
- The teaching of technical and procedural skills is readily adaptable to simulated learning environments.
- The challenge for the teacher is to remain mindful that he/she has achieved unconscious competence, whereas the learner is working from first principles.
- The four-step approach to teaching a skill is an excellent technique which ensures that learners develop an appropriate level of awareness before attempting a skill.
- When designing a skills teaching episode, establishing learning objectives defines a learning pathway which guides the learner and the teacher.
- A successful skills teaching episode will embrace elements of positive critiquing, allow initial, formative, and summative assessment, and will be subject to evaluative scrutiny to determine that it has met its objectives.

6.1 Introduction to teaching a clinical skill

The methodology around the teaching of clinical skills has experienced a substantial boost in prominence with both the development of simulation centres and as a result of what is arguably a revolution in medical education. The insights provided in the first edition of this book represented the best of what was available at the time—best practice if you like. Little has changed in the interim. Accordingly, the techniques described are as relevant now as they were at the time of the first edition but with several additional features; such as the development of fresh frozen cadaver technologies to provide more realistic tissue handling and consideration of virtual reality (see Chapter 31). Many of the principles described here emphasize surgical skills but the same axioms apply to all clinical skills.

6.2 **Adult learning**

The teachers who have had the greatest impact on us achieved that effect not necessarily because they were the best surgeons or physicians in their fields. Rather, they were good teachers because they may have made a difficult concept seem straightforward, a boring subject interesting or relevant, or may even have imparted a level of inspiration to those they were teaching.

Adult learning is substantially different from childhood education for a variety of reasons. The following key aspects of adult learning should be taken into account when teaching an adult a new clinical skill:

- Adult learners retain 90% of skills learnt by **doing rather than by watching**.
- Adult learning needs to be **immediately relevant**.
- Adults need to be **actively involved**.
- Adult learners have a surprisingly **short concentration span**.
- Adult learners need **clear goals and objectives**.
- Adult learners need **feedback**.
- Adult learners need an opportunity for **reflection**.

> The most important features of successful adult learning include the identification of clear goals, relevance to practice, and the opportunity for reflection.

6.3 **Apprenticeship model**

The teaching of clinical skills has of recent times undergone somewhat of a paradigm shift. Historically, the model has followed the traditional master–apprentice relationship and at times has been akin to 'learning by osmosis'. The concept of 'see one, do one, teach one' though can no longer be argued as adequate. There have been a number of factors influencing this change. Strong drivers include an increasingly focused student and junior doctor body demanding teaching and a consequent alignment towards student-centred learning versus the historical teacher-centred approach. Accordingly, this has necessitated a somewhat different approach to teaching skills.

Picture the historical vignette of the teaching ward round. The white coat resplendent senior consultant and his entourage sweep through the ward. The patient has been brought into the hospital two days before her operation in order for there to be an adequate exposure for the team's medical students. The students might clerk the patient, the consultant (faculty) attends for the teaching ward round and examines the patient, demonstrating the signs to the students, before proceeding to discuss the case over the patient at the bedside.

Student: 'Sir, why is the potassium level raised in renal failure?'

Consultant: 'Because it always has been, and always will be.'

Table 6.1 Apprenticeship versus structured programme participation

Apprenticeship	Structured programme
Art and craft	Science and craft
Long working hours	Shift work
Low technology, low cost	High technology, high cost
See and do	Formal skills training
Problem-driven accountability	Evidence-based accountability
Moderated by peer pressure	Moderated by peer pressure
Mentor evaluation	Objective evaluation
Assessment based upon traits	Competency-based assessment

Reproduced from 'Acquiring surgical skills', J.M. Hamdorf and J.C. Hall, *British Journal of Surgery*, 87(1), pp. 28–37, DOI: 10.1046/j.1365–2168.2000.01327.x Copyright (c) 2000, John Wiley and Sons.

There is a move towards reducing the length of training programmes and with this attention needs to be drawn towards ensuring that trainees are adequately exposed to appropriate learning opportunities allowing them to achieve the broad competencies required at graduation. The essential differences between the time-honoured apprentice model and the structured-programme approach are summarized in Table 6.1.

6.4 **Simulated learning environments**

The teaching of technical and procedural skills is readily adaptable to simulation using inanimate substrates such as knot-tying jigs, silicone co-polymer skin substitutes, torso trainers for laparoscopy, etc. Yet, synthetic substitutes are relatively expensive and may not simulate human tissue as reliably as animal tissue. The aims of using simulations in such training situations are first to allow trainees to learn a skill without the need to expose a patient to the increased risk of the novice operator and second to allow for the teaching of skills in a planned and timely fashion without having to wait until a patient arrives with a particular pathological process.

Simulation-based training should employ a reproducible systematized approach to demonstration and teaching. This allows for courses to be repeated in the future and in different venues with a minimum of further effort. It also provides a framework on which other skills courses may be based. The other advantage is that a robust reproducible process will allow the supervision of the course to be undertaken by others, perhaps less senior, while ensuring that the same learning objectives and teaching methods are embraced.

6.5 **Unconscious competence**

Teaching a skill is undoubtedly more challenging than one considers at first glance. The teacher is an expert, having achieved mastery in his/her craft, and performs such skills on a daily basis as a part of his/her professional practice. Where this is a complex technical skill

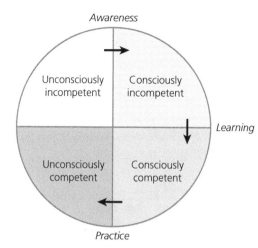

Fig. 6.1 The learning cycle modified from Peyton.

Reproduced from Peyton, Rodney, 'The learning cycle', in Rodney Peyton, ed., *Teaching and learning in medical practice*, pp. 13–19 Copyright © 1998, Manticore Europe Limited.

like surgical anastomosis or interpreting an ECG, the skilled clinician will display 'unconscious competence' in performing the task. Senior clinicians carry with them significant past experience and this is borne out by a high level of pattern recognition. The novice, on the other hand, is clearly not competent and perhaps may really not be aware of this—'unconscious incompetence'. The learning cycle (see Figure 6.1) reminds us of the stages the novice needs to negotiate in order to achieve competence.

The challenge for the teacher is to remain mindful that he/she has achieved unconscious competence, whereas the learner is working from first principles.

6.6 **Teaching a skill in four easy steps**

Consider the last time you taught someone a new skill outside the medical field. It may have been relatively simple like changing a tap washer or it may have been a more complex task. When new skills are taught we innately break the skill down into a series of steps. You might have demonstrated the skill in real time first and then demonstrated the skill in slow motion while commenting on the important steps before allowing the person that you are teaching an opportunity to try it themselves. An analogous approach can be applied to teaching a clinical skill. Peyton[2] has formalized and popularized this into a four-step approach to teaching a skill (see Table 6.2).

This process ensures that the learner has first observed the skill at a level of competence, then comprehends the component steps, and finally is able to perform the skill under supervision. This fulfils the learning paradigm in Figure 6.2.

The process allows for steps that are not successfully completed to be reviewed and repeated before proceeding to the next step. Another aspect that is frequently not considered is providing the opportunity for the trainee to practise the skill learnt and, certainly, teaching hospitals and jurisdictions need to remain mindful of the obligation to ensure that the newly acquired skill may be utilized lest it be lost.

Table 6.2 A four-step approach to teaching a skill

1. Demonstration	Trainer demonstrates at normal speed without commentary
2. Deconstruction	The task is broken down into its component steps and the trainer demonstrates while describing these steps
3. Comprehension	Trainer demonstrates while learner describes steps
4. Performance	Learner demonstrates while learner describes steps

Source: data from Peyton, Rodney, 'The learning cycle', in Rodney Peyton, ed., *Teaching and learning in medical practice*, pp. 171–180, 1998, Manticore Europe Limited.

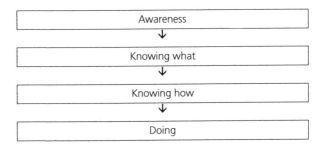

Fig. 6.2 Learning paradigm.

This approach takes a little practice in real life and the tendency may be for teachers to talk themselves through the first demonstration. This should be avoided.

> Before presenting a skills course you should practise breaking down both complex and simple tasks into their component steps.

6.7 Designing a skills teaching episode

6.7.1 Learning objectives

When designing a teaching episode consider addressing the three broad aspects of planning, content, and closure[3]. Specifically, consider the following questions.

6.7.1.1 Is it clear what the learners are going to learn?

Establishing learning objectives defines a learning pathway that guides both the learner and the teacher. In particular, the context and goals of the teaching programme need to be considered. Learning objectives for a bowel anastomosis workshop might then include:

◆ To employ previously learnt safe surgical techniques.

◆ To understand the principles of handling tissues and employ optimal suture placement in the formation of an intestinal anastomosis.

◆ Further objectives might include the ability to form specific suture placements such as mucosal-inverting vertical mattress sutures, extramucosal techniques versus full thickness anastomoses, etc.

6.7.1.2 Am I designing this lesson at the right level?

A learner embarking on a bowel anastomosis workshop should have previously achieved competence in a number of skills prior to presentation, such as safe handling of instruments and sharps, suture placement, formation of surgical knots by hand, and using an instrument tie technique, etc.

6.7.1.3 Is there immediate relevance to the learners' current clinical practice?

As noted previously, effective adult learning needs to be immediately relevant.

6.7.1.4 Will they be able to put the new skill into action in the near future?

Timely practice under supervision allows trainees to reinforce motor pathways and establish durable neural networks that ultimately allow them to become independently competent.

6.7.2 **Learning environments**

6.7.2.1 Is the environment conducive to the learning experience?

Many hospitals now have specific training workshops and access to larger dedicated skills facilities. Accordingly, the environment will generally be adequate for the workshop's purpose. There does need to be adequate lighting and the bench or table height needs to allow for a safe and comfortable posture for the learners. If learners are to spend a half or whole day learning a new technical skill then they will need to be comfortable, so matters such as heating/cooling of the workshop and avoidance of work distractions need to be considered. Have they arranged for someone else to carry their bleeper/pager? Have mobile phones been turned to silent?

6.7.2.2 What simulation will be used for the workshop?

Animal parts will often be readily available and relatively cost effective for use in technical skills courses. Examples which are frequently used include pig bellies for suturing and trotters for tendon repair (see Figure 6.3), legs of lamb or turkey for debridement of contaminated wounds, lamb thoraces for tube thoracostomy, etc. In addition to the advantage of availability, the tissue-handling characteristics are often most akin to the human form.

Special considerations apply to the use of animal parts or viscera. Planning needs to be given to surface protection from contamination and for the disposal of tissue. Some participants may express conscientious or religious objection to the use of animal tissues and synthetic substrates may need to be available. Participants handling animal tissues will need to be provided with adequate contamination barriers, a minimum of which would include gloves, plastic apron, and protective spectacles. In addition, the supply of the tissues should be reliable.

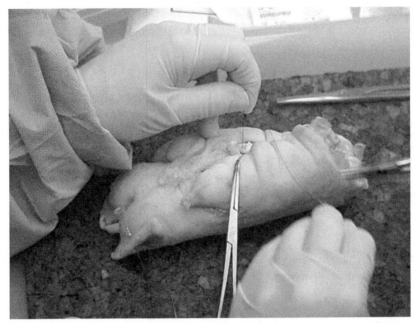

Fig. 6.3 Pig's trotters provide an excellent model for tendon repair.
Reproduced by kind permission of Jeff Hamdorf. Copyright © 2015 Jeff Hamdorf.

More advanced facilities will utilize human cadaver tissue for surgical courses. This is a most expensive and rare resource. Yet, the fresh cadaver is an excellent teaching model highly representative of the living open surgical scenario where advanced trainees and newly qualified consultants can improve their operative confidence and consequently patient safety in surgery. Considerable care must be taken to ensure the safety of participants in surgical simulation employing human tissue with respect to the risk of infection from body fluids; cadaver tissue should be considered as infective as an unknown patient in an emergency room.

Significant resources must be invested for this resource to be employed both ethically and with some modicum of cost-efficiency.

6.7.2.3 Are instruments and consumables available for the course?

Many training workshop facilities have relied on the goodwill of recently retired surgeons to supply their instruments. Other sources include replaced instruments from the operating theatres. Often, instruments may be purchased on the receipt of seed funding from health services and private benefactors. Whatever the source of supply of the instruments used it is important that the instruments are at least in good working order and they are size matched.

Sutures and ligatures should match those that the learners will use in practice.

6.7.2.4 Are there any foreseeable barriers to the course proceeding successfully?

Barriers to running a successful course fall into a variety of categories. Junior doctors may face challenges in being released from their service commitments, although there has been an encouraging recent trend towards quarantined training time for junior doctors. Equally, a junior doctor who has 'swapped into' a night shift in order to be able to attend a workshop is unlikely to perform and learn at his/her best. Heavy clinical commitments, as well as concern for, or preoccupation with, sick patients may impact on the attendance and commitment of faculty members.

Course participant and teacher numbers need to be carefully planned to ensure that there is an optimal teacher:learner ratio. Basic courses in which the learners are embracing fundamental skills should be planned with a ratio of 1:4, whereas this may be eased to 1:6 or 1:8 where the learners are acting more independently.

6.7.2.5 Is the programme achievable?

Can I take this group of surgical trainees from a pre-task level of basic suture placement to anastomosis formation in this session? The determination as to whether the learning objectives can be achieved in the allotted time is one that can be challenging. One way of helping to ensure that the learner is ready to 'hit the ground running' might be to make arrangements for pre-learning of the cognitive aspects pertinent to the skills to be taught. This may be presented and assessed as an online module. There will always be a spectrum of performance among learners and, accordingly, the teachers will need to monitor the progress of their learners and be prepared to offer more assistance to those whose progress does not meet the programme expectations. To that end, use of continuous formative assessment can be very valuable in this situation. Whether there is a need for a summative assessment is dependent on programme objectives and will be discussed a little later in this chapter.

Formative assessment is of immediate benefit to the learner, providing the critiquing is performed in a positive manner and is timely.

6.8 Critiquing, assessment, and evaluation

6.8.1 Positive critiquing

Critiquing a student's performance of a task is a skill in itself. Positive critiquing is very valuable to a trainee's outcome, while arguably a negative critique may markedly reduce the value of an educational experience. Critiquing using a participant-driven method described here will allow the learner to reflect on performance. After the participant has completed the skill, the following four-step approach to critiquing is applied:

1 What the student thought went well.

2 What the other learners, or teacher, thought went well.

3 Opportunities for improvement identified by the learner.

4 Opportunities for improvement identified by the teacher.

Naturally, if opportunities for improvement have been identified then ideally these will be exploited during the course.

6.8.2 **Assessment**

To gauge a learner's progress requires assessment. This can take various forms.

6.8.2.1 Initial assessment

Initial assessment is conducted prior to a learning exercise to establish a baseline from which progress can be measured.

6.8.2.2 Formative assessment

Formative assessment is generally performed concurrently with instruction and typically involves feedback on a student's performance. As an example one might include a simple score as to how well a learner is able to complete a new task:

♦ no errors observed

♦ occasional errors but corrected by participant

♦ occasional errors uncorrected by the participant

♦ frequent errors

♦ unable to proceed without step-by-step instructions

The most important aspect of formative assessment using a model such as this is that the learner's performance is judged against his/her own progress, not against an external standard or peer-performance standard.

Careful and considerate assessment of the learners will allow identification of those requiring remedial attention and directly benefit the learner.

6.8.2.3 Summative assessment

Summative assessment is quite different from formative assessment. Summative assessment is where the learner's performance is judged against a standard set as part of the learning programme; e.g. in the case of bowel anastomosis, the standard might include the distance between adjacent sutures, a judgement as to the tension of the knots formed, and even the watertightness of the anastomosis (see Figure 6.4).

The following points should be taken into account when we consider fair summative assessment of learners in the workshop environment:

♦ The purpose and manner of assessment should be well stated (transparency of assessment).

♦ The assessment should be clinically relevant—e.g. a bowel anastomosis that will be used again in practice.

♦ There should be an adequate time allowed for the assessment to take place.

♦ The assessment should be a multiple-level process—previous knowledge should be included as well as material from the current course and perhaps from extended experience. This allows the excellent students to excel.

♦ The assessment process should meet student expectations.

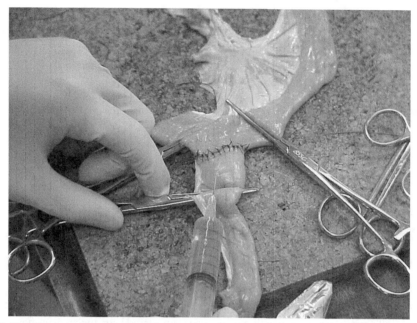

Fig. 6.4 Benchtop testing of an intestinal anastomosis.
Reproduced by kind permission of Jeff Hamdorf. Copyright © 2015 Jeff Hamdorf.

◆ Provision of assessor checklists or a defined way of identifying how the assessment is to proceed.

◆ Assessment may be competency-based and, therefore, a decision needs to be made about what to do by way of remediation.

◆ Consider global assessment versus an objective-structured approach.

6.8.3 **Evaluation**

Evaluation is an assessment of an educational programme. It is the process of determining the value of a course to its participants and offers an opportunity for reflection on the merit of the education or training episode. The evaluation process should address the following considerations:

◆ The course meets its aims and objectives.

◆ The needs of the target group are met; i.e. the course is 'pitched' at the right level.

◆ There is a mechanism for implementation of changes suggested by the evaluation process.

Methods of evaluation include:

◆ **Observation**: of faculty and participants by trained observers (educators). This can be distracting.

- **Written**: commonest method. This utilizes entry and exit questionnaires with space for free text comments. Questions are aimed to gauge the participants' opinion of the extent to which a workshop has met their expectations. A Likert scale is usually used to allow comparative grading between different courses. The Likert scale seeks for the respondent to identify their level of agreement with a statement, e.g.:

The links between basic science and clinical practice have been highlighted in the course:
1. strongly disagree
2. disagree
3. neither agree nor disagree
4. agree
5. strongly agree

While there are some limitations, Likert scale scores may be analysed to inform further course development and enhancement.

6.9 **Conclusion**

A structured learning programme that incorporates principles of adult learning and is designed around specified learning objectives is the most effective way of teaching of a clinical skill. Such a programme will often utilize a simulated learning environment.

References

1 Hamdorf JM, Hall JC. Acquiring surgical skills. Br J Surg 2000;**87**:28–37.
2 Peyton JWR. The learning cycle. In: Peyton JWR, editor. Teaching and learning in medical practice. Rickmansworth: Manticore Europe Limited; 1998, 13–19.
3 Lake FR, Hamdorf JM. Teaching on the run tips 5: teaching a skill. Med J Aust 2004;**181**:327–328.

Chapter 7

Teaching in clinical settings

Fiona Lake

Overview

- The clinical setting, when teachers and trainees are caring for patients, is very important for learning and offers opportunities to integrate the various domains necessary for a practice as a competent clinician.

- Many clinicians find themselves teaching in both simulated and clinical settings, the latter bringing challenges of needing to facilitate learning while providing quality care, dealing with unpredictable availability of learning material and the need to teach trainees at different levels.

- Effective clinical teachers need to combine being a competent clinician, supportive supervisor, and interested mentor with being a teacher.

- Adult learning principles, useful guides to consider when teaching, require understanding the learner's motivation, ensuring the learning is meaningful, experience-centred, set at the appropriate level, has clearly set goals, involves the learners, and provides feedback and time for reflection.

- Teaching or facilitating learning, whether in a discrete session done 'on the run' in the workplace (e.g. inpatients, outpatients, handover meetings) or tutorial setting, or across a clinical attachment, requires planning.

- The learning cycle provides a useful framework for considering learning, from both the teachers and learners viewpoints and moves from defining outcomes, through to planning learning/teaching, doing it, providing assessment and feedback, which then allows revisiting of the outcomes the trainee needs to address.

- Outcomes should be clear, achievable, and measurable, and should cover all aspects of competence including clinical management, communication, and professionalism.

- A framework for planning an educational encounter should include **set** (what are the outcomes, the methods and environment), **dialogue** (using a variety of teaching methods and questions to engage, consider the patient), and **closure** (provide a summary, link to future learning).

Overview *(continued)*

- In the clinical setting, frameworks such as the one-minute teacher and SNAPPS (where the learner probes the teacher on areas they do not understand), are useful.

- Assessment, defined as a judgement as to whether performance reaches a certain level against defined criteria, usually external, can be both summative, where the decision can affect a trainees progress, or formative, used to guide the trainees learning plans. Assessment is part of the learning cycle but to be done well require observation on many occasions by many members of the team.

- Feedback should use constructive critique, by first asking the trainee and then providing your feedback on first what is going well and second what could be improved. Feedback should be specific, incorporate a plan for improvement, occur frequently, and in sufficient time for trainees to try to improve.

- Evaluation of the learning experience should happen after all encounters and is key to improving teaching and learning. A variety of methods including reflection on what went well and what could be improved, gathering verbal or written feedback from trainees, or asking for peer review on discrete sessions or clinical attachments should be used.

7.1 Introduction to teaching in clinical settings

Learning in the simulation setting offers the opportunity to closely plan educational encounters, provides a safe environment, ensure trainees receive detailed feedback, and provides repetition allowing consolidation of skills. Trainees learn from making mistakes, and in the simulation setting, such mistakes when combined with reflection provide a powerful learning opportunity. The point of the learning under simulation is to increase confidence and safety when the skills and knowledge are used with patients. Clinicians, be they doctors, nurses, or clinical educators, often teach in both high- or low-fidelity simulated settings and in the clinical setting while caring for patients.[1] Unless thought is put into how skills are taken from simulated to clinical settings, there is some evidence that learning is not transferred.[2]

Learning in the clinical setting requires different planning; it is often chaotic; safe patient care must be assured, and the clinical team consists of different people with different needs. Mistakes need to be anticipated and minimized but when they do occur, a supportive no-blame environment where trainees can reflect is important. Often in this clinical environment, teaching and learning need to be done 'on the run'.

A good teacher must not only be a good doctor but have educational knowledge and skills and the flexibility to apply them under varying circumstances which may arise. Although this unpredictability may occur more commonly in the clinical setting, such flexibility may also be required in the simulation setting, when a trainee unexpectedly performs at a different level to the rest of the trainees, or equipment fails. Being able to teach on the run requires significant planning, with stored 'scripts' that can be grabbed at the right moment, and the confidence to use educational knowledge and skills to suit the circumstances. This chapter will detail key steps in learning from a teacher's perspective, namely planning, teaching, assessing, providing feedback, and finally evaluating their own skills as a teacher. It will focus on a teacher who is responsible for both facilitating learning in the workplace and running discrete teaching sessions. The term 'trainee' is used to cover anyone from undergraduate, through to specialist training.

7.2 Teachers, learners, the educational environment, and the learning cycle

7.2.1 Clinical teachers

Clinical teachers are expected to teach in the clinical environment in which they work, for example:

- while providing clinical care—inpatient or outpatient settings, on clinical rounds, during procedures, when the teacher and trainee may jointly or separately see the patient
- in clinical meetings or handover
- in small group interactive tutorials
- in large group (lecture) sessions

A clinical teacher needs to consider not only the effectiveness of a session (such as how much learning occurred during a ward round or clinic), but also a complete attachment, such as the three or six months a trainee spends on a unit. The same cycle of planning, teaching, assessment, feedback, and evaluation can be applied to short sessions and long attachments.

An effective clinical teacher needs to be all of the following:[1]

- clinician—competent, caring and professional, a role model
- supervisor—who can ensure support is given when caring for patients and who provides feedback
- mentor—who shows interest and provides career and personal advice
- teacher—understands the learner and their needs and plans and ensures effective learning

The relationship one has with the learner, such as knowing their name, needs and abilities, is key to whether the learning experience is effective. In some studies the interpersonal factors can account for up to 50% of the variance in teaching effectiveness.

7.2.2 Learners

Trainees are adults who want to learn but also want input into that learning. They come with a whole range of prior skills and knowledge that must be built on. The features of an

Table 7.1 Adult learning principles

i	Learner's motivation—do they want to improve care or pass an exam?
ii	Meaningful—the topic should be relevant to the trainee's current or future work
iii	Experience-centred—simulation, by definition, is experience-centred. In the clinical setting, trainees want learning to be linked to work they are doing or to patient care
iv	Set at the appropriate level—for their stage of training
v	Clear goals are articulated—with the outcomes for the session or attachment defined
vi	Involvement of the learner—active in the learning process through being questioned, seeing patients, or performing procedures
vii	Feedback provided—so trainee knows how they are performing
viii	Reflection—ensuring sufficient time is allowed

adult learner have been explored as principles (see Table 7.1) and are useful 'models of assumption about learning'. They are sensible and should be considered when planning or used as a starting point for reflecting on sessions.[3]

Shifting from thinking about what needs to be taught to what learners need to know, shifts from a teacher-centred to learner-centred approach, which requires the teacher to have a clear concept about what needs to be learnt (outcomes) and what knowledge or skills the learner comes with or lacks (what is their prior knowledge level?). The learning is facilitated with this information in mind. Finally, it requires an ongoing review of what learning is occurring (what are they still confused about?). Built into the teaching strategy has to be a way to find out about the knowledge level of the learner or their needs through, for example, observing and questioning.

7.2.3 **Teaching and learning styles[4]**

Learning is about creating gaining new knowledge and skills by integrating new information with old, an active process which challenges the learner's prior knowledge. As learners progress, there is often a shift from being dependent (the learner needs significant input and direction), to interest, where the learner needs some guidance, to someone who is self-directed, taking personal responsibility for their own learning. In addition, learners come with their own learning style (i.e. deep, superficial) and instructional preference (written, verbal, visual, interactive, didactic).

The strategies used by a teacher needs to take into account their own teaching preferences and abilities (an authority, a motivator or facilitator, a delegator), as well as the learner stage and learner preference. Expecting a struggling junior doctor to define their own needs, or presenting a mini-lecture to a mature and enquiring registrar will demotivate both. Some mismatch can be a good thing and challenge the learners. Shifting teaching styles from authoritarian (telling them) to delegating (getting them to tell us) shifts the workload away from the teacher and can make it more fun. Flexibility, however, is key as everyone likes to learn, and teach, in different ways at different times.

7.2.4 Educational environment

When the aim of learning is to become a well-rounded competent clinician, the clinical workplace is ideal as it requires the integration of clinical competence, communication, and professional behaviour required for optimal care. In becoming a clinical expert, recent reviews suggest it is not only how much experience trainees get (by seeing many patients) but how this exposure occurs (what is the emphasis, what feedback is given) which contributes to efficiency in learning.[5,6] As opposed to the old apprenticeship model of learning, which is often unstructured and involves 'observation' of the expert, so-called 'deliberate practice' focuses more on the needs of the learner by:

♦ defining outcomes which are important to focus on

♦ having an opportunity to repeat tasks and improve

♦ having good supervision and feedback

This is more than reflective practice. Rather than presuming by immersing trainees in clinical work they will optimally learn, consideration of elements of deliberate practice (Is feedback occurring? Are they getting enough exposure?) should inform what the teacher should do.[5,6]

Two other aspects about the educational environment are important. First, one learns more from what one doesn't know, than from reinforcing what one does know. Encouraging problem solving, rather than focusing on factual recall, can facilitate the learner working out what they don't know. You then want to inspire (or cajole) them into doing something about that lack of knowledge. Second, this will only occur if an environment where it is acceptable to demonstrate a lack of knowledge and not feel embarrassed and inadequate, is fostered. So a supportive and safe environment is key.

The three most important words in education are 'I don't know', either from the teacher or learner.

David Pencheon, UK Public Health Physician
Reproduced from 'Thoughts for new medical students at a new medical school',
Richard Smith, *British Medical Journal*, 327 (7429), p. 1430, doi: http://dx.doi.org/
10.1136/bmj.327.7429.1430 (published 18 December 2003), Copyright (c) 2003,
BMJ Publishing Group Ltd. With permission from BMJ Publishing Group Ltd.[7]

7.2.5 The learning cycle

A framework for thinking about how trainees learn, and how teachers can facilitate learning, whether in a single session or over a lengthy attachment, is embodied in the learning cycle (see Figure 7.1).[1,8] The cycle involves planning, teaching, assessing, and providing feedback, and finally an evaluation of the effectiveness of your teaching for learning. Although these processes occur continuously and simultaneously (a trainee should receive feedback throughout the term), it is helpful to consider each part in turn.

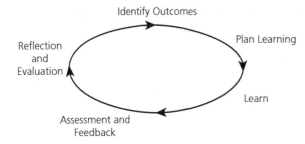

Fig. 7.1 The Learning Cycle—
the learner's viewpoint.
Adapted from Peyton JWR
(1998). 'The learning cycle'. In:
Peyton JWR, editor. *Teaching
and learning in medical practice.*
Rickmansworth, UK: Manticore
Europe Limited, 13–19.

7.3 **Teaching and learning in clinical attachments**

7.3.1 **Planning**

The first stage of planning requires definition of what outcomes the teacher wants the learner to achieve.[9] Outcomes may be provided by someone else, such as the university or college, or be developed by you as the teacher. Experienced clinicians often have a good idea as to what is important but need to consider what is occurring elsewhere in training, to avoid repetition or gaps.

Outcomes should be:

◆ specific—clearly described

◆ achievable—during that attachment or session

◆ measurable—in that the learner can be assessed to determine competence

There are a range of domains that a training doctor needs to address to ensure competent practice. The CANMEDS Framework provides a comprehensive guide incorporating at what stage in training competencies should be met (see <http://www.royalcollege.ca/portal/page/portal/rc/common/documents/canmeds/framework/canmeds2015_framework_series_II_e.pdf>).

The key areas are:

◆ medical expert

◆ communicator

◆ collaborator

◆ leader (formerly manager)

◆ health advocate

◆ scholar

◆ professional

Outcomes for an attachment or session usually cover a number of these domains in different ways, through explicit teaching or role modelling. A fault of teachers is to try to cover too much, so focus on a manageable number of important outcomes and guide learners to additional outcomes, which can be used to guide self-directed learning.

Trainees will also have their own personal learning needs, based on interests or weaknesses, which should be addressed.

The second consideration is how these outcomes are going to be achieved. The traditional apprenticeship model of training where an attachment with (hopefully) plenty of unstructured exposure allows a bright trainee to gradually meet the outcomes. Using an approach of **deliberate practice**, the focus is not just on what or how much a trainee sees[6,8] but through good supervision, feedback, and encouragement of self-reflection, a trainee can determine their progress on key outcomes such as performing a history and examination, formulating a problem list, or writing a relevant discharge summaries. This means the clinician teacher has to add structure to ensure observation and feedback occurs around important outcomes.

An **orientation**[10] at the beginning of the attachment is important for detailing what outcomes trainees would be expected to cover and how, as well as covering basic issues such as what is expected of the trainee in the job, administrative arrangements, what teaching they can expect from you, and their clinical and other responsibilities. How they are going to be assessed and when feedback will be provided should be defined. Trainees should be directed to resources (websites, handbooks, people).

7.3.2 Teaching and learning

When trainees are busy caring for patients, it is hard for them to recognize what learning is occurring. As outlined with the concept of deliberate practice, emphasizing learning by providing feedback and encouraging self-reflection are important.

In thinking about specific learning opportunities, research shows in the clinical setting trainees value informal and formal registrar teaching, formal and informal consultant teaching (although this occurs less frequently), simulation, clinical skills sessions, and tutorials.[10,11] Ward rounds and clinics in the community or hospitals when patients are discussed are valued, whereas unit meetings, grand rounds, and computer programs were not found to be valuable.[11] Although not shown to be the best method to stimulate thinking and knowledge transfer, trainees like tutorials—perhaps a reflection of the need to have a break and meet with friends and colleagues.

In teaching in these clinical settings, over time clinical teachers build up 'teaching scripts' related to diagnosis, management, ethics, and so forth (e.g., management of pneumonia, interpretation of an electrocardiogram or introducing ideas of palliation). Using the patient as the starting point, teachers can draw on these scripts to ensure they teach essential points. Even though much of the teaching is 'on the run', it needs to be planned and by knowing the topics that recurrently come up, teachers can be ready for a five-minute grabbed moment, a 30-minute interactive tutorial, or a one-hour lecture, as required.

In any teaching session, from 5 to 60 minutes, a framework consisting of **set** (what you need to be considered before), **dialogue** (what happens during), and **closure** (how you finish off) is useful.[12] The essentials of **set** include:

- Outcomes: as noted achievable in the time available, relevant and important for the learner, and set at the right level. Trainees like frameworks rather than facts.

- Environment: whether the seating, the room (not busy, noisy, public, or uncomfortable), the patient or the teaching 'props' are adequate. Not all 'moments' are good if you or the learners are tired or hungry or have other pressing duties.

The **dialogue** involves interaction between the learner and the teacher and this could appropriately be one way (didactic), interactive, or a mixture. The attention span of an adult is short (10–15 minutes) and varying methods of delivery to break up a session can significantly increase factual recall in learners. Using questions, eye contact, and names can engage learners, keep them all involved, and allow checking of understanding.

The **closure** should provide a summary, suggest further learning, and be an opportunity for clarifying what is not understood. The session should finish on time. This is also the time to evaluate the session by asking what went well and what should be changed.

In applying this to learning around patients, the structure can ensure the focus is not just on what is wrong with the patient or what needs to be organized, but can check knowledge and encourage thinking. The aim is to make the trainee's knowledge and reasoning transparent, ensure feedback is given, and further learning planned. Models which are based around discussions of clinical cases include the one-minute teacher[13] and SNAPPS,[14] where the trainee:

Summarizes the case

Narrows the differential diagnosis

Analyses the differential diagnosis

Probes (the learner asks the teacher about areas they don't understand)

Plans management

Selects an issue for self-directed learning

The probing is a change from usual teaching, where by getting the trainee to ask the questions, they can focus on what they don't know, rather than the teacher reinforcing what they do know. This structure can also allow teachers to look for one of the commonest diagnostic errors in young doctors: premature closure—that is, the failure to consider alternate diagnoses. A focus on where common errors occur, such as with premature closure, patient instructions, medication charts, and communication with other doctors, can encourage reflection and prevent mistakes.

Patients are frequently part of teaching encounters and evidence shows they like being involved.[15] It increases the time doctors spend with patients and studies have shown they are more satisfied with their inpatient stay. Frequently, it is an opportunity to educate patients and have their concerns addressed, as well as allow teachers to observe how trainees interact with patients. Problems arise when patients' rights are not recognized, when they have medical or psychiatric conditions not appropriate to discuss in front of a group, or the discussion is upsetting or confusing. Essentials are asking for the patient's consent before the session, introducing everyone to the patient, being approachable, asking for questions, and providing clear explanations.

Applying set, dialogue, and closure to more formal sessions[12] such as tutorials is relatively easy. As noted previously, the most common mistake made is to try to cover too much in a session, with too many outcomes or too many facts. A framework is valued more. In keeping in mind the attention span of an adult learner, a variation in pace or method (didactic **versus** interactive, video- **versus** paper-based stimulus) has been shown to improve retention. With easy access to electronic presentation, this medium is frequently allowed to overwhelm the message, with significant loss of value. As with any other aspect of a teaching session, it is essential to consider the purpose of visual aids being used and make sure they are simple, clear, and add to the session.

The use of questions[10] can provide a stimulus for learners, promote their thinking, and allow the teacher to assess the knowledge level of the learner. Simple yes/no questions or closed questions (looking for a single answer or fact) may not be as powerful as open questions (where there is not one correct answer, but reasoning can be probed) in determining the knowledge level of a trainee and encouraging thinking. Questions starting 'What do you think?', or 'What are you uncertain about?' are useful. Providing an environment where trainees feel comfortable to explore their thinking and demonstrate a lack of knowledge is essential.

In working in a small group, group dynamics need to be addressed, in particular making sure all are involved (by keeping an eye on who hasn't spoken, by directing questions to all), dealing with different levels of learners (redirect basic questions to more senior trainees), that disruptors are re-engaged (by sitting or standing near them, directing a question to them), and ensuring the topic is relevant and they are not getting confused (check by asking them).

7.4 **Assessment and feedback in clinical attachments**

7.4.1 **Assessment**[16]

Determining how a trainee is going and whether they are learning should be reviewed continuously as it is critical for allowing trainees to reflect on and plan further learning and for teachers to adjust their teaching programme. Additionally, clinicians at work are frequently involved in assessment for external bodies at undergraduate, prevocational, and vocational levels.

Assessment is a judgement about whether someone's performance reaches a certain level, measured against defined criteria, usually external. **Summative** assessment is used to decide on the progress of trainees in their career whereas **formative** assessment is used to 'inform' the learner, so they develop an educational plan to address deficiencies. Assessment tools may include written (essay, multi-choice), structured clinical (OSCEs—Objective, Structured Clinical Examination, mini-CEX—structured short case reviews), 'in-training' (based on observation in the workplace by a supervisor over a period of time), or multifaceted assessment, such as the 360° assessment by multiple colleagues and patients, gathered into a portfolio. All have their own profile of reliability, validity, and feasibility.

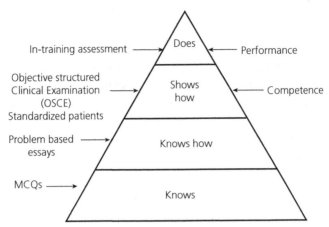

Fig. 7.2 Framework for clinical assessment.
Adapted from *Academic Medicine*, 65(9), 'The assessment of clinical skills/competence/performance', G. Miller, pp. S63–67, Copyright (C) 1990, Association of American Medical Colleges.

Workplace assessment can be improved by the assessor:

◆ knowing the outcomes expected to be achieved and at what level (as shown in Millar's Pyramid[17]: knows, knows how, shows how, or does (see Figure 7.2))

◆ finding 'assessable' moments and actually observes the trainee

◆ observing on multiple occasions

◆ collecting observations by multiple people

7.4.2 **Feedback**

A mark of a good supervisor is they are supportive and provide regular feedback. Receiving feedback on how they are doing and helping plan ways to address concerns makes it more likely trainees will pass their assessment or be fulfilled in professional life. However, there is evidence that feedback is often not provided, is given too late or given in such a fashion that it is useless. In a study where medical students had to solicit written feedback once every two weeks from a senior and junior clinicians (instead of the usual setting where students wait for seniors to say something), more feedback was received than usual. However, only 10% of the feedback was determined to be effective as most was too general to allow the students to understand what they did well or what they should change. Feedback should be balanced (allows the trainee to understand what they did well and what they need to improve) and constructive (gives guidance as to how they can address areas where they are performing poorly). As shown in Table 7.2, ineffective feedback is too non-specific to allow the trainee to understand what area they need to focus on or what strategy they can use to overcome the deficiency. More thinking about and analysing what has gone well and what needs to change should occur before a feedback session.

Table 7.2 Effective and ineffective feedback

Poor-quality feedback (non-specific, all negative or positive, no plan on how to improve)
'You did a great job.'
'Excellent, have you thought about doing respiratory medicine?'
'That was hopeless, you really need to do more work on this.'
'Poor case history.'
Effective feedback
'You need to learn about sterile technique when putting in an IV cannula.'
'Your history taking was very good, you were organized, you were clearly thinking about what was happening and your questions led to your diagnosis.'
'Your physical examination revealed the main finding, which was good. It was disorganized, however, and was stressful for the patient as you had them sitting up and down all the time. Best to start in the front and move to the back. Look at the proforma in the *Core Clinical Methods* book, and practice that on family members till you can do it without thinking. Let us check your technique at the next tutorial.'

In providing that feedback, teachers should use the framework of **constructive feedback**[18]:

- Ask the learner what they did well.
- You discuss what they did well.
- Ask the learner what they could improve.
- You discuss what they could improve (and how).

This encourages reflection and self-assessment, as well as balances good and poor. Importantly, it is constructive, so discussing what and how they could improve rather than what they did badly implies a plan of action to guide efforts. The feedback should be **specific** and achievable; for example, on a particular area or topic rather than a broad learning topic (see Table 7.2). For example, in reviewing a trainee's letters to general practitioners (GPs), the feedback may provide a framework for covering important areas a GP is interested in, as a basis for writing letters next time. Feedback should be provided at the time the observation has been made, and occur on an almost daily basis. An overall review should occur at formal times during the term (mid-term), with a date agreed on during the orientation. Feedback must be provided in time for trainees to address concerns before the end of the attachment.

7.4.3 Self-assessment[10,16]

Good doctors underestimate their abilities; poor doctors overestimate their abilities. We can get better at self-assessment by benchmarking with feedback from experienced clinicians. Challenges arise when doctors do not accept a view of their deficiencies. A marker of professional misconduct is an inability to accept or act on any advice from supervisors. When faced with this challenge, patience is required. The teacher should focus not on the person but the issues and provide clear examples. If the issues are important, they need to be addressed and not avoided, which may mean seeking help from more senior supervisors or directors of the educational programme.

7.4.4 Evaluation[1,19]

Evaluation as a term is often used interchangeably with assessment. Evaluation usually focuses more on the teacher or the programme, and is the trainee's judgement of how well the session or programme was delivered and met their needs. It should be an integral part of any teaching programme. Teachers should gather information, usually in a variety of ways, so they can review and revise as required. Information could focus on both the teaching (content, session organization, and format) and learning (did they learn what they were meant to learn; what is still causing confusion). Methods for gathering data could include:

- verbal feedback—asking what went well and what should be changed
- written feedback—from complex surveys to a quick jot on a scrap of paper
- peer observation of teaching with feedback

There can be conflict between a clinical teacher trying to obtain useful feedback in an evaluation, when they are also the trainee's assessor. A trainee is unlikely to give an honest but negative opinion of teaching, if they know the assessment will be completed by the same person. Separating the two processes or gathering the information in an anonymous form may be important.

7.4.5 Flexibility

Flexibility in teaching in clinical settings is required to cope with the varied needs of learners at different levels, the broad outcomes which need to be met, including clinical competence, communication, and professionalism, and the fluid nature of the clinical environment. However, planning which takes into consideration what needs to be covered, the many ways it can be covered, and how assessment and feedback will occur puts structure into this environment. Finally, it is worth considering the responsibilities of the learner and what part they will play in allowing the educational programme to be implemented. By sharing the load, it is far more likely to be successful.

References

1 Lake FR. Teaching on the run tips: doctors as teachers. Med J Aust 2004;**180**(8):415–416.
2 Heaven C, Clegg J, Maguire P. Transfer of communication skills training from workshop to workplace: the impact of clinical supervision. Patient Educ Coun 2006;**60**:313–325.
3 Kaufman DM. ABC of learning and teaching in medicine: applying educational theory in practice. BMJ 2003;**326**:213–216.
4 Vaughn L, Baker R. Teaching in the medical setting: balancing teaching styles, learning styles and teaching methods. Med Teacher 2001;**23**:610–612.
5 Peyton JWR. The learning cycle. In: Peyton JWR, ed. *Teaching and learning in medical practice*. Rickmansworth: Manticore Europe Limited, 1998: 13–19.
6 Schuwirth LWT, van der Vleuten CPM. Challenges for educationalists. BMJ 2006;**333**:544–546.

7 **Smith R**. Thoughts for new medical students at a new medical school. BMJ 2003;**327**:1430–1433.

8 **Ericsson KA**. Deliberate practice and the acquisition and maintenance of expert performance in medicine and related domains. Acad Med 2004;**79**(10):S70–81.

9 **Prideaux D**. The emperor's new clothes: from objectives to outcomes. Med Educ 2000;**34**:168–169.

10 **Gordon J**. ABC of learning and teaching in medicine: one-to-one teaching and feedback. BMJ 2003;**326**:543–548.

11 **Dent AW, Crotty B, Cuddihy HL, et al**. Learning opportunities for Australian prevocational hospital doctors: exposure, perceived quality and desired methods of learning. Med J A 2006;**184**:436–440.

12 **Lake FR, Ryan G**. Teaching on the run tips 3: planning a teaching episode. Med J Aust 2004;**180**(12):643–644.

13 **Furney SL, Orsini AL, Orsetti KE, et al**. Teaching the one minute preceptor. A randomised controlled trial. J Gen Intern Med 2001;**16**:620–624.

14 **Wolpaw TM, Wolpaw DR, Papp KK**. SNAPPS: a learner-centred approach for outpatient education. Acad Med 2003;**78**:893–898.

15 **Howe A, Anderson J**. Involving patients in medical education. BMJ 2003;**327**:326–328.

16 **Lake FR, Ryan G**. Teaching on the run tips 8: assessment and appraisal. Med J Aust 2005;**182**: 580–581.

17 **Millar GE**. The assessment of clinical skills/competence/performance. Acad Med1990;**65**(9):S63–67.

18 **Pendelton D, Schofield T, Havelock P, Tate P**. *The consultation: an approach to learning and teaching*. Oxford: Oxford University Press,1984.

19 **Morrison J**. ABC of teaching and learning in medicine. Evaluation. BMJ 2003;**326**:385–387.

Chapter 8

Teaching and learning through the simulated environment

Iris Vardi

Overview

- Teaching for learning in the simulated environment requires sound planning, good teaching, and evaluation that supports improvement.

- Planning involves the development of learning objectives, tasks, activities, and assessments.

- Good teaching in the simulated environment focuses on learning through doing, and involves sound management of sessions, clear delivery of information, and attention to students' needs and styles of learning.

- When evaluating to improve, it is important to draw from various perspectives including those of the teachers, the students, experts in the field, and educational experts.

8.1 Introduction to teaching and learning through the simulated environment

The simulated environment offers learners many opportunities that extend far beyond the traditional lecture, classroom, tutorial, or laboratory setting. They can take on a new role, learn by doing, experiment, solve problems, and make decisions within a safe context that mimics the workplace.

In the real-life context, we have no control over the nature of the problems or conditions that present. This sometimes leaves learners to deal with situations when they have not yet developed the necessary skills. With simulation, this can be overcome. It is the educators, rather than the presenting patients, who determine the nature of the learning experience including the difficulty and complexity of the task. In such a controlled environment, learners can be given the time and space to learn from the actions they took and the decisions they made without the pressure of the daily work environment and its associated accountabilities.

However, in order to fully realize the potential of simulation, we need to do more than simply place learners within a simulated environment and provide them with varied experiences. Realizing the full potential of the simulation lies in the planning, execution, and follow-up to the learning experience.

8.2 Planning for learning in the simulated environment

Planning is an essential part of the teaching process. At the most basic level, you need to know how many sessions to run, what will be covered in each session, and how long they should run for. However, there is much more to plan. You need to determine what needs to be taught, the best ways to teach and sequence activities for maximum learning, how and when feedback should be provided, how to assess, and how to support transference to the workplace.

8.2.1 Determining the learning objectives

In order to plan properly, your first task is to determine what the participants need to learn. There are so many different types of skills and abilities that can be learnt through simulation. Students could increase their core knowledge, develop practical manual skills, improve their abilities to read, analyse, and interpret clinical signs and symptoms, solve problems, make decisions, and work effectively in a team—to name but a few.

Deciding which skills and abilities to develop is, to a large degree, dependent on your audience and the reasons for providing the learning experience in the first place. Neophytes in any given area may well need to start with core knowledge and practical manual skills. But experienced practitioners probably need something different. For instance, they may have the manual skills, but need to develop their teamwork or decision-making skills.

Clearly articulating your aims for the students provides a set of parameters for your planning. These are usually expressed in the form of learning objectives, also known as learning outcomes (see Box 8.1).

You can see that these learning objectives focus on both the **content** that will be covered (unconscious patients, VF, VT, and asystole) and the **behaviours** that learners will be able to demonstrate with that content within a workplace context (recognize and appropriately manage). Matching learner behaviours with content is the key to providing active learning

Box 8.1 Examples of learning objectives/outcomes for a course

By the end of this course, the student will be able to:

♦ Recognize and appropriately manage an unconscious patient

♦ Recognize and appropriately manage ventricular fibrillation (VF), ventricular tachycardia (VT), and asystole experiences which make use of the simulated environment. It will also help you to design activities in which the students think and act through practising, evaluating what they have done, analysing situations, and making decisions. This is in stark contrast to simply listening to others telling them about good practice.

When putting learning objectives together, try to progress beyond basic skill development to more challenging outcomes. For example, you may focus on some of the Accreditation Council for Graduate Medical Education core competencies (see <http://www.acgme.org>): patient care, medical knowledge, practice-based learning and improvement, interpersonal and communication skills, professionalism, and systems-based practice. These can be addressed, for instance, through incorporating objectives that require:

♦ protocols to be followed

♦ differential diagnosis and appropriate selection of treatment

♦ evaluation of critical incidents

♦ working effectively as a team during a crisis

8.2.2 Tasks and activities for learning

Your learning objectives set the scene for determining what will occur in the course. Start by designing real-life complex tasks that your students could do in the simulated environment which would demonstrate their achievement of the learning objectives. We will refer to these as the learning objective tasks. Let's have a look at some complex simulation tasks that would demonstrate the learning objectives given previously (see Table 8.1).

As these examples show, the learning objective tasks will generally be too difficult for your students to achieve at the start of the course. These become the **summative tasks** that allow you to evaluate the sum of knowledge and skills that the students have gained by the end of the course. To successfully achieve these tasks, you need to think about the types of prerequisite knowledge and skills that the students would need. For example, to be able to manage an unconscious patient in a team setting, each of your students will first need to be able to: (i) establish an airway and commence breathing; (ii) check pulse and establish circulation; and (iii) work effectively as part of a team. This prerequisite knowledge can be taught first, often in smaller, less complex support tasks. These are often referred to as the **formative tasks** in which students learn and practise using the underlying skills and knowledge required for the summative task.

Table 8.1 Examples of complex tasks that demonstrate learning objectives

Learning Objective	Learning Objective Task
Recognize and appropriately manage an unconscious patient	Initial team management of an unconscious patient using ABC in a number of different scenarios with differing patient histories
Recognize and appropriately manage VF, VT, and asystole	Team assessment and management of life-threatening arrhythmias in a number of different scenarios with differing patient histories

Formative support tasks are extremely important in ensuring that your students will be successful when they finally attempt the more complex summative learning objective task. There are so many different types of support tasks that you could design. For instance, in addition to practising manual skills, your students could make and justify differential diagnoses based on evidence/data they collect, design and trial safe protocols or working environments, or even trial and evaluate different treatment procedures. Whatever you decide, these tasks will need to be sequenced so that knowledge and understanding is built and reinforced.

Remember, people learn in different ways. Some are listeners and watchers, some learn by doing, some like to work on their own, and others like to work in groups. Often, people like a little bit of each. Cater for different learners by building in listening, speaking, doing, reading, writing, working alone, and working together into each task. Students rarely learn everything the first time. Building in these different types of activities into each task supports and reinforces learning as students engage with the same information in different ways. Use building activities before, during, and after each task.

8.2.2.1 Before the task

Prior to any task, there is usually background information that each participant needs to know. This could include understanding how the simulators operate, how the environment works, and essential medical knowledge. Such background information could be developed in various ways. First, you may decide to give a short talk, lecture, or practical demonstration. These types of activities provide learners with an opportunity to listen and watch. It has been found that most people can listen effectively for about 20 minutes, so plan accordingly.

However, there are also activities that your students could do before the task. Your students come with a range of experiences and knowledge to think about, share with the group, and build on. Such thinking and talking activities could include, for example, brainstorming, short multiple-choice quizzes to attempt and then discuss, and asking participants to share practices within their particular medical context. Some of these activities could be done individually, some in pairs, and others with the group as a whole. As the aim is to prepare for the task, design these to be quick and short. 10–15 minutes is a good time frame to aim for.

8.2.2.2 During the task

The task provides the opportunity for the participants to actually do activities that simulate the work environment. This also requires careful detailed planning. Think about:

- what the students are required to do and why;
- the context or the patient history that requires this action;
- the information that the students will need in order to successfully complete the task;
- whether the students will work alone or in groups;
- whether the students will need a practical demonstration first; and
- whether a checklist would be helpful for the students when they practise.

Addressing the mechanics of the task in this way will provide you with the basis for developing a set of steps and materials that will support the students in their learning. Remember to (i) build in plenty of opportunities for the students to practise, and (ii) to design materials that will support students in making their own decisions and being able to check how they are progressing.

8.2.2.3 After the task

Designing the simulated task is not, however, the end of the planning. You also need to plan post-task activities. The aim of these activities is to provide the students with an opportunity to reflect on the actions they took in the simulation, explore other options and possibilities, and extend their learning. Reflecting on actions requires a framework, or set of standards or behaviours against which students can evaluate and discuss. Design activities in which students recall what happened, rate, or examine their actions and discuss how they could improve. This could occur through the completion of self-evaluation checklists, small group discussion, and/or large group discussion or debriefing.

These after-task activities are critical for learning. Through these activities, students can learn from one another, and set their own goals for improvement. Opportunities for discussion also provide a time for the teacher to confirm and reiterate the important 'take home' messages. They also allow the teacher to make sure that no-one leaves with any misconceptions or misunderstandings.

8.2.3 Documenting your planning

Teaching within a simulated environment often requires extensive coordination between the teachers in the course, the technicians, and the administrative staff. A well-constructed teaching plan provides all concerned with a clear understanding of how the course is to proceed.

Teaching plans often include:

- the tasks and their associated learning activities
- assessment tasks
- how long each assessment, task, and activity will take
- equipment needed including medical equipment, models, multimedia devices, cadaveric material, handouts, worksheets, checklists, and so forth
- scenarios and case studies appended to the plan. See Duke University's scenario template at <http://anesthesiology.duke.edu/?page_id=825706>
- the core competencies being addressed, also appended to the plan

Table 8.2 shows a sample teaching plan based on the learning objective 'Recognize and appropriately manage an unconscious patient'. It incorporates the learning objective task as well as the support tasks which develop the prerequisite knowledge and understandings required. It also shows how pre- and post-activities for each task can be incorporated.

Table 8.2 Sample teaching plan

Course Name:

Session Name: ABC and the unconscious patient		Session Time: 8.30 a.m.–12 noon
No. of participants: 20		
Start	**Task/Activity**	**Equipment**	**Time**
8.30 a.m.	Introduce course Students brainstorm—what needs to be done with an unconscious patient?	– Whiteboard and markers – PowerPoint presentation	15 mins
8.45 a.m.	**Support Task 1: Establish airway and commence breathing**		**45 mins total**
8.45 a.m.	(i) Before Task 1 5 groups of 4. Teachers explain and demonstrate AB.	– 5 Mannequins/models – 20 handouts on ABC – 5 pocket masks	15 mins
9.00 a.m.	(ii) Task 1 In pairs students practice AB. One student practises, while other marks the checklist and provides feedback. Students swap roles. 5 minutes practice each.	– PowerPoint with task details – 10 mannequins/models – 20 checklists of AB behaviours – 20 pocket masks	15 mins
9.15 a.m.	(iii) After Task 1 Students complete self-evaluation form. Teacher facilitates group discussion, discusses implications for the workplace and summarizes main 'take home' messages.	– 20 self-evaluation forms – PowerPoint slides – Whiteboard and markers	15 mins
9.30 a.m.	**Support Task 2: Check pulse and establish circulation**		**35 mins total**
9.30 a.m.	(i) Before Task 2 5 groups of 4. Teachers explain and demonstrate C.	– 5 mannequins/models – 5 backboards	10 mins
9.40 a.m.	(ii) Task 2 In pairs students practise C. One student practises, while other marks the checklist and provides feedback. Students swap roles. 5 minutes practice each.	– 10 mannequins/models for practice – 20 checklists with C behaviours – 10 backboards	15 mins
9.55 a.m.	(iii) After Task 2 Teacher facilitates group discussion. Students write personal goals for improvement in the workplace.	– PowerPoint slides – whiteboard and markers	10 mins

continued

Table 8.2 (continued) Sample teaching plan

Course Name:

Session Name: ABC and the unconscious patient		Session Time: 8.30 a.m.–12 noon	
No. of participants: 20			
Start	**Task/Activity**	**Equipment**	**Time**
10.05 a.m.	Break		20 mins
10.25 a.m.	**Learning Objective Task 3: Initial team management of unconscious patient**		
10.25 a.m.	Revision—ABC multiple choice quiz (3 mins). In pairs, students compare and discuss answers (4 mins). Group shares and discusses answers (8 mins).	– 20 ABC multiple choice quizzes – Whiteboard and markers	15 mins
10.40 a.m.	(i) Before Task 3 Teacher introduces task. Students brainstorm the characteristics of good teamwork. Teacher shows slides on good teamwork.	– Whiteboard and markers – PowerPoint slides	15 mins
10.55 a.m.	(ii) Task 3: Part 1 5 groups of 4. Each group has a different scenario.	– 5 different scenarios (blocked/unblocked airway, adequate/inadequate breathing, with/without pulse) 5 copies of each – 5 mannequins/models prepared as per scenarios – 5 rooms/cubicles	15 mins
11.10 a.m.	(iii) After Task 3: Part 1—debrief Students group evaluation checklist. Each group discusses their clinical and group skills in the scenario. Students write individual goals for improvement.	– 20 group evaluation checklists covering ABC and group behaviours – Whiteboard and markers – 5 separate rooms/cubicles	20 mins
11.30 a.m.	(ii) Task 3: Part 2 Same groups, students swap rooms and scenarios.	– 5 scenarios as before. 5 copies of each – 5 mannequins/models each prepared as per scenarios – 5 rooms/cubicles	15 mins
11.45 a.m.	(iii) After Task 3—debrief All groups together. Discuss what was learnt and important 'take home' points.	– Whiteboard and markers	15 mins
12 noon	Lunch		

As you look through the sample teaching plan in Appendix 8, take note of features important for good teaching and learning. First, note how the plan is focused on student activity: talking, thinking, and doing. Teacher talk is limited to the essentials that wrap around the learning activities: introductions, explanations and demonstrations, clarification, and summing up of important points.

Next, note how information is recycled, checked, and reinforced. This is carefully built into the plan through the use of the formative support tasks, pre-task activities, and quick revision activities. In this plan, teaching starts from the students' own knowledge base by probing what they already know. It then moves to teaching and practising first AB and later C. As you look carefully through the plan, you will see that knowledge and skills are developed, checked, and reinforced through the systematic incorporation of: (i) modelling; (ii) practice; (iii) checklists for peer feedback and evaluation; (iv) self-evaluation forms; (v) group discussion; and (vi) a quick revision activity. All of this formative activity occurs before the students attempt the complex summative task that reflects the learning objective for the course. Designing a course in this way supports your students in their learning and helps them to be successful.

8.3 Facilitating learning

While a solid plan lays the foundation for good teaching and sound learning experiences, it is the teachers who bring the plan to life and create the learning experiences. Teachers take on many roles for students. They are session organizers, mentors, guides, sources of expertise and knowledge, motivators, and confidence builders. Each of these roles reveals itself in different ways as teachers and students interact. The manner in which this interaction proceeds determines whether learning occurs at all, is impeded or is progressed.

8.3.1 Managing the session

Students will only be able to complete all the activities and tasks, and meet the learning objectives for the course, if you manage the session well. This involves sound management of tasks, activities, time, and participants. The teaching plan lays out the nature of the tasks and activities, and the time frame in which they need to be completed. It is important that you adhere to these times as planned.

Manage the session and your students by:

- Being succinct in your explanations and instructions.
- Letting students know how much time they have to do a task, e.g. 'You have five minutes to . . .'
- Explaining what needs to be accomplished in that time frame, e.g. 'By the end of this activity you should have eight examples of . . .'
- Letting students know how much time they have left, e.g. 'You have just one more minute before you need to swap over.'

◆ Circulating between groups, resolving any problems, and keeping your participants on task.

◆ Thanking talkative participants for their input and letting everyone know that due to time constraints you may need to limit discussion time.

8.3.2 Conveying information clearly

To manage a session and develop knowledge well, it is important to convey instructions and knowledge in a clear, logical, and succinct manner. Not only does clarity help students to understand, it also shows that the teacher clearly knows what s/he is doing. In fact, in surveys of what adult learners value in their teachers, 'clear explanations' rate very highly indeed.

Within the simulated environment, students need to be clear about many things:

◆ the background knowledge they need in order to be successful;

◆ the task or activity they are to complete;

◆ how to use the equipment;

◆ which skills and abilities they need to demonstrate;

◆ how skills and abilities will be evaluated; and

◆ the important points they can take into their practice in the 'real world'.

Sometimes, actions speak louder than words and it can be far easier to show how something is done rather than just explain it. This also requires careful thought and planning. Often, when we are expert at carrying out a procedure or executing a skill, we do it automatically without thinking about how we accomplished the task. During the planning stage, deconstruct the steps you take in a task before you try to teach it to others. Think about why you do it this way. Now you have a set of steps or points to guide your students through. As before, you will only have a limited time to model, so highlight the most important aspects for your participants. The finer details can come later as you guide your students while they practise.

Whenever you are modelling, make sure that everyone can see what you are doing, and direct their attention to the details that you want them to focus on or notice. For example, 'See how I am . . .' and 'Notice the way that . . .'

8.3.3 Focusing on the student

Imparting knowledge in a clear and enthusiastic way is important, but gives us no idea how much the student has actually learnt. In fact, whenever we simply impart information, no matter how clearly, we do not really know whether that information was new to the student, whether it covered all that they needed to know, whether they understood it correctly, or even whether they could use it effectively within the work environment. Asking 'Do you understand?' may also not yield sufficient information, particularly when students are too embarrassed to confess their lack of understanding or when they mistakenly believe that they have understood.

To guide, mentor, and progress student learning, you need to go beyond imparting information to focusing on the students, their needs, and their understanding. A good teaching plan should provide you with multiple opportunities to check student understanding and ascertain their needs as knowledge and skills are repeatedly brought to bear in different activities. As you work with students, be alert to their strengths, weaknesses, gaps, and misconceptions, and then tailor your teaching to meet needs.

8.3.3.1 Facilitating learning

The different tasks and activities in the teaching plan require more than your organization. They also require you to actively facilitate the learning for each student. How to do this, however, will vary from student to student. Make sure that you and everyone in the teaching team circulates and attends to each and every participant. Tailor your teaching to best match your student needs at that time. This requires you to do more listening and watching, and less talking and directing. Think about when to step in and guide learning, and when to let the participants be. As you observe your students, be alert to student differences and provide support, input, and advice as required.

Also make sure you provide additional support for students for whom English is a foreign language:

- Provide notes that summarize what you have said.
- Provide short video demonstrations that students can view on their own.
- Put your instructions for tasks and activities in writing on the whiteboard.
- Provide students with time to gather their thoughts in English before they speak.
- Keep your sentences short and clear and do not speak too rapidly.

Many of these extra supports may also prove helpful to all your participants.

8.3.3.2 Providing feedback

Guiding learning requires the ability to give useful feedback at the right time. Verification and corrective feedback is very useful. **Verification** feedback lets students know what they are doing correctly and how well they are doing it; for example, 'Your use of the . . . is extremely good. Keep it up.' **Corrective** feedback helps students to improve and develop their knowledge and skills.

When providing corrective feedback, make sure that you focus on only one or two main points at a time. Don't try to correct everything at once. As you work with individual participants on their activities or tasks, make sure that your corrective feedback is direct and unambiguous. Prompt students to recall something that was taught earlier; for example, 'Do you remember . . .', and use their response as basis for guiding or correcting what they are doing. Or, you could simply tell the student what to do and how to do it; for example, 'Pull the . . . back'. Provide praise as they get it right; for example, 'Yes, that's it!'

Whenever providing feedback, or in fact whenever you are teaching, you also need to be aware of your students' state of mind. This is where your role as a confidence builder and motivator comes into play. Students will come to your course with various levels of confidence.

Some may be concerned about revealing a lack of knowledge, failure, or mistakes in front of their colleagues, and see it as a loss of face. This requires sensitivity on your part in where, when, and how you speak to your students. Look out for the quiet students. They may prefer to chat separately with you about their learning, whereas others may be happy to speak up, learn, and receive feedback in front of others. It is important that you create a safe environment for all students to discuss how they are going, where they need help, and how to improve.

No matter what context, or for what purpose you are providing feedback, always strive to be encouraging, respectful, and supportive to your students. This will help them participate, try things out for the first time, and remain motivated.

8.4 Evaluating for improvement

Once a course is over, it is important to evaluate how it went. Evaluation should help you determine what went well and how to improve. These can range from participant perceptions of the course to comprehensive evaluations that gain the insights of others, such as experts in the field, the teaching staff, and educational experts. The depth of evaluation you need depends on the context. If you are running a course for the first time, you will need different types of information than if you are running or reviewing an established course. Remember, it usually takes a few iterations to get a course to the stage where you will be satisfied with how it runs. It is very rare indeed that everything goes so well the first time that no improvement is needed.

Evaluating for improvement can cover a number of different areas including quality of the course, the teaching, and the learning.

8.4.1 Quality of the course

An important aspect to examine when looking to improve is the course itself—its content, learning objectives, tasks, activities, and assessments:

- Is the course complete and up to date?
- Are the activities well structured and well sequenced?
- Does everyone have sufficient time and opportunity to participate and practise?
- Do the assessments accurately capture student learning?
- Does the set-up of the room and the equipment allow for sound observation and learning?

As you consider these types of questions, think about what needs to be modified for improvement.

8.4.2 Quality of the teaching

No matter how good the planning and set-up are, without good teaching it all goes to waste. Hence, evaluation of teaching is enormously important:

- Were sufficient teaching staff available?
- Did they have the necessary skills and expertise?

- Did they provide useful feedback?
- Were they respectful, encouraging, and sensitive to students' needs?

Think about improvements, and the types of teacher or facilitator training that might be of benefit to you and other staff.

8.4.3 **Quality of learning**

Of course, student learning and reaction to the teaching and course should lie at the heart of your evaluation. There is no point in running a simulation course if students leave without being positive about what they learnt and without being able to take away safe practical skills and abilities that they can apply in the workplace. So, it is important to ascertain what students learnt, what they didn't learn, and how they felt about it. There are a number of aspects to consider:

- How did the students change in their skill and knowledge set from the start of the course to the end of the course?
- What were their reactions to instructions, activities, tasks, and the amount of time given?
- What were their reactions to the styles of the different teaching staff?
- Did all the students participate and were they engaged?

As you examine the student learning experience, consider what you would have liked them to have learnt, whether this was achieved, and what you would do differently next time.

8.4.4 **What and how to evaluate**

It is important to gather information from a variety of different sources to ensure reliability and accuracy of your findings. First, gather information from the participants themselves. Their satisfaction and perceptions of their own learning, relevance to their workplace, and quality of the content, activities, tasks, and teaching can be gathered through questionnaires and/or focus groups.

Another important source of information is from the assessments you ran. How well did they perform on these assessments? Did they learn the knowledge and skills you set out for them to learn at the start of the course? How well did they achieve the learning objectives?

Assessments, however, are not the only sources of information about learning. Structured observations, based on observation forms or checklists, can also provide important information. Observations can be collected from the teaching staff and/or external observers.

Also of importance are your discussions with your teaching staff. A debrief at the end of a course allows teachers to share their general observations and put together suggestions for improvement. These could cover a range of matters including:

- the content, layout, equipment and structure of the course;
- the nature and design of the tasks, activities and assessments; and
- how student learning progressed.

These sessions are also useful for sharing with staff the participants' perceptions of the course, their learning, and the teaching that they received.

8.5 **Where to from here?**

Evaluation is not the end of the process. Often, it takes you right back to the beginning. Teaching and learning is a complex process with so many different variables which come together in differing ways: the students, the teachers, and the course itself.

This chapter has attempted to provide you with a framework and a basis from within which you can view teaching and learning. From here you can only learn more. The following chapters will provide you with more techniques, insights, and ideas. Use, practise, and experiment with these. With sound planning, implementation, and evaluation, your course, your teaching, and your students' learning can only improve and grow.

8.6 **Recommended reading**

Biggs J. (1999) *Teaching for quality learning at university: what the student does.* Buckingham: Society for Research into Higher Education and Open University Press.

Cannon R. (1992) *Lecturing.* Campbelltown, NSW: Higher Education Research and Development Society of Australasia.

Chalmers D, Fuller R. (1996) *Teaching for learning at university: theory and practice.* London: Kogan Page.

Kember D, Kelly M. (1993) *Improving teaching through action research.* Campbelltown, NSW: Higher Education Research and Development Society of Australasia.

Ladyshewsky R. (1995) *Clinical teaching.* Campbelltown, NSW: Higher Education Research and Development Society of Australasia.

MacDonald R. (1997) *Teaching and learning in small groups.* Birmingham: SEDA.

Ramsden P. (1992) *Learning to teach in higher education.* London: Routledge.

Vardi I. (2012) *Effective feedback for student learning in higher education.* Milperra, NSW: Higher Education Research and Development Society of Australasia.

Chapter 9

Simulation in nursing education and practice

Joseph S Goode Jr and John M O'Donnell

Overview

- Simulation in nursing education has become a standard practice in many parts of the world, but there remain issues related to instructor preparedness, resources, and appropriate curricular integration.

- A variety of educational theories, models, or frameworks are available to guide the development of nursing simulation educational and research programmes, but no single model predominates. Potential barriers are the lack of standardized nomenclature and the lack of a predominant theoretical model.

- Clinical experiences for nursing students are becoming increasingly difficult to arrange, especially in specialty and high-acuity areas. With appropriate curricular integration, simulation can be a viable approach to supplement clinical experiences with targeted learning in areas such as critical thinking/clinical reasoning, safety skills, communication, competency evaluation, and management of high-risk procedures.

- The body of evidence supporting the replacement of some clinical experience with simulation is growing. What remains to be determined is the exact mix of 'live' versus 'simulated' clinical exposure.

9.1 The state of the nursing simulation science

The use of simulation as either a primary educational approach or as a supplement for both didactic teaching and clinical experience has now become standard practice across much of the world. Most nursing educators now have at least some familiarity with the methodology and, in fact, there is a tradition of using simple simulation events in the profession. Role-playing and other forms of non-patient interaction have long been used with static mannequins such as 'Mrs. Chase' from the early 1900s foreshadowing the evolution of the current computer-controlled devices.[1] The acquisition of affordable, advanced simulators has encouraged widespread exploration and adoption of the approach. Instructor preparedness, placement of simulation modules within a curriculum, substitution of simulation for actual clinical time, and the transfer of learning from the lab to the bedside remain ongoing issues. Aspects of simulation as basic as development of a standard nomenclature to describe roles and activities have continued to act as barriers to shared understanding and smooth adoption.

In 2003, the National League of Nursing in the United States and the Laerdal Corporation formed the NLN/Laerdal partnership. This partnership led to the development of online resources (Simulation Innovation Resource Center (SIRC)) intended to spur faculty development in simulation educational methods.[2] At the same time, a large number of national and international simulation societies (e.g. Society for Simulation in Healthcare, US and Society in Europe for Simulation Applied to Medicine, Europe) emerged with the goal of supporting healthcare simulation training around the world. In 2010 the International Nursing Association for Simulation and Clinical Learning (INASCL, US), a nursing-focused society, initiated a standards development process with expertise drawn from around the world. Seven standards for simulation terminology and educational methodology were published in 2013. These standards include: Terminology (I), Professional Integrity (II), Participant Objectives (III), Facilitation (IV), Facilitator (V), Debriefing Process (VI), and Participant Assessment and Evaluation (VII).[3-10]

The INACSL standards parallel the reviews of simulation best practices that have been conducted by Issenberg et al., Bremner et al., McGahie et al., and Cook et al., all of which summarized key design or curricular components associated with high-quality simulation education and improved outcomes.[11-15]

9.2 Models or frameworks used in nursing simulation education and research

A variety of models and constructs have been used to provide the theoretical support for nursing simulation educational interventions. Advantages in adopting a valid theoretical model include the ability to consolidate nomenclature and identify causal or predictive relationships. Additionally, a model provides an educator-focused tool to organize development and implementation of student-centred simulation curricula and can be an important guide for research efforts. No single theoretical model predominates in the simulation literature and no theory to date has shown itself to be easily applied to real-world simulation processes. Nursing simulation educators and researchers often don't identify a theoretical framework when publishing their work.[16-23] The majorities of the frameworks mentioned are either based on structured process models or are dependent on educational theory. In this section we discuss prominent examples of both types, as well as others, which currently appear within the nursing literature.

9.2.1 **Structured model: the nursing process construct**

A desire to describe and define the underlying work of nursing drove the first descriptions of nursing as a 'process' in the late 1950s, which evolved into a six-step process in the 1973 American Nurses Association (ANA) standards. Nursing oversight bodies in the US, Canada, and the UK were quick to integrate these process steps into Nurse Practice Acts. The steps of the nursing process typically include: Assessment, Diagnosis, Planning/Outcomes, Implementation, Evaluation (ADPIE).[24] This construct has been used as a model for structuring nursing simulation course content. Burns et al. describe using this structure to teach freshmen undergraduate students the steps of the process. Interestingly, they added a sixth step, Communication, to make the rubric ADPIE-C. These authors reported changes in knowledge, attitude, and skill with respect to evaluating a series of patients.[25] McCausland also described the use of the nursing process to develop both objectives and evaluation tools for a heart failure simulation.[26]

A weakness in using the Nursing Process within interprofessional courses is the Diagnosis step. A Nursing Diagnosis is supposed to be a standardized description of the patient state matched with both antecedent conditions and potential nursing actions. Lists of standardized Nursing Diagnoses are approved and published by NANDA International Inc., a for-profit organization.[27] The nursing diagnosis concept has evolved because the scope of practice of bedside nurses does not typically include making a medical diagnosis. Advocates purport that Nursing Diagnosis statements are designed to empower nurses, standardize hospital language, and provide clarity. Unfortunately, no other profession in healthcare teaches this language. Del Bueno suggests that this has created confusion and contributed to a lack of clear communication between nurses and other providers.[28] This is critical, as Leonard points out, because failure in communication is a core component of adverse outcomes.[29] The Joint Commission sentinel event programme continues to cite communication failures among the top five most common factors in the evolution of sentinel events. Because of this disconnect we have eliminated the use of Nursing Diagnoses in our work and encourage use of standard clinical terminology or physiologic descriptors as being more appropriate, especially if interprofessional education is planned.

9.2.2 **Benner's model: the process of moving from novice to expert**

In attempting to define how the work and scope of nursing is distinct from that of doctors and other healthcare providers, the nursing profession has developed theories and models. More recent models that have become prominent have focused on observable behaviour and parallel accepted educational and social science theory. An example is the 'Novice to Expert Model' proposed by Benner. Progression across the spectrum of clinical proficiency is emphasized, with five levels from novice to expert level practice identified.[30, 31] Benner does not specifically define how a trainee might gain expertise or how more rapid progression to higher levels of practice could be facilitated. Simulation activities have the potential to address these elements and several authors have used the Benner model as a theoretical construct to inform the design of their simulation activities.[32–34]

9.2.3 Process mapping: Hierarchical Task Analysis (HTA)

While models and educational theory may be useful in designing simulation curricula, the ability to connect simulation and real-world outcomes remains problematic. As simulation moves into the high stakes areas of competency verification, certification, and licensure, metrics must be reproducible and accurately correlate with real-world performance. One approach toward accurately describing clinical activities is systematic task analysis. Task analysis is the process of defining either a job or the particular task or set of tasks within a job.[35] A sub-type is the Hierarchical Task Analysis (HTA), which lists each step in a particular task, analyses the steps, and attempts to place them in the order in which they should or could be performed. Because HTA involves detailed descriptions of processes it is a powerful approach when attempting to create simulations of complex tasks.[35] Task analysis methodology has demonstrated effectiveness in healthcare simulation education as well as practice. This approach has demonstrated utility in mapping process and in generating substantial change in knowledge, skill, and attitudes in both simulated and clinical settings.[36–38]

9.2.4 The NLN/Jeffries framework

In 2003, the NLN/Laerdal partnership with Dr Pamela Jeffries acting as Project Coordinator supported development of an exemplar model for simulation education in nursing. This model was 'intended to provide a context for relating a variety of likely variables' that might be incorporated into simulation course development and measurement.[39] The model draws on the Chickering and Gamson seven principles for good practice in undergraduate education and includes active learning, prompt feedback, student/faculty interaction, collaborative learning, and high expectations.[40, 41] Jeffries notes that simulation training done without a good supporting model results in difficulties identifying what does and doesn't work. The NLN/Jeffries model is accurate in that instructor, student, and educational factors clearly interact. However, the way these and other factors interact, the nexus of interaction, and the role and timing of self-reflection and structured debriefing are not made clear. Wilson et al. tried to use the model to design simulations for postgraduate nurses in the acute-care setting. They reported that functional utility of the model was lacking.[42] The NLN/Jeffries model provides a good foundation from the perspective of educational theory, but how the components fit together in a functionally relevant whole or how they might work together in real-world processes has not been established.[43, 44]

In 2010, Ravert et al. performed a structured literature review to determine if the NLN/Jeffries model was being widely used in the five years post publication. Five teams focused on the construct areas of participant, teacher, simulation design, educational practices, and learning outcomes. These reviews found that the model has not yet been widely adopted in educational and research applications.[16–19, 21, 22]

9.3 **Supplementing clinical experiences**

9.3.1 **Curricular integration**

Attempts at integrating simulation into nursing curricula are increasingly being re-ported.[39, 45–48]. Challenges remain as some nursing faculty remain unfamiliar with the methods and are unsure of how to blend the simulation experience into the traditional educational model. Cross-referencing curricular maps with accreditation requirements, competencies, or standards of practice can inform this process. Educators continue to focus on the use of simulation activities to help attain isolated key clinical educational benchmarks or provide students with a surrogate experiential learning opportunity for rare but critical (or crisis) events.[49–52] A different approach would be to embed simulation throughout a curriculum where appropriate, instead of viewing a simulation exercise as an independent set-piece.[53–56] Vertical and horizontal integration of simulation in a curriculum can help to achieve this goal.

Vertical integration means that a single core simulation course or scenario can be used across the spectrum of novice to expert learners. This model requires development of level-specific objectives, an increasing degree of complexity of the core scenario, and matching of the level of autonomy of action within the scenario to the expected capability of the student. An example of this vertical model would be a single obstetric scenario such as care of the postpartum patient. From this base scenario, level-specific objectives and clinical activities can be designed so that multiple levels of learners can use the same core scenario.

In the same vein, horizontal simulation-programme development would reflect object-ives designed to meet the needs of an interprofessional team within a simulation course or scenario. The horizontal development approach supports the ability for contemporaneous or combined simulation courses between nurses and other healthcare professionals. An example is rapid response or medical emergency team (RRT/MET) simulation where doctors, nurses, and other providers share a common overall objective while concurrently meeting profession specific objectives.[57]

9.3.2 **Critical thinking, clinical judgement, and clinical reasoning**

Critical thinking is valued as an important attribute of expert nurses. The ability of a nurse to use critical thinking to make a correct clinical decision is thought to be important to patient safety and eventual outcomes.[58, 59] Another reason for the focus on critical thinking is the disconnect that has been identified between the preparedness of nursing programme graduates and the expectations of the clinical setting.[60–62]

Critical thinking is defined as a thought process that involves imposing intellectual standards to situations.[63] As a nurse moves from the novice to expert level of practice, critical thinking skills should concurrently improve. Many approaches have been advocated for development and assessment of 'critical thinking'. Development approaches have included the traditional clinical practice setting as well as computer simulations, video-taped vignettes, role-playing, and simulation. Many standardized critical thinking assessment tools have been published and 'validated'.[17, 64–68] However, no educational approach (including simulation) has been proven effective in consistently improving critical thinking skills among nurses or nursing students.[69–72] This suggests that the conceptualization of the construct may be incorrect or that the tools being utilized are not actually valid for the concept being assessed. New concepts, which are surrogate endpoints for critical thinking, have been proposed. These concepts are clinical judgement and clinical reasoning. Lasater describes the measurement of confidence, aptitude, skill, and experience as they relate to development of clinical judgement through simulation. He emphasizes that improved clinical judgement should reflect improved critical thinking.[73]

Clinical judgement and clinical reasoning have both been defined as the **application** of critical thinking in a practice setting.[63] Because the outcomes of clinical decisions can be defined, these concepts should be easier to measure and amenable to intervention. In 2010, Lapkin et al. performed a systematic review that was inconclusive regarding the effectiveness of using simulators to teach clinical reasoning although they reported improvement in knowledge acquisition, critical thinking, and identification of at-risk patients. While these surrogates for the concept of critical thinking continue to be explored, they have not as yet been shown to be easily measureable or amenable to improvement.

9.3.3 **Safety and competency**

Simulation can be used to teach a variety of safety skills for nursing students and practising professionals. Organizations such as the Joint Commission, the Institute of Medicine, and the World Health Organization have focused on development of safety skills within the health professions. In 2005, a multi-institutional study funded by the Robert Wood Johnson Foundation focused on Quality and Safety Education for Nurses (QSEN). The safety areas that were identified were patient-centred care, teamwork and collaboration, evidence-based practice, quality improvement and informatics, and safety. Simulation experiences have been used to evaluate attainment of these QSEN skill sets. In 2013, Paully-O'Neill et al. used paediatric simulation and clinical activities to determine how often students were able to deploy the QSEN skills they had been taught.[74]

Communication issues are at the heart of patient safety and are ripe for evaluation and intervention using simulation. It is clear that lack of development of structured communication skills at both the trainee and practitioner levels remains a problem. The Joint Commission continues to identify communication as one of the top three variables implicated in healthcare errors.[75, 76] In a 2013 review, Theisen and Sandau analysed new graduate nurse skill deficits. They suggested that training programmes should add structured communication elements within their curricula utilizing simulation scenarios.[77] Simulation training provides an opportunity for practising the language of effective communication in a realistic healthcare setting. The hope would be to more permanently impact subsequent improvement in real-world communication.[50, 78–81] Additionally, the simulation setting, because of its ability to replay a process or scenario over and over, can be used to identify and avoid common communication errors within professions and across multidisciplinary teams.[50, 78–82]

Nurses are increasingly being required to demonstrate competency in the workplace and for the purposes of credentialing and certification. Nursing professional associations, credentialing bodies, and recertification agencies are moving this agenda forward and simulation is one solution as many competency objectives can only be verified through demonstration. However, acceptance of simulation as a method to evaluate competency is mixed, with one study indicating that only 41.9% of surveyed undergraduate and 34.9% of graduate nursing programmes agree with doing so.[83] Given the rapidly changing health-care environment and the ongoing momentum of the national and international patient safety movements, it is likely that pressure to move toward competency-based training and education for nurses using simulation will continue.[84–86]

9.3.4 Difficult to access, rare, and critical clinical events

Difficult to access, rare, and critical clinical events are frequently targets within simulation-training curricula. Robertson describes the use of human simulation scenarios in combination with a birthing simulator in offering undergraduate students a realistic obstetric experience.[87] Cioffi et al. investigated the impact of simulation training on mid-wifery student performance with improvements noted in ability to collect data, increased confidence, and more rapid decision-making during subsequent simulation scenario testing.[88] There are now a significant number of reports of obstetric crisis team training using simulation with improvement in team performance. Several investigators have conducted post-simulation retrospective analysis of the incidence of actual adverse events demonstrating improved clinical performance and patient outcomes.[89, 90]

Several authors have reported integration of simulation content into acute care and critical care undergraduate courses with focus placed on development of patient care skill, communication ability, and patient safety behaviours.[88, 89] Marsch et al. reported improvement in the ability of first responders to adhere to algorithms of cardiopulmonary resuscitation using a simulated cardiac arrest in an intensive care environment.[91] These authors also were able to diagnose problems in the functions of resuscitation teams. Hoffman et al. described the integration of human simulation educational modules within an undergraduate critical care course and used the Basic Critical Care Knowledge Assessment Test, Version 6 (BKAT-6) to compare knowledge gain in simulation and clinical versus clinical alone. Student knowledge gain in the simulation arm was significant in 6/8 BKAT subscales.[92] Another approach to preparing nurses for critical events is termed 'Just in Time' training. In 2009, Niles et al. reported 420 'just-in-time' training sessions with PICU staff over a 15-week period. They were able to demonstrate that time to achieve CPR success was significantly faster for PICU staff that had 'refreshed' more than two times per month.[93]

9.4 Replacing clinical experiences

Nursing programmes around the world face an increasing challenge in finding appropriate clinical opportunities. Simulations have potential to provide realistic 'hands-on clinical training' in these areas and in some cases may represent the only opportunity for students to manage patient problems independently. Some nursing education programmes have reported use of simulation experiences as a replacement for clinical time.[83] In an attempt to more fully address this issue, the US National Council of State Boards of Nursing (NCSBN) conducted a multisite prospective study that compared replacement of up to 10% (control) vs 25% vs 50% of actual clinical time with simulation activities. The study included structured simulation experiences in all domains of undergraduate clinical experience. Knowledge, attitude, and competency of participants were assessed with evaluations conducted at the end of the undergraduate programmes and also at one-and-a-half, three, and six months postgraduation. Sample sizes were robust with a total of 666 participants. The results demonstrated no significant differences in knowledge or nursing licensure pass rates between the three groups. Clinical competence was assessed by course instructors, clinical preceptors, and nurse managers (postgraduation) with no significant differences reported. The 50% simulation group did experience a higher dropout rate and there were some differences in performance between groups in specific practice domains. Further, the 50% simulation group had a lower incidence of being assigned to charge duties at six months. This study is the first large-scale evidence that simulation in undergraduate nursing education can replace clinical practice hours without a drop-off in key outcome areas. The authors caution that attention to variables they have defined as important to high-quality simulation activities is necessary to achieve a comparable outcome.[94, 95]

9.5 Summary and future directions

Over the last two decades, nursing education in the US and across the world has undergone a remarkable evolution. Moving from static, classroom-based education approaches to more immersive and interactive environments, leading nursing educators have embraced practices that reflect a more student-centric approach to the teaching-learning environment. Simulation is now a core nursing educational approach and is considered to be a best educational practice. In combination with structured models that support the development of both educational and research methodology we can begin to better understand what works and what does not. These factors hold promise to deepen our understanding of how learning translates from the classroom to the laboratory and ultimately to clinical practice, thus supporting the higher concept of patient-centric simulation education. Emerging evidence suggests that simulation can be effectively used in support of and even as a replacement for actual clinical experiences with similar knowledge, licensure success, and clinical performance outcomes. These findings make a powerful statement underlining the importance of simulation to the future of nursing education.

References

1 Herrmann EK. Mrs. Chase: a noble and enduring figure. American Journal of Nursing 1981;**81**(10):1836.

2 Nursing NLf. Simulation Innovation Resource Center (SIRC): National League for Nursing; 2014 [cited 31 October 2014]. Available from: <http://sirc.nln.org/>.

3 Boese T, Cato M, Gonzalez L, Jones A, Kennedy K, Reese C, et al. Standards of best practice: simulation standard V: facilitator. Clinical Simulation in Nursing 2013;**9**(6):S22–S5.

4 Decker S, Fey M, Sideras S, Caballero S, Rockstraw L, Boese T, et al. Standards of best practice: simulation standard VI: the debriefing process. Clinical Simulation in Nursing. 2013;**9**(6):S26–S9.

5 Franklin AE, Boese T, Gloe D, Lioce L, Decker S, Sando CR, et al. Standards of best practice: simulation standard IV: facilitation. Clinical Simulation in Nursing 2013;**9**(6):S19–S21.

6 Gloe D, Sando CR, Franklin AE, Boese T, Decker S, Lioce L, et al. Standards of best practice: simulation standard II: professional integrity of participant(s). Clinical Simulation in Nursing 2013;**9**(6):S12–S4.

7 Lioce L, Reed CC, Lemon D, King MA, Martinez PA, Franklin AE, et al. Standards of best practice: simulation standard III: participant objectives. Clinical Simulation in Nursing. 2013;**9**(6):S15–S8.

8 Meakim C, Boese T, Decker S, Franklin AF, Gloe D, Lioce L, et al. Standards of best practice: simulation standard I: terminology. Clinical Simulation in Nursing 2013;**9**(6):S3–S11.

9 Sando CR, Coggins RM, Meakim C, Franklin AE, Gloe D, Boese T, et al. Standards of best practice: simulation standard VII: participant assessment and evaluation. Clinical Simulation in Nursing 2013;**9**(6):S30–S2.

10 The IBoD. Standard IV: facilitation methods. Clinical Simulation in Nursing 2013;7(4):S12–S3.

11 Issenberg SB, McGaghie WC, Petrusa ER, Lee Gordon D, Scalese RJ. Features and uses of high-fidelity medical simulations that lead to effective learning: a BEME systematic review. Med Teach 2005;**27**(1):10–28.

12 McGaghie WC, Issenberg SB, Petrusa ER, Scalese RJ. A critical review of simulation-based medical education research: 2003–2009. Med Educ 2010;**44**(1):50–63.

13 Cook DA, Hamstra SJ, Brydges R, Zendejas B, Szostek JH, Wang AT, et al. Comparative effectiveness of instructional design features in simulation-based education: systematic review and meta-analysis. Medical Teacher 2013;**35**(1):e867–898.

14 Cook DA, Brydges R, Hamstra SJ, Zendejas B, Szostek JH, Wang AT, et al. Comparative effectiveness of technology-enhanced simulation versus other instructional methods: a systematic review and meta-analysis. Simul Healthc 2012;**7**(5):308–320.

15 Bremner MN, Aduddell K, Bennett DN, VanGeest JB. The use of human patient simulators: best practices with novice nursing students. Nurse Educ 2006;**31**(4):170–174.

16 Groom JA, Henderson D, Sittner BJ. NLN/Jeffries simulation framework state of the science project: simulation design characteristics. Clinical Simulation in Nursing 2014;**10**(7):337–344.

17 O'Donnell JM, Decker S, Howard V, Levett-Jones T, Miller CW. NLN/Jeffries simulation framework state of the science project: simulation learning outcomes. Clinical Simulation in Nursing 2014;**10**(7):373–382.

18 Ravert P, McAfooes J. NLN/Jeffries simulation framework: state of the science summary. Clinical Simulation in Nursing 2014;**10**(7):335–336.

19 Jones AL, Reese CE, Shelton DP. NLN/Jeffries simulation framework state of the science project: the teacher construct. Clinical Simulation in Nursing 2014;**10**(7):353–362.

20 Jeffries RG, Frankowski BJ, Burgreen GW, Federspiel WJ. Effect of impeller design and spacing on gas exchange in a percutaneous respiratory assist catheter. Artif Organs 2014;**38**(12):1007–1017.

21 Hallmark BF, Thomas CM, Gantt L. The educational practices construct of the NLN/Jeffries simulation framework: state of the science. Clinical Simulation in Nursing 2014;**10**(7):345–352.

22 Durham CF, Cato ML, Lasater K. NLN/Jeffries simulation framework state of the science project: participant construct. Clinical Simulation in Nursing 2014;**10**(7):363–372.

23 LaFond CM, Van Hulle Vincent C. A critique of the National League for Nursing/Jeffries simulation framework. J Adv Nurs 2013;**69**(2):465–480.

24 **Association AN**. The Nursing Process Washington, DC: American Nurses Publishing, American Nurses Association; 2014. Available from: <http://www.nursingworld.org/EspeciallyForYou/What-is-Nursing/Tools-You-Need/Thenursingprocess.html>.

25 **Burns H, Hoffman R, O'Donnell JM, editors**. Enhancing nursing knowledge acquisition through an innovative curricular approach using high-fidelity human simulation. 23rd Quadrennial International Council of Nurses (ICN) Congress; 2005; Taipei, Taiwan: ICN.

26 **McCausland LL, Curran CC, Cataldi P**. Use of a human simulator for undergraduate nurse education. International Journal of Nursing Education Scholarship 2004;**1**(1):1–17.

27 **NANDA**. NANDA International Philadelphia 2007 [cited 9 June 2007]. Available from: <http://www.nanda.org/>.

28 **del Bueno D**. A crisis in critical thinking. Nursing Education Perspectives 2005;**26**(5): 278–282.

29 **Leonard M, Graham S, Bonacum D**. The human factor: the critical importance of effective teamwork and communication in providing safe care. Quality & Safety in Health Care 2004;**13**(1): i85–90.

30 **Benner PE**. From novice to expert: excellence and power in clinical nursing practice. Menlo Park, CA: Addison-Wesley Pub. Co., Nursing Division; 1984: xxvii, 307.

31 **Benner P**. From novice to expert . . . the Dreyfus Model of Skill Acquisition. Am 1982;**82**:402–407.

32 **Larew C, Lessans S, Spunt D, Foster D, Covington BG**. Innovations in clinical simulation: application of Benner's theory in an interactive patient care simulation. Nurs Educ Perspect 2006;**27**(1):16–21.

33 **Nicol M, Freeth D**. Assessment of clinical skills: a new approach to an old problem. Nurse Education Today 1998;**18**(8):601–609.

34 **Nicol MJ, Fox-Hiley A, Bavin CJ, Sheng R**. Assessment of clinical and communication skills: operationalizing Benner's model. Nurse Education Today 1996;**16**(3):175–179.

35 **Stanton NA**. Hierarchical task analysis: developments, applications, and extensions. Applied Ergonomics 2006;**37**(1):55–79.

36 **Phipps D, Meakin GH, Beatty PCW, Nsoedo C, Parker D**. Human factors in anaesthetic practice: insights from a task analysis. British Journal of Anaesthesia 2008;**100**(3):333–343.

37 **O'Donnell JM, Goode JS, Jr, Henker R, Kelsey S, Bircher NG, Peele P, et al**. Effect of a simulation educational intervention on knowledge, attitude, and patient transfer skills: from the simulation laboratory to the clinical setting. Simul 2011;**6**(2):84–93.

38 **O'Donnell JM, Goode JS, Henker RA, Kelsey S, Bircher N, Peele P, et al**. An ergonomic protocol for patient transfer that can be successfully taught using simulation methods. Clinical Simulation in Nursing 2012;**8**(1):e3–e14.

39 **Jeffries PR**. A framework for designing, implementing, and evaluating simulations used as teaching strategies in nursing. Nursing Education Perspectives 2005;**26**(2):96–103.

40 **Jeffries PR, Jeffries PR**. Technology trends in nursing education: next steps. Journal of Nursing Education 2005;**44**(1):3–4.

41 **Chickering A, Gamson Z**. Seven Principles for good practice in undergraduate education. The Wingspread Journal 1987;**9**(2).

42 **Wilson RD, Hagler D**. Through the lens of instructional design: appraisal of the Jeffries/National League for Nursing Simulation Framework for use in acute care. J Contin Educ Nurs 2012;**43**(9):428–432.

43 **Schiavenato M**. Re-evaluating simulation in nursing education: beyond the human patient simulator. J Nurs Educ 2009;**48**(7):388–394.

44 **Young PK, Shellenbarger T**. Interpreting the NLN Jeffries Framework in the context of nurse educator preparation. J Nurs Educ 2012;**51**(8):422–428.

45 O'Donnell JM, Fletcher J, Dixon B, Palmer L. Planning and implementing an anesthesia crisis resource management course for student nurse anesthetists. Crna 1998;**9**(2):50–58.

46 Haskvitz LM, Koop EC. Students struggling in clinical? A new role for the patient simulator. J Nurs Educ 2004;**43**(4):181–184.

47 Parr MB, Sweeney NM. Use of human patient simulation in an undergraduate critical care course. Crit Care Nurs Q 2006;**29**(3):188–198.

48 Hayden J. Integrating simulation throughout the curriculum: tales from the NCSBN National Simulation Study. Clinical Simulation in Nursing 2012;**8**(8):e407.

49 Liaw SY, Chen FG, Klainin P, Brammer J, O'Brien A, Samarasekera DD. Developing clinical competency in crisis event management: an integrated simulation problem-based learning activity. Adv Health Sci Educ Theory Pract 2010;**15**(3):403–413.

50 Flanagan B, Nestel D, Joseph M, Nestel DP, Kneebone RFM, Kidd JP, et al. Making patient safety the focus: crisis resource management in the undergraduate curriculum. Medical Education 2004;**38**(1):56–66.

51 Fallacaro MD. Untoward pathophysiological events: simulation as an experiential learning option to prepare anesthesia providers. Crna 2000;**11**(3):138–143.

52 O'Donnell J, Fletcher J, Dixon B, Palmer L, O'Donnell J, Fletcher J, et al. Planning and implementing an anesthesia crisis resource management course for student nurse anesthetists. Crna 1998;**9**(2):50–58.

53 Masters K. Journey toward integration of simulation in a baccalaureate nursing curriculum. Journal of Nursing Education 2014;**53**(2):102–104.

54 Howard VM, Englert N, Kameg K, Perozzi K. Integration of simulation across the undergraduate curriculum: student and faculty perspectives. Clinical Simulation in Nursing 2011;**7**(1):e1–e10.

55 Starkweather AR, Kardong-Edgren S, Starkweather AR, Kardong-Edgren S. Diffusion of innovation: embedding simulation into nursing curricula. International Journal of Nursing Education Scholarship 2008;**5**:Article13.

56 Moody ML, Slakey K, LaVelle B. Integration of high-fidelity patient simulation into CRNA curriculum: student perception. AANA Journal 2007;**75**(5):375.

57 DeVita MA, Schaefer J, Lutz J, Wang H, Dongilli T. Improving medical emergency team (MET) performance using a novel curriculum and a computerized human patient simulator. Quality and Safety in Health Care 2005;**14**(5):326–331.

58 Turner P. Critical thinking in nursing education and practice as defined in the literature. Nursing Education Perspectives 2005;**26**(5):272–277.

59 Paul RW, editor. Critical thinking. Santa Rosa, CA: Foundation for Critical Thinking; 1993.

60 JCAHO. Healthcare at the crossroads: strategies for addressing the evolving nursing crisis. Joint Commission on Accreditation of Healthcare Organizations, 2002.

61 Kenward K, Zhong EH. Report of findings from the practice and professional issues survey—fall 2004. July 2006. Report No.

62 Li S, Kenward K. A national survey on elements of nursing education—fall 2004. July 2006. Report No.

63 Victor-Chmil J. Critical thinking versus clinical reasoning versus clinical judgment: differential diagnosis. Nurse Educator 2013;**38**(1):34–36.

64 Goodstone L, Goodstone MS, Cino K, Glaser CA, Kupferman K, Dember-Neal T. Effect of simulation on the development of critical thinking in associate degree nursing students. Nursing Education Perspectives 2013;**34**(3):159–162.

65 Shinnick MA, Woo MA. The effect of human patient simulation on critical thinking and its predictors in prelicensure nursing students. Nurse Educ Today 2012;**5**:5.

66 Fero L, O'Donnell JM, Zullo T, Dabbs A, Kitutu J, Samosky JT, et al. Critical thinking skills in nursing students: comparison of simulation-based performance with metrics. Journal of Advanced Nursing 2010;**66**(10):2182–2193.

67 Brooks KL, Shepherd JM. The relationship between clinical decision-making skills in nursing and general critical thinking abilities of senior nursing students in four types of nursing programs. Journal of Nursing Education 1990;**29**(9):391–399.

68 Seldomridge LA, Walsh CM. Measuring critical thinking in graduate education: what do we know? Nurse Educator 2006;**31**(3):132–137.

69 Chau JP, Chang AM, Lee IF, Ip WY, Lee DT, Wootton Y. Effects of using videotaped vignettes on enhancing students' critical thinking ability in a baccalaureate nursing programme. Journal of Advanced Nursing 2001;**36**(1):112–119.

70 Peterson MJ, Bechtel GA. Combining the arts: an applied critical thinking approach in the skills laboratory. Nursing Connections 2000;**13**(2):43–49.

71 Jenkins P, Turick-Gibson T, Jenkins P, Turick-Gibson T. An exercise in critical thinking using role playing. Nurse Educator 1999;**24**(6):11–14.

72 Weis PA, Guyton-Simmons J. A computer simulation for teaching critical thinking skills. Nurse Educator 1998;**23**(2):30–33.

73 Lasater K. The impact of high-fidelity simulation on the development of clinical judgment in nursing students: an exploratory study [Ed.D.]: Portland State University; 2005.

74 Pauly-O'Neill S, Prion S, Nguyen H. Comparison of Quality and Safety Education for Nurses (QSEN)-related student experiences during pediatric clinical and simulation rotations. Journal of Nursing Education 2013;**52**(9):534–538.

75 Joint Commission T. Sentinel event data root causes by event type 2004—2Q 2014: Joint Commission; 2014 [updated 10 January 2014; 7 November 2014]. Available from: <http://www.jointcommission.org/>.

76 Joint Commission T. Sentinel event statistics, 2006.

77 Theisen JL, Sandau KE. Competency of new graduate nurses: a review of their weaknesses and strategies for success. Journal of Continuing Education in Nursing 2013;**44**(9):406–414.

78 Wakefield A, Cooke S, Boggis C. Learning together: use of simulated patients with nursing and medical students for breaking bad news. International Journal of Palliative Nursing 2003;**9**(1):32–38.

79 Kneebone R, Kidd J, Nestel D, Asvall S, Paraskeva P, Darzi A. An innovative model for teaching and learning clinical procedures. Medical Education 2002;**36**(7):628–634.

80 Blum RH, Raemer DB, Carroll JS, Dufresne RL, Cooper JB. A method for measuring the effectiveness of simulation-based team training for improving communication skills. Anesth Analg 2005;**100**(5):1375–1380.

81 Donovan T, Hutchison T, Kelly A. Using simulated patients in a multiprofessional communications skills programme: reflections from the programme facilitators. Eur J Cancer Care (Engl) 2003;**12**(2):123–128.

82 Choi J-I, Hannafin M. Situated cognition and learning environments: roles, structures, and implications for design. Educational Technology Research & Development 1995;**43**(2):53–69.

83 Nehring WM, Lashley FR, Nehring WM, Lashley FR. Current use and opinions regarding human patient simulators in nursing education: an international survey. Nursing Education Perspectives 2004;**25**(5):244–248.

84 Kohn LT, Corrigan JM, Donaldson MS. To err is human: building a safer health system. Washington, DC: National Academy Press; 1999.

85 JCAHO. 2006 national patient safety goals. Joint Commission on Accreditation of Healthcare Organizations, 2005.

86 **Berwick DM**. IHI proposes six patient safety goals to prevent 100,000 annual deaths. Qual Lett Healthc Lead 2005;**17**(1):11–12, 1.

87 **Robertson B, Robertson B**. An obstetric simulation experience in an undergraduate nursing curriculum. Nurse Educator 2006;**31**(2):74–78.

88 **Cioffi J, Purcal N, Arundell F, Cioffi J, Purcal N, Arundell F**. A pilot study to investigate the effect of a simulation strategy on the clinical decision making of midwifery students. Journal of Nursing Education 2005;**44**(3):131–134.

89 **Siassakos D, Crofts JF, Winter C, Weiner CP, Draycott TJ**. The active components of effective training in obstetric emergencies. BJOG: An International Journal of Obstetrics & Gynaecology 2009;**116**(8):1028–1032.

90 **Draycott TJ, Crofts JF, Ash JP, Wilson LV, Yard E, Sibanda T, et al**. Improving neonatal outcome through practical shoulder dystocia training. Obstetrics & Gynecology 2008;**112**(1):14–20.

91 **Marsch SC, Tschan F, Semmer N, Spychiger M, Breuer M, Hunziker PR**. Performance of first responders in simulated cardiac arrests. Critical Care Medicine 2005;**33**(5):963–967.

92 **Hoffmann R, O'Donnell JM, Kim Y**. The effects of human patient simulators on basic knowledge in critical care nursing with undergraduate senior baccalaureate nursing students. Simulation in Healthcare: The Journal of the Society for Simulation in Healthcare 2007;**2**(2):110–114.

93 **Niles D, Sutton RM, Donoghue A, Kalsi MS, Roberts K, Boyle L, et al**. 'Rolling refreshers': a novel approach to maintain CPR psychomotor skill competence. Resuscitation 2009;**80**(8):909–912.

94 **Hayden JK, Smiley RA, Alexander M, Kardong-Edgren S, Jeffries PR**. The NCSBN National Simulation Study: a longitudinal, randomized, controlled study replacing clinical hours with simulation in prelicensure nursing education. Journal of Nursing Regulation 2014;**5**(2):S1–41.

95 **Kardong-Edgren S, Willhaus J, Bennett D, Hayden J**. Results of the National Council of State Boards of Nursing National Simulation Survey: Part II. Clinical Simulation in Nursing 2012;**8**(4):e117–e23.

Chapter 10

Incorporating simulation into the medical school curriculum

Randolph H Steadman, Maria D D Rudolph, Christine C Myo-Bui, and Rima Matevosian

Overview

- This chapter reviews the rationale, evidence, and expanding role for simulation-based learning in undergraduate medical education.

- Successful medical student simulation programmes demonstrate the clinical application of didactic content introduced elsewhere in the curriculum, providing an early exposure to clinical material and promoting critical thinking.

- Students appreciate simulation sessions with well-chosen objectives that are meaningful in the context of the overall curriculum.

- For faculty, simulation provides an opportunity to develop unique skills that facilitate discovery and understanding. Instructors who encourage student discovery, rather than provide answers, optimize the experiential learning opportunity.

- Simulation programme leadership must set objectives, plan and pilot content, budget equipment and personnel, evaluate effectiveness, and secure institutional support in order to sustain a successful programme.

- An outline of the undergraduate medical simulation curriculum at the authors' institution is presented.

10.1 Introduction: definition and scope of simulation-based medical education

Simulation for medical students encompasses a wide array of interactive, experiential learning techniques, including:

- standardized patients (actors coached to portray a patient);
- screen-based computer programs (realistic physiology and/or pharmacology incorporated into a clinical scenario);

- part-task trainers (models for intravenous catheter insertion, prostate examination, newborn delivery, etc.);

- computerized, life-sized, interactive manikins that breathe, have pulses, produce an electrocardiogram, and respond to medications; and

- complex scenarios, perhaps including training in non-technical cognitive skills such as leadership, communication, and coordination with a multidisciplinary healthcare team.

The common aspect unifying these modalities is the reproduction of a state that allows the learner to systematically and deliberately rehearse tasks and/or thought processes associated with clinically relevant objectives. The role of deliberate practice, or rehearsal, common in domains such as athletics and music, has been identified as important for medical training. Accrediting bodies have expressed support for simulation as a risk-free, standardized modality that promotes practice.

Models that permit novice students to learn from their mistakes have an intrinsic appeal, as such experiences are difficult, if not unethical, to teach in the clinical setting. It is expected that the public will, over time, come to expect a certain level of proficiency in the simulated environment before a trainee is permitted to approach the bedside.

Simulation permits medical students to experience decision-making challenges generally reserved for interns, residents, and fully trained practitioners. The planned simulation experience also includes a structured opportunity for reflection, feedback, and repetition—something that the demands of the clinical setting seldom allow.

Simulation-based learning benefits students at every level of training. In this chapter we will review the rationale for implementing a four-year simulation curriculum for medical students, outline practical issues that affect a programme's success, consider appropriate simulation-based learning objectives for students in the pre-clinical and clinical years, and define the core elements of a successful programme. We include a review of the evidence supporting simulation as an educational tool for medical students.

10.2 **Rationale for starting a simulation programme**

The primary reason for starting a simulation programme is to provide experiential interactive learning opportunities and simulated clinical training in a low-stakes environment with no risk to patients. The simulated procedure or scenario can be standardized to permit a reliable, reproducible experience. Such consistency is important for training, and mandatory if the simulated experience is to be used for summative assessment.

A successful programme increases departmental visibility, both within and outside the institution. Prospective applicants are often interested in the simulation programme and the institutional commitment to learning that it represents. Simulation broadens career choices by exposing students to clinicians earlier in their education.

From the standpoint of the instructor, simulation-based training is an opportunity to observe students as they apply knowledge, without the need to intervene that exists in the clinical setting. The open-ended format identifies gaps in knowledge that are obscured by explicit direction in clinical settings. Without the distractions of the clinical environment, instructors can focus on teaching. Students appreciate the attention and frequently reward instructors with laudatory evaluations.

10.3 **Practical issues**

A thorough knowledge of the existing course schedule is mandatory when incorporating simulation-based medical education (SBME); proper timing of the material is key. Simulation exercises that trail, or precede, the topic in the course curriculum are considered poorly integrated by the students and will be viewed as parenthetical offerings. In particular, if testing on the topic has already occurred, the simulation-based exercise is viewed as irrelevant.

The fidelity of the simulated procedures or cases may be higher (for example, using computerized manikins that can be manipulated to show varying physiological responses to the actions of students) or lower (for example, using a large doll to represent a patient), but in all instances the sophistication of the equipment should be aligned with the learning objectives.

The medical terms used during the simulation-based sessions should be standardized with the terms used within the remainder of the course, particularly for first-year courses, when knowledge of medical terminology is scant. For instance, first-year students may not recognize 'pump failure' as congestive heart failure. Understanding such details requires coordination with lecturers and textbooks.

Deciding where to prioritize simulation in the School of Medicine curriculum can be a difficult decision. The Dean of Education and the Medical Education Committee (termed Curricular Committee by some schools) may suggest specific courses to target. Course directors for poorly received courses frequently welcome liaisons that update their teaching methods. Additionally, student representatives (most schools have students from each year on the curricular committee) will provide information regarding opportunities for improvement.

Before offering a new simulation-based session, ensure that the learning objectives are clearly defined and appropriate (from the course director's and students' perspective), and that the scenario has been piloted to eliminate ambiguities. We have been consistently impressed by students' willingness to approach complicated simulated scenarios with zeal (and a disregard for the possibility of exposing knowledge gaps) when such experiences afford them the opportunity to exercise their clinical reasoning ability in a risk-free environment.

Similarly, the faculty perspective must be considered and addressed prior to imposing a new, touted technique on experienced teachers. Requiring that instructors leave behind the comfort of a well-rehearsed slide show for the unpredictability of simulation puts new demands on instructors. Rarely will scenarios evolve in as foreseeable a manner as a slide-based lecture. Instructors must not only be comfortable with the application of the subject matter, but also comfortable with the technical nature of the equipment.

Instructors appreciate a professional development programme that includes an instructor-training course. The hardest, and most foreign, aspect for the instructor is standing by while the student flounders or commits frank errors. Yet, it is this experience that is so powerful for the student, as it illustrates the consequences of their decisions. Instructors who use simulation must have an understanding and appreciation of the power of self-reflection and the importance of self and peer-led discovery.

10.4 Learning objectives of a simulation-based programme for medical students

Simulation-based programmes offer a chance for clinicians to teach applied physiology and pharmacology to pre-clinical students, complementing the course material developed by the school's basic science departments. The application of knowledge in these areas places complex material into a practical framework, and introduces first-year students to the clinical relevance of the subject matter. Students can experience the clinical setting before they see their first patient and develop clinical reasoning and problem-solving skills. For specific topics and an example of the structure and format of the simulation curriculum at the authors' institution, see Table 10.1. Other institutions have published their pre-clinical simulation curriculum.[1]

For students in their final (clinical) years of medical school, the number of appropriate topics is extensive. Ideal topics to consider are the diagnosis and treatment of vital sign

Table 10.1 The UCLA David Geffen School of Medicine simulation curriculum. The simulation centre serves approximately 720 medical students (180 students per class year). The number of students per simulation session is smaller during the clinical years (6–8 students) than during the pre-clinical years, reflecting the goal of increased student autonomy during the later years. Students take turns in the 'hot seat' while their colleagues observe. Students are debriefed using case checklists specific to each scenario. An orientation to the manikin and the session's objectives is included for each session.

Year	Scenarios/Workshop	Learning objectives
Recruitment/ Interview Day	Cardiac arrest on an airplane	Introduce the prospective students to the simulation lab
First Year	Shock scenarios	Interpret vital signs and physical exam; how to differentiate cardiogenic, hypovolemic, distributive shock
	Hypoxemia scenarios	Interpret vital signs, physical exam, and diagnostic studies in hypoxemic patients
	Acid-base scenarios	Interpret blood gases in COPD exacerbation; acute asthma; acute cardiac arrest; primary hyperaldosteronism
	Acute care scenarios	Critical thinking skills
	Ultrasound workshop	Physics of ultrasound; use of gain; cardiac, GI, and musculoskeletal imaging; correlates with anatomy
	Standardized patient encounters	Physical examination and communication skills
	Objective, structured clinical exam (OSCE) with standardized patients	Summative evaluation after each organ system block

continued

Table 10.1 (continued) The UCLA David Geffen School of Medicine simulation curriculum. The simulation centre serves approximately 720 medical students (180 students per class year). The number of students per simulation session is smaller during the clinical years (6–8 students) than during the pre-clinical years, reflecting the goal of increased student autonomy during the later years. Students take turns in the 'hot seat' while their colleagues observe. Students are debriefed using case checklists specific to each scenario. An orientation to the manikin and the session's objectives is included for each session.

Year	Scenarios/Workshop	Learning objectives
Second Year	Cardiovascular pathophysiology scenarios	Interpret history, physical, vital signs, diagnostic studies Learning to diagnose and manage respiratory distress and shock
	Pediatrics, gynaecology, obstetrics, and urology pre-clerkship workshops	Specialty-specific physical examination skills
	Cardiac/pulmonary/renal case-based scenarios	Pathophysiology of shock, ARDS, and COPD; CV pharmacology
	Acute care scenarios	Critical thinking skills
	Ultrasound workshop	Transthoracic and transesophageal cardiothoracic imaging
	Standardized patient encounters	Physical examination and interpersonal communication skills
	OSCE with standardized patients	Summative evaluation after each organ system block
Third Year	Scenarios introducing clinical clerkships	Identify dysrhythmias; defibrillator use; basics of airway management
	OB/Gyn clerkship scenarios	Orient students to clinical OB; perform an uncomplicated vaginal delivery
	Neurology clerkship workshop	Lumbar puncture procedure
	Surgery clerkship scenarios	Recognize post-op complications; learn differential diagnosis of surgical disease
	Standardized patient and task-trainer-based clinical performance exam	Summative assessment of history-taking, physical examination, differential diagnosis, and patient counselling skills
Fourth Year	Common scenarios in primary care, surgery, and acute care	Diagnose and manage common clinical problems
	Anesthesia sub-internship scenarios	General anesthesia: induction, maintenance, and emergence
	ICU sub-internship scenarios	Diagnose and manage common critical care scenarios
	Evening seminar scenarios	Diagnose and manage specialty-based clinical problems
	Boot camp	Preparation for internship

abnormalities (hypotension/hypertension, bradycardia/tachycardia, and dysrhythmias), hypoxaemic states, situations incorporating equipment (physiological monitors, bag-valve mask devices, intravenous lines, ventilators, defibrillators), infusions of vasoactive medications, and teamwork skills, to name a few.

The University of Pittsburgh has described a third- and fourth-year medical school curriculum that uses simulation to teach clinical skills such as the evaluation and management of patients with respiratory distress and cardiovascular events (chest pain, arrhythmias, and pulselessness).[2] Similarly, a 'one-hour on-call' simulation provided third-year medical students an opportunity to prioritize, perform typical tasks in real-time, and through debriefing, allowed students to reflect on their experience and consolidate their skills.[3] Simulation has even been used effectively to teach students to use electronic health records.[4]

10.5 Essential elements for a medical student simulation programme

The following elements are suggested for a successful programme:

- an experienced educator skilled in simulation-based techniques, who serves as the liaison to the course director;
- instructors trained in the theory and practice of simulation-based education;
- content experts who set the objectives of the simulation exercise;
- technical support personnel who are able to assist clinicians in scripting, programming, and running the simulator during the session(s);
- educational objectives that are coordinated with course content, have an appropriate degree of complexity for the level of the trainee, and utilize the simulator's capabilities;
- a script that specifies an appropriate group size (all students are involved to varying degrees);
- clinically relevant equipment; and
- a standardized orientation to the environment, including the simulator.

Supplemental elements (to be added as the programme grows):

- dedicated rooms for orientation, the simulation encounter, and the debriefing; and
- capability of videotaping, which allows reflection and analysis of performance.

Though there is no proven benefit to the learner, videotaping allows research to be conducted without the need for data collection on the fly.[5, 6] Videotaping is also invaluable for instructor standardization.

10.6 Evidence supporting simulation-based learning for medical students

SBME is widespread. In 2011, the Association of American Medical Colleges (AAMC) conducted a survey of simulation in medical schools. Of the 90 medical schools that responded, 84% of first-year students and 91% of second-year students used simulation for clinical skills/doctoring, introduction to clinical medicine, and physical diagnosis. The survey also reported that 94% of third-year and 89% of fourth-year students used simulation for learning content in specific disciplines. In all, 86 of the 90 medical schools indicated that simulation was used for clerkships.[7]

Teaching critical thinking skills with simulation can address limitations of the lecture format, such as: difficulty demonstrating cognitive and psychomotor skills, clinical decision-making, integrity, and empathy; a lack of engagement due to the non-interactive nature of lectures; and the inability to assess whether students can incorporate the material into patient care.[8, 9] In addition, the infrequency of acute events limits opportunities for undergraduates to train from real-world experience. Simulation addresses these limitations and provides a safe environment in which to develop and practice clinical skills.

An important question is whether simulation has an impact on patient outcomes. A review of the data on translational outcomes demonstrates that simulation may improve patient outcomes when implemented at the postgraduate level.[10] At the undergraduate level, the most compelling studies are those examining internship 'boot camps' for fourth-year medical students, which show clear evidence that such experiences improve the clinical performance and self-efficacy of these students once they become interns (see section 10.6.7).[11, 12]

As described in the following sections, there are numerous types of simulation with varying levels of cost and sophistication, and extensive research has shown that simulation-based methods improve students' short-term and long-term skill levels, as well as improving students' and instructors' comfort with students performing tasks in clinical settings.

10.6.1 Surveys addressing the value of simulation

Numerous published surveys have shown that medical students value simulation. Specifically, students have found the simulated learning environment realistic and capable of meeting their learning objectives.[13, 14, 15] Other surveys found that 85% of students rated the session excellent or very good, 80% thought simulator-based training should be required for medical students, and 94% felt simulation should be incorporated permanently into their clerkship.[16, 17] Important aspects of simulation sessions identified during surveys include 'being put on the spot' and the debriefing session at the completion of the scenario, which allows for 'capturing of learning' and 'discharging of emotions'.[17, 18]

10.6.2 Simulation with simulated and standardized patients

Simulated patients are actors who play the role of patients for educational purposes. Simulated patients have been used in medical education for decades to teach and test clinical skills. Simulated patients who are trained to interact and respond consistently and reliably to students' verbal and non-verbal interventions are referred to as standardized patients. Standardized patients may also be trained to report or give feedback on their experience as 'patients'.[19]

Either simulated or standardized patients may be used for formative assessment; for example, to teach physical examination skills. For high-stakes, summative assessment (e.g. Objective Structured Clinical Examinations or OSCEs), standardized patients should be used.[20] The previously cited AAMC survey reported that 94% of the responding medical schools use standardized patients to varying degrees (the range of contact hours was more than fourfold).[7]

10.6.3 Screen-based simulation for medical students

Screen-based simulation, including the use of 'virtual patients', is used in 60% of medical schools, as reported in the 2011 AAMC survey.[7] Computer-based simulation has been used for medical students in a number of areas, including histology,[21] teaching trauma skills (no improvement compared with seminar-based training),[22] pharmacokinetics (improvement over a control group that had less contact time with material),[23] and cardiac arrest (improved performance on a high-fidelity simulator following screen-based simulation).[24] An advantage of computer-based technology is that it can be 'the equivalent of a teacher's best day' in the classroom.[25] Virtual patient simulation may be used for both learning and assessment, and may enable students to achieve higher examination scores even on traditional examinations.[26]

Students who desire a more extensive exposure to a particular topic can use screen-based simulation to supplement classroom material. For a recent review of the wide scope and growing sophistication of virtual patient simulation in medical education, see Kononowicz and Hege's chapter in *E-learning Experiences and Future*.[27]

10.6.4 Simulation for procedural skills acquisition

The AAMC survey found that 93% of medical schools use partial task trainers for procedural skills acquisition.[7] The repetition of procedures has been documented to improve competency. Forty-seven tracheal intubations, 60 brachial plexus blocks, and 90 epidurals were needed for novices to achieve an 80% success rate in the respective procedure.[28] Some studies have shown that medical students who are assessed following simulation-based training perform better than their peers who have trained using only traditional approaches.[29, 30]

One half of all adverse medical events are a result of an invasive procedure.[31] It follows that trainees desire procedural skills training with simulators. In a survey of 158 trainees, of which approximately one-third were medical students, chest tube insertion, central line placement, and tracheal intubation were felt most likely to benefit from simulation (procedures rated less highly, in decreasing order, were peripheral intravenous line insertion, arterial blood gas sampling, nasogastric tube insertion, bladder catheterization, and venipuncture).[32] Naylor et al. showed that third-year medical students trained on a simulator could achieve proficiency in knot-tying and bladder catheterization, as evidenced by both subjective and objective ratings of skills ability.[33] In a study comparing medical students' intracorporeal knot-tying and suturing skills to those of senior surgical residents, simulator-trained students achieved equivalence in the number of needle manipulations, with nearly a similar number of errors.[34] In another study comparing 'best practice skills lab' training (individual instruction, feedback, and practice on manikins) for nasogastric tube placement and intravenous cannulation with the traditional 'see one, do one' approach, the students who had trained on the simulator scored significantly higher immediately after training and retained significantly more performance ability at three and six months follow-up. The superiority of skills lab over traditional training was greater for the more complex skill of intravenous cannulation.[30]

Similarly, in another study, fourth-year medical students performed comparably to senior general surgery residents following simulation-based training with deliberate practice of end-to-end vascular anastomosis.[35] Medical students trained with a high-fidelity simulation perform better on obstetric skills assessment, which included interpreting foetal heart rate tracings, identifying foetal and maternal structures during vaginal examination, and obstetric decision-making compared with peers who trained on lower-fidelity models.[36]

10.6.5 Manikin-based simulation for medical students

The AAMC survey found that 95% of medical schools use full-scale manikins in simulation training.[7] Investigations of the effect of SBME with manikins on clinical knowledge and skill of undergraduate medical students have shown benefits. One study showed that simulation training had a modest impact on 291 senior medical students' ability to diagnose acute coronary syndrome when compared with students who had not experienced simulation education.[37]

Manikin-based simulation exercises can be useful in the pre-clinical curriculum as well. A study involving second-year medical students showed students who received additional training on the simulator achieved higher scores on a written post-test (on altered mental status) and reported greater self-efficacy compared with students who learned only through classroom exercises.[38]

A study comparing low- and high-fidelity manikin simulators reported that medical students trained on a high-fidelity simulator felt greater satisfaction and confidence than students who trained on a low-fidelity simulator. However, the low- and high-fidelity manikin simulators facilitated similar levels of objectively measured outcomes of teamwork or integrated skills station performance.[39]

10.6.6 Using simulation for medical student assessment

Simulation may be used for either formative (low stakes) or summative (high stakes) assessment, such as in an OSCE. Indeed, the AAMC survey cited above reported that medical schools surveyed used assessment to evaluate patient care (78% of respondent schools), psychomotor tasks (64%), and decision-making (61%).[7] The reliability and validity of simulation-based assessment was examined in a study of acute care skills in 40 medical students and interns.[40] Reliability and validity of the assessment was good, although the considerable variability in any individual's scores between the various scenarios suggests that examinees should undergo a number of assessments to evaluate overall ability. In another study from the University of Toronto, the construct validity of simulation-based testing was demonstrated, as the scores of fully trained anesthesiologists and residents were higher than those of medical students.[41] These researchers also noted considerable inter-case variability in scores.

In another investigation, medical students who had been taught the assessment and management of shock using simulation showed better comprehension of shock management as evidenced by superior examination scores compared with the group that had been taught through case-based discussion.[42] Nevertheless, the same study showed no difference in examination questions on patient evaluation or invasive monitoring.

10.6.7 Simulation for internship preparation: 'boot camps'

Simulation may also be used as part of a 'boot camp' curriculum to prepare graduating medical students for internship. One study found that such training was highly valued by students. Five to seven months after fourth-year students completed a one-week multimodal course of simulated patient care scenarios, the former students, now interns, were surveyed. Eighty-nine per cent of the respondents reported that the boot camp had been the most helpful course in preparation for internship.[12]

Another study compared the clinical skills of interns who had completed a two-day (16-hour) boot camp prior to graduation to prior years' interns who had not completed a boot camp. The study found that interns who had competed the boot camp performed significantly better in every clinical skills assessment: cardiac auscultation, paracentesis, lumbar puncture, ICU clinical skills, and code status discussions. As in the previous study, students valued the boot camp experience highly and reported increased confidence going into their internship.[11]

10.6.8 Simulation for interprofessional education

Interprofessional education (see also Chapter 12) is defined as 'occasions when two or more professions learn from and about each other to improve collaboration and the quality of care'.[43] The most recent Joint Commission sentinel event data report notes that human factors, as well as failures of leadership and communication, remain the leading root causes of sentinel events.[44] Interprofessional simulation-based education (IPSE) provides a platform for improving communication and collaboration on healthcare teams, leading to better delivery of healthcare.

Simulation has been successfully used to implement interprofessional education across specialties. There has been increasing evidence that IPSE results in significant improvements in team performance. One study using pre- and post-assessment of 149 medical, nursing, pharmacy, and physician assistant students participating in a one-hour didactic and three-hour simulation session found significant improvement in attitudes toward team communication, motivation, utility of training, and advocacy of patients.[45] Another study of 28 medical, 20 nursing, and 18 nurse anesthetist students showed that using high-fidelity simulation for interprofessional team training in the operating room improved subjective and objective ratings of team-based competencies and performance.[46]

Similarly, a recent review of the literature conducted by Gough et al. concluded that IPSE is a useful teaching tool at the undergraduate level.[47] The most common positive outcome measures related to increased confidence, knowledge and leadership, teamwork, and communication skills. Noted barriers to introducing IPSE were practical considerations, such as distance, timing, and costs.

10.7 Conclusions

As the acuity of hospitalized patients continues to increase, the role of students on the healthcare team has been diminished. Patients with less acute problems, who were traditionally assigned to students, are now cared for in ambulatory settings, and are less available to students. Both of these trends have resulted in fewer learning opportunities. Simulation addresses these shortcomings and provides students a risk-free setting in which to apply physiology and pharmacology and to learn clinical skills, including teamwork. As safety initiatives change patients' expectations, it is unlikely that trainees will continue to be directed to the bedside of patients to learn using the apprenticeship methods of the past.

The evidence supporting simulation continues to accrue, although it is not yet clear that proficiency in simulated settings consistently translates to proficiency in clinical settings or improved patient outcomes. Nevertheless, educators support the concept of deliberate rehearsal and practice for skill acquisition and students recognize and appreciate the opportunity that simulation affords. Prospective students may reasonably expect that the medical school's curriculum will incorporate simulation-based learning, albeit to varying degrees.

Simulation is becoming a mainstay of medical education. As the technology evolves, more life-like and realistic replicas of human anatomy, physiology, and behaviour will be ushered into undergraduate medical education. Accrediting agencies and specialty societies have already embraced the idea that simulation is a necessary component of training. As educators further define the role and scope of rehearsal in medical training, the integration of simulation into undergraduate medical education will undoubtedly continue.

References

1 **Euliano TY**. Small group teaching: clinical correlation with a human patient simulator. Adv Physiol Educ 2001;**25**(1–4): 36–43.

2 **McIvor WR**. Experience with medical student simulation education. Crit Care Med 2004;**32**(2 Suppl):S66–69.

3 **Lumley S**. An hour on call: simulation for medical students. Med Educ 2013;**47**(11):1125.

4 **Milano CE, Hardman JA, Plesiu A, Rdesinski RE, Biagioli FE**. Simulated electronic health record (Sim-EHR) curriculum: teaching EHR skills and use of the EHR for disease management and prevention. Acad Med 2014;**89**(3):399–403.

5 **Sawyer T, Sierocka-Castaneda A, Chan D, Berg B, Lustik M, Thompson M**. The effectiveness of video-assisted debriefing versus oral debriefing alone at improving neonatal resuscitation performance: a randomized trial. Simul Healthc 2012;**7**(4):213–221.

6 **Savoldelli GL, Naik VN, Joo HS, Houston PL, Graham M, Yee B, et al**. Evaluation of patient simulator performance as an adjunct to the oral examination for senior anesthesia residents. Anesthesiology 2006;**104**(3):475–481.

7 **Passiment M, Sacks H, Huang G.** Medical simulation in medical education: results of an AAMC survey 2011 September 2011 [cited 29 October 2011]. Available from: <https://www.aamc.org/download/259760/data/medicalsimulationinmedicaleducationanaamcsurvey.pdf>.

8 **Rogers PL.** Simulation in medical students' critical thinking. Crit Care Med 2004;**32**(2 Suppl):S70–71.

9 **Khan K, Pattison T, Sherwood M.** Simulation in medical education. Med Teach 2011;**33**(1):1–3.

10 **McGaghie WC, Issenberg SB, Barsuk JH, Wayne DB.** A critical review of simulation-based mastery learning with translational outcomes. Med Educ 2014;**48**(4):375–385.

11 **Wayne DB, Cohen ER, Singer BD, Moazed F, Barsuk JH, Lyons EA, et al.** Progress toward improving medical school graduates' skills via a 'boot camp' curriculum. Simul Healthc 2014;**9**(1):33–39.

12 **Laack TA, Newman JS, Goyal DG, Torsher LC.** A 1-week simulated internship course helps prepare medical students for transition to residency. Simul Healthc 2010;**5**(3):127–132.

13 **Cleave-Hogg D, Morgan PJ.** Experiential learning in an anaesthesia simulation centre: analysis of students' comments. Med Teach 2002;**24**(1):23–26.

14 **Weller JM.** Simulation in undergraduate medical education: bridging the gap between theory and practice. Med Educ 2004;**38**(1):32–38.

15 **Zirkle M, Blum R, Raemer DB, Healy G, Roberson DW.** Teaching emergency airway management using medical simulation: a pilot program. Laryngoscope 2005;**115**(3):495–500.

16 **Gordon JA, Wilkerson WM, Shaffer DW, Armstrong EG.** 'Practicing' medicine without risk: students' and educators' responses to high-fidelity patient simulation. Acad Med 2001;**76**(5):469–472.

17 **McMahon GT, Monaghan C, Falchuk K, Gordon JA, Alexander EK.** A simulator-based curriculum to promote comparative and reflective analysis in an internal medicine clerkship. Acad Med 2005;**80**(1):84–89.

18 **Stafford F.** The significance of de-roling and debriefing in training medical students using simulation to train medical students. Med Educ 2005;**39**(11):1083–1085.

19 **Adamo G.** Simulated and standardized patients in OSCEs: achievements and challenges 1992–2003. Med Teach 2003;**25**(3):262–270.

20 **Barrows HS.** An overview of the uses of standardized patients for teaching and evaluating clinical skills. AAMC. Academic Medicine 1993;**68**(6):443–451.

21 **Nelson D, Ziv A, Bandali KS.** Going glass to digital: virtual microscopy as a simulation-based revolution in pathology and laboratory science. J Clin Pathol 2012;**65**(10):877–881.

22 **Gilbart MK, Hutchison CR, Cusimano MD, Regehr G.** A computer-based trauma simulator for teaching trauma management skills. Am J Surg 2000;**179**(3):223–228.

23 **Feldman RD, Schoenwald R, Kane J.** Development of a computer-based instructional system in pharmacokinetics: efficacy in clinical pharmacology teaching for senior medical students. J Clin Pharmacol 1989;**29**(2):158–161.

24 **Bonnetain E, Boucheix JM, Hamet M, Freysz M.** Benefits of computer screen-based simulation in learning cardiac arrest procedures. Med Educ 2010;**44**(7):716–722.

25 **McGee JB, Neill J, Goldman L, Casey E.** Using multimedia virtual patients to enhance the clinical curriculum for medical students. Medinfo 1998;**9**(2):732–735.

26 **Botezatu M, Hult H, Tessma MK, Fors U.** Virtual patient simulation: knowledge gain or knowledge loss? Med Teach 2010;**32**(7):562–568.

27 **Kononowicz A, Hege I.** Virtual patients as a practical realisation of the e-learning idea in medicine. In: Soomro S, editor. E-learning experiences and future, InTech. 2010. Available from <http://www.intechopen.com/books/e-learning-experiences-and-future>.

28 **Konrad C, Schupfer G, Wietlisbach M, Gerber H.** Learning manual skills in anesthesiology: is there a recommended number of cases for anesthetic procedures? Anesth Analg 1998;**86**(3):635–639.

29 **Okuda Y, Bryson EO, DeMaria S, Jr, Jacobson L, Quinones J, Shen B, et al.** The utility of simulation in medical education: what is the evidence? Mt Sinai J Med 2009;**76**(4):330–343.

30 Herrmann-Werner A, Nikendei C, Keifenheim K, Bosse HM, Lund F, Wagner R, et al. 'Best practice' skills lab training vs. a 'see one, do one' approach in undergraduate medical education: an RCT on students' long-term ability to perform procedural clinical skills. PLoS One 2013;8(9):e76354.

31 Leape LL, Brennan TA, Laird N, Lawthers AG, Localio AR, Barnes BA, et al. The nature of adverse events in hospitalized patients. Results of the Harvard Medical Practice Study II. N Engl J Med. 1991;324(6):377–384.

32 Greene AK, Zurakowski D, Puder M, Thompson K. Determining the need for simulated training of invasive procedures. Adv Health Sci Educ Theory Pract 2006;11(1):41–49.

33 Naylor RA, Hollett LA, Valentine RJ, Mitchell IC, Bowling MW, Ma AM, et al. Can medical students achieve skills proficiency through simulation training? Am J Surg 2009;198(2):277–282.

34 Van Sickle KR, Ritter EM, Smith CD. The pretrained novice: using simulation-based training to improve learning in the operating room. Surg Innov 2006;13(3):198–204.

35 Nesbitt JC, St Julien J, Absi TS, Ahmad RM, Grogan EL, Balaguer JM, et al. Tissue-based coronary surgery simulation: medical student deliberate practice can achieve equivalency to senior surgery residents. J Thorac Cardiovasc Surg 2013;145(6):1453–1458; discussion 8–9.

36 Scholz C, Mann C, Kopp V, Kost B, Kainer F, Fischer MR. High-fidelity simulation increases obstetric self-assurance and skills in undergraduate medical students. J Perin Med 2012;40(6):607–613.

37 DeWaay DJ, McEvoy MD, Kern DH, Alexander LA, Nietert PJ. Simulation curriculum can improve medical student assessment and management of acute coronary syndrome during a clinical practice exam. Am J Med Sci 2014;347(6):452–456.

38 Sperling JD, Clark S, Kang Y. Teaching medical students a clinical approach to altered mental status: simulation enhances traditional curriculum. Med Educ Online 2013;18:1–8.

39 Curran V, Fleet L, White S, Bessell C, Deshpandey A, Drover A, et al. A randomized controlled study of manikin simulator fidelity on neonatal resuscitation program learning outcomes. Adv Health Sci Educ Theory Pract 2015;20(1):205–218.

40 Boulet JR, Murray D, Kras J, Woodhouse J, McAllister J, Ziv A. Reliability and validity of a simulation-based acute care skills assessment for medical students and residents. Anesthesiology 2003;99(6):1270–1280.

41 Devitt JH, Kurrek MM, Cohen MM, Cleave-Hogg D. The validity of performance assessments using simulation. Anesthesiology 2001;95(1): 36–42.

42 Littlewood KE, Shilling AM, Stemland CJ, Wright EB, Kirk MA. High-fidelity simulation is superior to case-based discussion in teaching the management of shock. Med Teach 2013;35(3):e1003–1010.

43 Education CftAoI. The definition and principles of interprofessional education 2002 [cited 2014; 15 October 2014]. Available from: <http://caipe.org.uk/about-us/the-definition-and-principles-of-interprofessional-education/>.

44 The Joint Commission. Sentinel event data—root causes by event type 2004–2002Q 2014: Joint Commision Resources; 2014 [cited 2014; 15 October 2014]. Available from: <http://www.jointcommission.org/assets/1/18/Root_Causes_by_Event_Type_2004–2002Q_2014.pdf>.

45 Brock D, Abu-Rish E, Chiu CR, Hammer D, Wilson S, Vorvick L, et al. Interprofessional education in team communication: working together to improve patient safety. BMJ Qual Saf 2013;22(5):414–423.

46 Paige JT, Garbee DD, Kozmenko V, Yu Q, Kozmenko L, Yang T, et al. Getting a head start: high-fidelity, simulation-based operating room team training of interprofessional students. J Am Coll Surg 2014;218(1):140–149.

47 Gough S, Hellaby M, Jones N, MacKinnon R. A review of undergraduate interprofessional simulation-based education (IPSE). Collegian 2012;19(3):153–170.

Chapter 11

Interprofessional education

Robert P O'Brien and Jonathan Mould

Overview

- Interprofessional education (IPE) occurs when two or more professions learn about, from, and with each other to enable effective collaboration and improve health outcomes.

- Interprofessional learning (IPL) is the learning that arises from the interaction between members of two or more professions.

- IPE is important as it assists in the development of a collaborative practice-ready health workforce.

- The use of simulation in IPE assists in the development of skills such as communication, leadership, and teamwork, which underpin patient safety.

- Educational and logistical issues are the factors affecting the successful delivery of IPE.

- Ensuring that there are clear and achievable learning objectives for simulation-based IPL will contribute towards a successful programme.

11.1 Introduction to interprofessional education

Interprofessional education (IPE) occurs when two or more professions learn about, from, and with each other to enable effective collaboration and improve health outcomes.[1] IPE varies from interprofessional learning (IPL) in that IPL is the learning that arises from the interaction between members of two or more professions.[1]

IPE has gained traction and momentum since the World Health Organization (WHO) recognized its importance in its report Learning Together to Work Together for Health.[2] In this report there was a call for improved links between education and health systems to assist in ensuring that health workforce had the capacity to respond to the needs of the health system.

In this chapter, we discuss the rationale for the groundswell of support for IPE and discuss the challenges and methods of adopting IPE. It will focus on the utilization of simulation-based education in healthcare in delivering IPE and discuss the benefits associated with this type of learning and possible future impacts on clinical education and patient safety.

11.2. **Theoretical principles of interprofessional education**

In recent years there have been number of educational theories linked to IPL and IPE in an effort to underpin the rationale for the use of this educational structure. This has resulted in each educator utilizing their favoured theory to articulate their position.[3] This has been in response to the suggestions that IPL and IPE are often theory-less.[4-6] The theories that are most commonly used to discuss and potentially validate IPL are:

- adult learning theory[7]
- constructivist learning theory[8, 9]
- behaviourists learning theory[10]
- reflective practitioner theory[11]
- experiential Learning[12]

The curriculum development and educational context for the delivery of IPE has a bearing on the educational theory that is utilized to underpin simulation-based IPE activities. Like all simulation-based education, there is not one single theory that would underpin simulation methodology. The educational theory that is utilized may vary depending on the modality of education being used and the stage of learning of the participants. The objectives of the programme will also be central to driving the educational approach to the IPE activity.

11.3 **Why is interprofessional education important?**

The delivery of clinical care across the world has substantially changed with the importance of multidisciplinary team care for patients across most medical conditions. This has contributed to the need to adapt and change the methods of delivery of health professional education.

Further, there has been an increase in pressure on the development and delivery of IPE, which is line with growing pressures on the healthcare system for increased outputs and delivery.[13]

The use of interprofessional simulated clinical skills training has been found to be a highly effective, low-risk method of enabling students to enhance their clinical skills, which could later be consolidated in the clinical environment.[14] The use of simulation, especially when conducted in an interprofessional manner, also allows for the development of the skills of communication, teamwork, and leadership skills, which are seen as essential in all healthcare environments and underpin safe practice and improve patient safety.[15]

Perhaps the main purpose and the most important aim of IPE is to create a well-trained, collaborative workforce that is ready to work in a team-oriented approach to provide patient-centred care.

11.4 **Logistical consideration in conducting interprofessional education**

The increase in delivery of IPE raises some logistical issues, which need to be considered when planning, and integrating simulation as part of IPE-based programme. These fall under two broad categories:

◆ educational activity, including course design and teamwork; and

◆ system issues, including the environment and funding.

11.4.1 **Educational activities**

Generally, immersive simulation will use standardized patients (live actors), simulated patients (mannequins), and hybrid simulation to provide an appropriate level of fidelity and participant engagement.

Simulated patients (SPs) challenge students and experienced clinicians alike through the provision of a comprehensive clinical history and ability to verbalize symptoms in real time. SPs can exhibit and convey emotions when examined; forcing participants of simulation-based education to interact with them in a similar manner to real people seeking healthcare. The use of SPs also allows for the utilization by the participant of both clinical and non-clinical (professional or behavioural) skills during the clinical interaction.

When using IPE and simulation, many of the objectives and learning outcomes will remain the same for all professions. There will be some variation to the individual professions' remit and clinical guidelines but the objectives may include a healthcare assessment, a plan of care, evaluation of the care, and follow-up care. These objectives can only be achieved through sound communication, effective teamwork, and adherence to treatment protocols.

Below is an example of how immersive simulation can achieve these learning outcomes. It is a sequential scenario with several shorter immersive sections to it. This example has an SP being assessed during the immersive simulations. Actors may be employed as relatives. Hybrids may be used if an invasive procedure is needed—such as, achieving intravenous access, and a mannequin may be used to substitute the SP if the scenario evolves to an emergency event, such as a cardiac arrest. The scenario starts with:

◆ Paramedics are called to a patient. They need to perform and assessment; including taking a comprehensive history. When they arrive at the healthcare facility, they are greeted in a respectful and professional manner by the healthcare staff and they hand over the care of the patient. They may demonstrate excellent communication skills that may include any treatment and care they perform. The immersive scenario stops for the debriefing. Following the debrief, the next scenario commences, as follows.

◆ Nursing and medical staff take over the care of the patient; they perform further assessments and deliver treatment (see Figure 11.1). They may need to refer to another specialty and the above process should be repeated. The patient is admitted for ongoing care. The immersive scenario stops for the debriefing. Following the debrief, the next scenario commences, as follows.

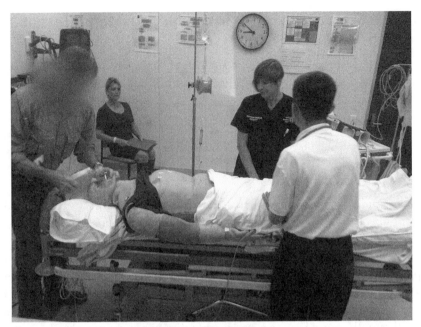

Fig. 11.1 Clinicians from multiple professions engaged in interprofessional education to assess and treat a patient (mannequin).

◆ Physiotherapy and occupational therapy staff are required and work with the nursing and medical staff. The patient may also need some additional support at home such that a social worker becomes involved. The immersive scenario stops for the debriefing.

Potentially, the above example can include more scenarios as necessary but it exemplifies how professions work together in clinical teams to assess and treat throughout the patient journey. The scenario is not unrealistic and provides an excellent environment for students, working with different professional groups, to develop their communication and assessment skills prior to clinical placements or prior to registration. If more experienced clinicians are participants, then emergency events may unfold to challenge those with increased knowledge and skills. For example, ventricular fibrillation may ensue or a distressed patient or relative may develop during an allied health interview.

For effective IPE, the scenarios need to meet the needs of all the participants in the programme and engage all of the professional groups. To meet the needs of these different groups, the objectives of the scenario must be clear. In the above example, communication techniques of each phase of the patient journey by the different professional groups may be an outcome. The scenario may also highlight the significance of roles in IPL and how a non-clinical role, such as caring for distressed relatives, is as important as other roles.

The logistical considerations for IPE through simulation are challenging. Using the above example, an ambulance may be needed but some form of receiving area, such as a triage bay or hospital bay, is required. A definitive care area is needed so that ongoing treatment can be provided. An interview or meeting area, where distressed patients and/or relatives can be interviewed, is also needed. This may be difficult for some simulation venues to provide. In addition, if SPs are employed, there is a duty of care from the providers to the SPs. These must include access to facilities as car parking and ramps, as some may have mobility needs. There also should be areas for the SPs to be briefed and debriefed, and be excluded from the participants throughout the programme, in order to maintain confidentiality of the scenarios for future participants on that day.

Using hybrid simulation includes simulated body parts placed so that they appear to be part of the SP. Commonly, a limb with an intravenous line *in situ* or a torso with an SP at the head of the bed in midwifery is often realistic. Hybrid simulation has many of the benefits of using SPs but can include invasive procedures such as venepuncture or intravenous infusion.

Considerations with hybrid simulation and IPL include the environment in which each professional group works. Having a static hybrid patient in bed may work well for nursing and medical staff but when a scenario involves SP transfers it presents challenges to maintaining the immersion. If the false limb or torso falls off or, is exposed, the realism and engagement of the participant is likely to be lost.

The value of using professional actors can be exceptional in immersive simulations as the participants/learners are exposed to a conscious patient to enhance communication skills between professional groups. A good example of this is a paramedic communicating with hospital professionals when they transfer a sick patient to hospital. If there is a conscious distressed patient present, they need to reassure the patient and at the same time give a concise history and description of the pick-up scene. If the patient is from an accident or crime scene, then this may involve the police. Building IPL activities with professions outside healthcare increases the fidelity of the scenarios and helps participants/students to have an increased understanding of each profession involved. However, this needs good coordination with each professional group to ensure that it occurs and that the experience for each profession is realistic and a reflection of their practice.

In addition to being an SP, live actors can play the role of relatives. The learning objectives for the scenario will dictate how the actors are instructed to respond and behave throughout the interaction with participants. How clinicians respond to, and interact with, relatives is extremely important. In immersive simulations, these additional members of the scenario may have the effect of increasing the stress levels of the participants but increase the reality of the situation. However, professional actors may be expensive to utilize for this purpose.

Despite the excellent experience gained by interacting with SPs, it is currently not possible to exhibit symptoms of a deteriorating patient or that of a patient needing airway support, including general anaesthesia, but hybrid simulation can be used for some invasive procedures such as suturing. For example, in a paediatric scenario, actors playing distressed parents should have a professional allocated to be with them during emergency treatment of the child. This role may be a social worker, a nurse, or a paramedic. If medical staff members are in the scenario, they too will need to communicate with the family. This challenges participants' communication skills with families but also how they may convey important information to and from the parents during an emergent situation. Actors who display realistic emotions can evoke feelings in the participants and needs to be acknowledged and discussed during debriefing.

Realistic scripts and prebriefing for simulated patients are important in simulation. If an appropriate prebriefing does not occur with setting of clear boundaries, and expectations of the simulated patient are not established, SPs with an acting background may take the scenario down a pathway that is not in line with the objective of the scenario. If staff members are used as actors, there is the danger they may overact which may result in derailing the scenario and an experience that does not meet the objectives. If SPs are used, it should be emphasized that they should only present symptoms that they have been given.

11.4.2 **System issues**

11.4.2.1 Institutional support

Ensuring that there is institutional support is integral to the success of IPE. This support is not only necessary when conducting simulations with an IPE focus; it is essential when designing simulation facilities. This includes the location and governance/management of the facility. There can be a perception of ownership of the facility if a single profession is provided with the remit of driving the process of integrating simulation into the health education and training curriculum. If the centre is in a specific area such as a nursing faculty or a postgraduate medical education centre, there may be an inference of ownership by a professional group.[16]

Another important consideration for effective IPE is to design the area as neutral as possible.[17] Professional groups may argue for particular fixtures such as nurse call bell or ceiling-mounted theatre lights. Permanent fixtures will restrict the usage of the space and may infer possession to other professional groups. Therefore, using portable facilities and equipment ensures the environments remain open to all professions. If the learning environment is generic it can reduce barriers to effective communication.[18] Creating an environment that is flexible and can have equipment and fixtures included for specific purposes on a temporary basis allows for greater utilization and inclusion from a wider range of professions.[18]

11.4.2.2 Funding

A major logistical issue when conducting IPE using immersive simulation programmes is that this methodology is often quite an expensive mode of delivery. Funding for multiple aspects of the programme is required to sustain the initiative. In the UK, there are simulation centres that are funded by health authorities to conduct IPE. Funding is 'ring-fenced', which means the centres are not reliant on participants in order for the programmes to run. Many of the courses offered are free to employees working within the health authorities and some offer courses to ward or department teams; including the ancillary staff. The investment includes covering ('backfilling') staff so that wards or departments are not penalized by shortages during education programmes. This is an excellent initiative and demonstrates a significant investment in IPE using simulation.[19]

Getting access to the facilities at an appropriate time may often be challenging.[20] It is suggested that flexibility is important for both timing and access to the teaching space available. In addition, it is argued that self-directed learning might be pertinent for IPE and those students be given access to the environments outside of usual teaching times.[20] A significant problem with this is security and care of, what is often, an extremely expensive capital investment.

It has, at times, been difficult to engage educators in immersive simulation per se. IPE may be more challenging for some centres but Steinert[21] and Chan[22] advocate convincing 'stakeholders' as to the benefits of this style of teaching and learning to guarantee its success. Therefore, engaging experts from all of the professional groups as champions in simulation may facilitate IPE and IPL. This also ensures that there is not a single champion but several interested parties, further enhancing sustainability should there be changes in staffing availability.[16]

There have been calls for simulation and IPE to be introduced in the first semester of university courses. Despite this, Chan[22] cautions that although early introduction of IPE into a curriculum may foster good working relationships, the participants do not have enough experience to actively engage in the scenarios. Anecdotally, this is a significant consideration.

Tullman[16] concurs with this in the report of nursing and medical student IPE. An IPL programme seemed to work best for third- and fourth-year students. Perhaps, core taught-units in an IPE forum facilitate students to meet but holding off from immersive simulation may be more appropriate until the students have had adequate clinical experience. Another factor that is thought to influence the success of IPE in early stages of professional entry education is that students may not have developed a sound sense of their professional identity, which may affect the way in which they interact with participants from other professions.

Even when delivering lecture material there are concerns about loss of specialist content during the rewriting stages. This may also be pertinent when scenarios are designed. Tullman[16] suggests these are important issues, which must be addressed, otherwise programmes are likely to fail.

Other potential problems include the hierarchy of professional groups. If inexperienced nurses, paramedics, or social work students work with medical students, then these groups may view the medical students as more senior. This may increase the pressure and discourage engagement with the simulation. This also puts unreasonable expectations on the medical students.

11.4.2.3 Releasing staff to attend interprofessional education

To ensure IPL is successful, good working relationships need to be fostered with service providers from all of the professions. This will help to ensure that students attend all sessions and not just those designed by their own professional group. Thus, there needs to be a commitment to meet and 'provide incentives' that may include rotations that have different craft groups featured each session.

Immersive simulation can be challenging for traditional educators. Therefore, they need to be part of planning to incorporate them into the simulations. Otherwise, what tends to occur is they revert back to 'chalk and talk' as there is a perceived loss of control. Sustaining IPE can be equally complex and requires supportive institutional policies and managerial commitment.[2]

11.5 Improving interprofessional education through the use of simulation-based learning

General feedback from students is that they want more interprofessional simulated events because the experiences are so positive.[16] Using immersive simulation in IPL is more realistic because many healthcare workers work interprofessionally. Arguably, working in an interprofessional team does not equate to working collaboratively.[2] If IPE immersive simulation can become the standard for healthcare education, it may equip the workforce with the skills needed to address the challenges of future healthcare users.

11.6 Using interprofessional education to improve professional/non-technical skills

More than 75% of errors in healthcare involve an element of poor communication and other human factors. Therefore, it is irrefutable that good, collaborative teamwork between all health professionals is vital; especially as clinicians are exposed to a rapidly changing healthcare environment with ever-increasing use of technology.[23] The use of simulation, including multiple professions focusing on human factors, allows for clinicians and students to become increasingly aware of the influence of human factors such as communication, situational awareness, leadership, and teamwork. These human factors can be discussed in the context of a clinical situation and highlight the need to be aware of the contribution of social interaction to high-quality healthcare. TeamSTEPPS® (<http://teamstepps.ahrq.gov/>) is one example of an evidence-based teamwork system developed to improve communication and teamwork skills among healthcare professionals.

As such, immersive simulation with participants from a different professional background is an important component in improving communication techniques and behaviours. Participants are afforded the opportunity to immediately reflect on their own, and fellow professionals', communication skills. This style of education and learning is more realistic for participants as the roles played are familiar to everyone. However, to reiterate the point, the scenarios must be well designed to meet these needs if simulated IPE is going to change the culture of healthcare and increase collaboration.

11.7 Challenges

Challenges to simulation-based IPE are no different to those experienced in other types of IPE.[21, 24] The learning methods must reflect the practice experiences of participants; therefore, the professional goals and objectives need to be understood by the entire faculty.

Regardless of the mode of simulation being utilized, the scenarios must meet the needs of the participant professions by being realistic and pertinent. For this to occur, the faculty needs to have a shared vision if IPE is going to be successful in any curriculum.

IPE is not a new concept and some countries have attempted to adapt this IPE in all healthcare education, but there is a reluctance to mandate this approach to education. Although parallels have been made between healthcare and the aviation industry, it is only pilots who have to return to a simulator if they have not completed three take-offs in a 90-day period. In healthcare, there is no mandated example of using simulation to continue to practise clinically if there has been an absence from practice. Even the Emergency Management of Anaesthetic Crises (EMAC) course, developed by the Australian and New Zealand College of Anaesthetists (ANZCA), is not a requirement for continuing practice in Australia and New Zealand.

11.8 **Conclusion**

The preceding information provides a snapshot of the evidence base and challenges associated with IPE. There is an increasing quantity of research and literature associated with IPE that demonstrates that the use of IPE and IPE simulation-based education is an imperative to enhancing the development of a safe and collaborative workforce. In a healthcare environment that is built on a team approach to patient-centred care, educating both future and current health professionals, with a focus on collaborative team-based care, should not be a choice but an expectation.

References

1 **Freeth D, Hammick M, Reeves S, Koppel I, Barr H.** Effective interprofessional education: development, delivery and evaluation. Oxford: Blackwell Publishing, 2005.

2 **World Health Organization.** Framework for action on interprofessional education and collaborative practice. Geneva: WHO, 2010.

3 **Hean S, Craddock D, O'Halloran C.** Learning theories and interprofessional education: a user's guide. Learning in Health and Social Care 2009;**8**:250–262.

4 **Freeth D, Hammick M, Koppel I, Reeves S, Barr H.** A critical review of evaluations of interprofessional education. London: LTSN-Centre for Health Sciences and Practices, 2002.

5 **Barr H, Koppel I, Reeves S, Hammick M, Freeth D.** Promoting partnership for health. London: Blackwell Publishing and CAIPE, 2005.

6 **Clarke P.** What would a theory of interprofessional education look like? Some suggestions for developing a theoretical framework for team training 1. Journal of Interprofessional Care 2006;**20**:577–589.

7 **Knowles MS.** The adult learner: a neglected species. Houston, TX: Gulf Publishing,1990.

8 **Dewey J.** Democracy and education. London: Collier Macmillan, 1966.

9 **Piaget J.** To understand is to invent. New York, NY: Grossman,1973.

10 **Skinner BF.** Science and human behavior. New York, NY: The Free Press, 1965.

11 **Schon DA.** The reflective practitioner: how professionals think in action. New York, NY: Basic Books, 2004.

12 **Kolb DA.** Experiential learning: experience as the source of learning and development. New Jersey, NY: Prentice-Hall, Hillside, 1983.

13 Nisbet G, Lee A, Kumar K, Thistlethwaite J, Dunston R. Interprofessional health education: a literature review. Sydney, NSW: University of Technology Sydney, 2011.

14 Bradley P, Postlethwaite K. Setting up a clinical skills learning facility. Medical Education 2003;37(1):6–13.

15 Robertson J, Bandali K. Bridging the gap: enhancing interprofessional education using simulation. Journal of Interprofessional Care 2008;22(5):499–508.

16 Tullmann DF, Shilling A, Goeke L, Wright E, Littlewood KE. Recreating simulation scenarios for interprofessional education: an example of educational interprofessional practice. Journal Interprofessional Care 2013;27(5):426–428.

17 Greenstock L, Brooks P, Webb G, Moran M. Taking stock of interprofessional learning in Australia. Medical Journal of Australia 2012;196(11).

18 Newton C, Bainbridge L, Ball VA, Wood VI. Health care team challenges: an international review and research agenda. Journal of Interprofessional Care 2013;27(6):529–531.

19 Montagu Clinical Simulation Centre: 2013, available at <http://www.montagusimulation.co.uk/Courses/Default.aspx> (accessed 11 November 2014).

20 Bradley P, Postlethwaite K. Setting up a clinical skills learning facility. Medical Education 2003;37(1):6–13.

21 Steinert Y. Learning together to teach together: interprofessional education and faculty development. Journal of Interprofessional Care 2005;S1:S60–S75.

22 Chan E. Reflecting on the essence of our problem-based learning discussions: the importance of faculty development and our continuous quest for applications of problem-based learning. Kaohsiung Journal of Medical Science 2009;25:276–281.

23 Institute of Medicine. Crossing the quality chasm: a new health system for the 21st century. Washington, DC: National Academy Press, 2001.

24 Jackson A, Bluteau P. At first its like shifting sands: setting up interprofessional learning within a secondary care setting. Journal of Interprofessional Care 2007;21(3): 351–353.

Chapter 12

Scenario design—theory to delivery

Chris Holland, Chris Sadler, and Nusrat Usman

Overview

- The object of good scenario design should be to provide students with a scenario or short course that is integrated with their whole curriculum and which they will see as relevant to their learning needs.

- The aviation industry has guidelines for designing flight simulation scenarios; these guidelines are also applicable to medical simulation scenario design.

- The initial definition of clear and unambiguous learning objectives, with the involvement of all stakeholders in the intended student audience's education, is imperative.

- Cognitive task analysis techniques can prove useful in breaking complex tasks performed by task experts into their constituent parts and therefore determining what some of the learning objectives should be.

- Scenarios should be written with the intention of allowing students to display the skills and behaviours that would indicate that the learning objectives have been achieved. The events that will trigger the performance of these actions must be written into the scenario in a credible fashion.

- Credibility is further enhanced by teaching students using evidence-based practice and this should be written into the scenario from the outset.

- Scenarios should be written to encourage the accumulation of deliberate practice and mastery learning.

- The scenario script should be as detailed, comprehensive, and unambiguous as possible. It represents the scenario lesson plan and should enable all competent simulator faculty to consistently provide the scenario to high standards.

- Once written, scenarios should be practised and modified as required. This process should continue, even after the scenario enters the student curriculum.

12.1 **Introduction to scenario design**

The scenarios used in simulation teaching are equivalent to a classroom teacher's lesson plan. Just as a high-school teacher would not start teaching for a new curriculum without creating new lesson plans, so scenario scripting should be accorded the attention it requires. In addition, the high-school teacher will want to ensure that their lessons fit into the whole curriculum in a logical way that will make their lessons relevant and necessary. If written well, a scenario will consistently provide students with multiple opportunities to practice technical and non-technical skills in a believable clinical situation. The better a scenario is the easier the students will find it to suspend disbelief and immerse themselves in the learning opportunity being afforded to them.

In this chapter, we discuss some educational theory and best practice for scenario design and the evidence supporting the process we advocate. We translate some of the lessons we have learnt from our own experience into practical guidance, illustrated through a worked example. Finally, we present a completed scenario as used in our simulation centre (Appendix 12.1). If the concepts and tools described below are employed then scenario design can be an intellectually stimulating and immensely creative exercise. The satisfaction of seeing a student benefit from a well-written and stimulating scenario designed with their precise needs in mind should not be underestimated.

12.2 **Theory**

As discussed in Chapter 1, the aviation industry has much to inform medical simulation, and so it is for scenario design. They describe five stages of flight scenario design (see Box 12.1).

Applying a similar evolutionary approach to medical simulation scenario design will ensure that students experience a carefully planned scenario, which has been created with specific learning objectives in mind and has content validity. Students will gain more from a learning opportunity they recognize as being relevant to them.

Box 12.1 Five stages of scenario design

1 Identification of primary crew resource management/technical training objectives.

2 Identification of possible incidents that will produce the training/learning objectives.

3 Specification and development of scenario event sets.

4 Evaluation and modification of the scenario as required.

5 Instructor training implementation and ongoing evaluation of scenarios.

Adapted from US Department of Transportation, Federal Aviation Administration (FAA), *Advisory Circular AC* 120-35C, (FAA, 2004), http://www.faa.gov/documentLibrary/media/Advisory_Circular/AC%20120-35C.pdf, accessed 01 Sep. 2014: 28–29.

When embarking on designing a scenario, consideration should be given to whether the scenario is to be part of a larger course that will, in part, occur external to the simulator and be delivered by other teachers, or if the whole course is to be provided by the simulator faculty. If it is to be the former then the learning objectives should be written jointly by simulator and non-simulator faculty. The scenarios must also sit comfortably within the objectives of the student's overarching curriculum; examination of a pre-existing formal curriculum can prove invaluable at this stage of the design process. When writing scenarios for qualified practitioners a training needs analysis will ensure that learning objectives are tailored to their specific requirements.[2] Close collaboration between simulator and non-simulator faculty will ensure that learning objectives are relevant and appropriately themed.

If the simulator faculty is not proficient in the subject matter to be taught then task experts should be consulted. These are practitioners who have performed the task many times, to the point that they can perform the uncomplicated task semi-automatically with little conscious thought and perform the task in more complex circumstances with obvious proficienc.[3] Involvement of proficient or expert practitioners will also raise the validity of scenarios from face to content validity. Cognitive task analysis (CTA) is a theoretically grounded method used for identifying the requisite knowledge, skills, and behaviours (KSBs) for effective task performance and there exists an extensive body of literature about CTA containing a large variety of techniques that can be employed.[4, 5] It is especially applicable when the analysed tasks are complex, such as in medicine, and it becomes important to understand the reasons behind experts observed behaviours. By using CTA, learning objectives can be linked to the desired KSBs and then embedded within scenarios. Lajoie describes the process of using CTA to inform the creation of educational resources for both aviation and medicine.[6]

Spending time and effort in the early stages goes a long way to making a scenario credible. The collaboration between task expert and simulator expert will help to ensure that learning environment fidelity is matched to the desired learning outcomes and what is achievable with available facilities. Higher fidelity does not automatically result in better real-world task performance and some complex skills can be taught using surprisingly low-fidelity teaching methods.[7, 8]

Scenario content should be written using a defensible evidence base. Technical skills required, clinical practice guidelines used, and the overall educational programme should be based on evidence of clinical effectiveness.[9] Additionally, consideration should be given to providing teaching on this evidence-based practice either before or after the course, or during the feedback session following the relevant scenario.[10] We encourage reflective and self-directed learning in our practice by providing candidates with a list of the references used in our scenario design.

McGaghie and colleagues have provided a Critical Review of Simulation-based Medical Education Research, which discusses 12 features and best practices to use in medical simulation for education. They suggest that the single most important aspect of simulator training to promote effective learning is the provision of feedback.[11] The aims and objectives of the feedback will be suggested by those of the scenario. Formative feedback will enable students to practise tasks and improve their performance. It should provide the opportunity to acquire new knowledge and fill in gaps exposed by their simulation experience and discuss behaviours and non-technical skills. When feedback is effective, students should not focus on the wrong objectives and will be encouraged to transfer new skills into clinical practice. When written as part of a course, repetition of skills in scenarios leading to repeated discussion in debriefing sessions will reinforce learning. The use of simulation for summative evaluations and high-stakes testing is also increasing. Scenarios designed for this purpose must be authentic and provide reliable data to assess students' competence.[7]

The move away from using experience as a substitute for competence to analyse performance should be reflected in educational programmes. Deliberate practice and mastery learning are powerful, evidence-based learning tools, which complement competency-based training.[11, 12] Deliberate practice is a highly structured activity with the specific goal of improving performance. It may be particularly useful for new skills, rare events, and emergencies. Deliberate practice relies on motivated students, well-defined learning objectives, tasks (both technical and non-technical) of an appropriate level of difficulty, focused and repeated practice of required skills with measurable outcomes, and access to informative feedback.[11] Mastery learning indicates a higher level of achievement than competence alone. To achieve a mastery standard, learning objectives and tasks within a scenario should be sequenced according to level of difficulty and rigorously evaluated against pre-set standards.[11] Issenberg et al. suggest that using scenarios with different levels of difficulty, utilizing different learning strategies, and capturing a wide variety of clinical variation will contribute to effective learning in medical simulators.[7]

12.3 Stages of scenario design

12.3.1 Identification of primary crew resource management/technical training objectives

Crew resource management skills can be compared to crisis resource management skills, anaesthetic non-technical skills, non-technical skills for surgeons, or anaesthetic non-technical skills for anaesthetic practitioners.[13] Technical training objectives are concerned with training students in the performance of a task using specific equipment. The explicit identification of technical and non-technical learning objectives means that all simulator faculty are likely to conduct the scenario and subsequent feedback with the same set of learning objectives and desirable observed behaviours as set endpoints. Salas and Burke[8] describe how simulation is most effective when scenarios are written with the required learning objectives embedded from the outset.

12.3.2 Identification of possible incidents that will produce the training/learning objectives

Identification of suitable incidents, or triggers, for scenarios will first require examination of the students' curriculum. Credibility is further enhanced when scenarios are designed using real events or critical incidents as triggers. A literature review should be performed in order to ensure best practice for management of the scenario.

12.3.3 Specification and development of scenario event sets

The trigger event, reactions, and the consequences of those actions is called an event set. By this stage we have the raw material to script event sets to embed within the scenario. We have used multiple sources of information to evolve a detailed concept of precisely what it is we want to teach, who our target audience is, and what the credible clinical background to the scenario will be. Task experts have helped to identify the triggers we will incorporate within the scenario, which should induce our students to display the desired behaviours.

Hamman[14] suggests a framework for conceptualizing an event set: topic, sub-topic, skill, and observable behaviour. This can be applied to both non-technical and technical skills. As the scenario is created using the learning objectives and storyboarding process outlined, overarching topics will be identified. Each topic will have multiple sub-topics and each sub-topic will require the exercising of specific skills. Each skill is demonstrated by the observation of certain behaviours. The data from any CTA already performed will naturally lend itself to this method of categorization.

For example, a scenario may be required to teach emergency airway management. One of the topics for that scenario will be patient safety. The topic would have multiple sub-topics, one of which would be reduction of aspiration risk. This would require skills and knowledge involving the anatomy of the upper airway. An observable behaviour demonstrating this skill would be utilization of cricoid pressure.

When designing a scenario, it is helpful to anticipate the different ways in which students could respond to each trigger event, and the best way to ensure that the simulated trigger event is credible and of sufficient fidelity. We also try to consider how the scenario will respond to as many conceivable student responses as possible and script for all eventualities where the scenario could end. By scripting a member of faculty into the scenario we are able to guide the learning experience to ensure that the original and intended learning objectives are never forgotten. This facilitator may interject with suggestions or provide technical support in a credible fashion to steer the scenario in the direction where learning objectives are achievable. Groups of students will naturally display different levels of competency and so achieve the desired outcomes with varying degrees of ease. We do not advocate prolonging scenarios once the desired outcomes have been reached as this then means the scenario is progressing to areas which have not been subjected to the rigorous design process outlined above and will, therefore, have less validity.

12.3.4 Evaluation and modification of the scenario as required

McGaghie et al.[11] recommend that once a scenario is written the script should explicitly describe the event sets, event trigger, and the related topics, sub-topics, skills, and observed behaviours for the benefit of those that will administrate the scenario. Once scripted in such a fashion it should undergo a 'dry-run' using at least two different groups of experts as candidates and involving the instructors who will administer the scenario. This will, hopefully, expose flaws in the scenario script and allow modifications to be made.

12.3.5 Instructor training implementation and ongoing evaluation of scenarios

An unambiguous version of the scenario that is to be used for teaching students can be published and the instructors can be trained in its administration. Frequently, even when the scenario is in use as a teaching tool, unexpected student behaviours are observed which require them to be modified to enhance the learning opportunities provided.

12.4 Worked example

So how does all this happen in reality? Our simulation centre was involved in the creation of a one-day simulation course for Foundation Programme 2 (FP2) doctors (see Appendix 12.1 for an example of a completed scenario). They had a detailed formal curriculum[15] covering six generic competencies as well as 16 competencies related to the care of the acutely unwell patient. This document provided explicit learning objectives and details of the KSBs required of this group of doctors.

We began by using a collaborative process involving simulator faculty, training scheme representatives, college tutors, educationalists, and clinicians to reach consensus on eight credible clinical events. These were used as storyboards into which the required event sets could be embedded. We sought a wide range of clinical problems and aimed to produce a set of scenarios with varying degrees of difficulty.

The FP2 curriculum core competencies were reviewed and appropriate trigger events in each of the clinical episodes identified; e.g. incorrect management of cardiac arrest in Appendix 12.1—storyboards could then be scripted in more detail. Each competency required at least one event set covering one topic. It was clear from the text of the formal curriculum document what the relevant sub-topics should be. Simulator faculty and experts in acute medicine contributed to the identification of the skills associated with the sub-topics and what explicit behaviours would provide evidence for possession of these skills; e.g. knowledge of new Advanced Life Support (ALS) guidelines in Appendix 12.1. Each scenario script had more detail inserted as the various layers of design were built up.

Once a script of sufficient detail was drafted, its component event sets were then mapped back onto a matrix. By ensuring that every topic was embedded into more than one scenario we were able to create opportunities for repetition of competencies and so observe each behaviour in more than one clinical situation. Issenberg's systematic review[7] identified that focused repetition of skills in a manner designed to engage the student was an important feature of effective learning in a high-fidelity simulation.

Clinical scenarios, covering acute medical emergencies ranging from cardiac arrest to epileptic seizure, were scripted using evidence-based guidelines. A facilitator was scripted into each scenario to play the role of a healthcare professional acting as an assistant and source of guidance to the student if required. In other courses we have scripted students

Box 12.2 Scenario template sections

1 Title (course title, patient details, and clinical diagnosis)

2 Synopsis (brief summary of case)

3 Learning objectives (event sets, topics, sub-topics, skills, and desired observed behaviours)

4 Environment set-up (set, props required)

5 Console (detailed initial and subsequent parameter settings)

6 Event trigger

7 Scenario progression

8 Patient details (history, past medical history, medications, allergies, investigations)

9 Candidate information/handover (information given to candidate at beginning of scenario)

10 Faculty characterizations (character list with required behaviours)

11 Scenario endpoints (desired observed endpoints to end scenario)

12 Suggested debriefing topics

13 References

to play the roles of healthcare professionals, such as theatre nursing staff. This presents an opportunity to teach the importance of non-technical skills such as interdisciplinary communication.

Our centre uses a standard template for scripting scenarios at this stage of development. It contains all the required information to run any scenario from set-up to debrief and can also be used to quickly orientate new faculty members. The template is organized under the following headings (see Box 12.2) (see Appendix 12.1 for a detailed example).

This unambiguous guide for running the lesson allows different teachers to conduct scenarios while still achieving the same learning objectives. Each section must be written carefully to ensure that it contains all the relevant information required by faculty members. For example, section 5 describing the console settings is the most important section for those in the control room. Here, the initial settings required for manikin, anaesthetic machine, etc. are specified. The actual variables stated will vary according to simulator fidelity, but should be detailed. Any parameter changes required as the scenario progresses, with the corresponding triggering observed behaviours, are also documented. If the scenario is not intended to progress to certain events such as cardiac arrest, faculty should not *ad lib*. When this section is detailed, concise, and unambiguous, the scenario is likely to run in a smooth and credible way without interruptions.

The amount of information the candidate is given just before going into the scenario or during patient handover will vary. Some scenarios require detailed handovers designed to direct the candidate to a certain course of action; others may have as an event trigger a poor-quality handover. Others may have no handover at all but simply require the candidate to respond to a crisis already in progress.

In faculty characterizations (section 10), we describe the roles and actions of faculty members participating in the scenario. Students may seek information from any character during the scenario. For this reason, all faculty should be aware of their own roles, the patient details, and learning objectives of the scenario. Some of our scenarios contain roles that are written to intentionally display challenging behaviours. The management of these behaviours will be one of the learning objectives for the scenario. We do not put candidates into scenarios where everyone is 'against them' and always have at least one member of faculty who will provide moral support if needed. For example, in Appendix 12.1, one of the learning opportunities is the management of poor performance in colleagues. We have written the scenario to include a member of faculty acting the role of a ward nurse who has recently completed basic life support (BLS) training. This faculty member is instructed to bolster the student's confidence in challenging the incorrect management of ventricular fibrillation by the surgical trainee, but only if the students are hesitant about doing so.

Debriefing topics are written with a certain degree of flexibility as we strongly believe that each debriefing must primarily deal with the behaviours observed and individual learning needs identified by those observations. If the scenario has been well designed and has run as expected then these will be exactly as planned. We do not advocate using just one scenario to cover all possible debriefing points. Repetition of skills in different scenarios within a course will allow for flexibility should one debriefing session become devoted to fewer topics for discussion than expected.

Once a scenario has been formatted to the described template we keep a secure master copy and a working copy for further development, updating the master copy as required. At this stage we start to circulate the scenario to the wider faculty to solicit feedback and evaluation of the proposed script. As the script reaches an ever wider audience, there has to be an agreed process of discussion and reaching consensus before changes to the script can be made, otherwise the careful embedding of planned learning objectives can become undone.

Once consensus has been reached the scenario is reviewed and the required props and accessories identified; for example, if patient notes are required to add to scenario fidelity then these must be written at this stage; credible investigation results must be sourced, including blood, ECG, and X-ray examinations. This also applies to requirements for appropriate manikin fidelity, such as wounded limbs or other findings on examination and the ability to perform practical procedures made necessary by the scripted clinical scenario.

Scenarios at this stage are now ready to be trialled. We try to run scenarios first as a rehearsal with stops whenever necessary to identify and resolve issues. This is followed by an uninterrupted dress rehearsal with a faculty member who has not been involved in the development of the scenario. The process needs to be repeated as often as required until the scenario runs smoothly along a credible path. Once required changes have been made, the final version of the scenario is distributed to simulator faculty in a timely fashion so that all participants can become familiar with their required roles and any faculty training requirements can be identified. Scenarios may also be pre-programmed at this stage of the process.

Now the scenarios are ready to be used for teaching purposes. The first few performances with students frequently result in further scenario refinements and reveal unexpected learning opportunities. Before making changes, however, faculty must not lose sight of the original learning objectives they set out to achieve. We have also learnt from experience that, occasionally, a scenario has to be simplified for its intended audience because the students do not have the skills or knowledge expected of them by the authors. If a scenario needs to be significantly edited to satisfy such learning needs, careful consideration has to be given as to whether the whole scenario is fit for purpose or if modification or embedding of additional event sets will be sufficient. Such insights can also arise from the feedback sessions following the scenario or from student evaluation forms at the end of each course. Over time, experience in scenario writing is accumulated and major rewrites become less and less frequent. In addition, it is best educational practice to review all scenarios frequently to ensure they remain fit for purpose.

Over the course of several years we have built up a library of scenarios sufficiently large that we frequently have 'off-the-shelf' solutions if asked to participate in ad hoc courses. We have also developed and maintain links with other simulator centres which have, on occasion, allowed us to source scenarios designed using the benefit of others' experiences.

12.5 **Conclusion**

The aviation simulation industry has a recommended procedure for scenario design and implementation. Planning scenarios in this way requires the initial, unambiguous definition of desired learning objectives. We advocate an inclusive process involving contributors with expertise in simulation, the skills and tasks being taught, and the overall requirements of the intended student audience. Students will expect to be taught to use evidence-based clinical practices and, if such evidence exists, it should also be incorporated into the scenario. If this approach is applied it ensures that scenarios are produced which are likely to have significant content validity. We have written many scenarios following this action plan and feel that it results in scenarios of excellent quality which stand up to rigorous scrutiny, are credible, and utilize the appropriate level of simulator fidelity. We have devised a template for scenario scripting so that every one of our scenarios is presented with the same degree of clarity. This adds to consistency of scenario provision when running different courses or when different faculty teach specific scenarios. We employ test runs, or dress rehearsals, using task experts as scenario candidates with subsequent modifications as required. These need to be run at a timely stage before course dates so that provision can be made for instructor training using the finished scenario before the scenario begins to be used as an educational tool.

Finally, evaluation data from students should be used in an iterative fashion and may uncover unanticipated learning needs requiring ongoing updating of a scenario library.

In addition, scenarios should be regularly reviewed to ensure they continue to teach best evidence-based practice and the learning objectives of the target audience.

References

1 US Department of Transportation. Advisory Circular 120–135c. Line operational simulations: line oriented flight training, special purpose operational training, line operational evaluation. Washington, DC: US Department of Transportation, Federal Aviation Authority; 2004.

2 **Alinier G.** Developing high-fidelity health care simulation scenarios: a guide for educators and professionals. Simulation & Gaming 2011;**42**(1):9–26. doi: 10.1177/1046878109355683

3 **Dreyfus HL, Dreyfus SE.** Mind over machine: the power of human intuition and expertise in the era of the computer. New York, NY: Free Press; 1986.

4 **Burke CS, Salas E, Wilson-Donelly K, Priest H.** How to turn a team of experts into an expert medical team: guidance from the aviation and military communities. Qual Saf Health Care 2004;**13**(1):96–104. doi: 10.1136/qshc.2004.009829

5 **Crandall B, Klein G, Hoffman RR.** Working minds: a practitioner's guide to cognitive task analysis. 1st edn. Cambridge, Boston: MIT Press; 2006.

6 **Lajoie SP.** In: Ericsson KA, ed. Development of professional expertise: toward measurement of expert performance and design of optimal learning environments. Cambridge, UK: Cambridge University Press; 2009, 61–83.

7 **Issenberg SB, McGaghie WC, Petrusa ER, Lee Gordon D, Scalese RJ.** Features and uses of high-fidelity medical simulations that lead to effective learning: a BEME systematic review. Med Teach Jan 2005;**27**(1):10–28.

8 **Salas E, Burke CS.** Simulation for training is effective when . . . Qual Saf Health Care Jun 2002;**11**(2):119–120.

9 **Grol R, Grimshaw J.** From best evidence to best practice: effective implementation of change in patients' care. Lancet 11 Oct 2003;**362**(9391):1225–1230.

10 **Lockyer J, Ward R, Toews J.** Twelve tips for effective short course design. Med Teach Aug 2005;**27**(5):392–395.

11 **McGaghie WC, Issenberg SB, Petrusa ER, Scalese RJ.** A critical review of simulation-based medical education research: 2003–2009. Medical Education 2010;**44**:50–63.

12 **McGaghie WC, Issenberg SB, Cohen ER, Barsuk JH, Wayne DB.** Medical education featuring mastery learning with deliberate practice can lead to better health for individuals and populations. Acad Med 2011;**86**:e8–e9.

13 Industrial Psychology Research Centre, University of Aberdeen: <http://abdn.ac.uk>.

14 **Hamman WR.** The complexity of team training: what we have learned from aviation and its applications to medicine. Qual Saf Health Care Oct 2004;**13**(Suppl 1):i72–79.

15 The Foundation Programme Committee of the Academy of Medical Royal Colleges. Curriculum for the Foundation Years in Postgraduate Education and Training. UK: Departments of Health, UK; 2005.

Example scenario

Foundation Year 2 Course

Harry Barlow; Patient identifier: 48372; Date of Birth: 21/09/1938

Scenario: Cardiac arrest and maintaining good medical practice

Synopsis

♦ *This scenario needs careful choreographing to run as intended.*

Harry is a 68-year-old man with ischaemic heart disease and coronary artery bypass 15 years ago. He was admitted for an elective inguinal hernia repair three days ago. He had an episode of chest pain in recovery post op and was kept in for cardiology follow-up. Troponin levels were negative and he is due for discharge today. Has VF arrest on ward. Surgical trainee attempts to lead arrest team but does so badly and using out-of-date guidelines.

Learning objectives

Candidates are expected to:

1 Know new ALS guidelines

  a Ventilate at 30:2 BVM ratio

  b Shock at 360 joules from initial shock

  c Shock is primary to giving adrenaline

2 Participate in cardiac arrest team

  a Follow initial directions from team leader

  b Effective BVM ventilation

  c Attach monitoring

  d Assess rhythm (VF)

3 Take over leadership of arrest team

  a Recognize poor leadership

  b Manage surgical doctor's poor leadership

4 Communicate with surgical trainee

Environment set-up

Ward-based, male manikin, ward staff nurse, surgical trainee (see Table A12.1)

Table A12.1 Initial monitoring required

	IN SITU	MONITORED
i. ARTERIAL LINE	ii. NO	
iii. NIBP	iv. NO	
PERIPHERAL LINE	v. YES	
vi. ECG	vii. YES	viii. YES VF
ix. SpO$_2$	x. NO	

In-room equipment

Cardiac arrest trolley, defibrillator, new ALS guidelines on wall.

Dressing over right inguinal area. Right inguinal drain with old blood minimal volume.

Drugs on prescription chart

Simvastatin 10 mg

Aspirin 75 mg OD (stopped for surgery)

Losartan 50 mg OD

Enoxaparin 20 mg BD changed to 60 mg BD post chest pain

Temazepam 10 mg nocte

Paracetamol 1 g QID

Ibuprofen 200 mg 8 hourly

Oromorph 20 mg 2–4 hourly

No known allergies

Console

Initial observations (see Table A12.2).

Table A12.2 Initial observations

HR	VF
xi. BP	xii. unrecordable
xiii. SpO$_2$	xiv. unrecordable
xv. RR	xvi. apnoea
ECG	xvii. VF

If after first shock at 200 joules candidates have still not recognized that surgical trainee does not know new guidelines then rhythm becomes VT and surgical trainee gives at-ropine to treat it.

Table A12.3 Observations after one correct cycle of ALS algorithm

xviii. HR		xix. 68b/m	
xx. BP		xxi. 94/56	
xxii. SpO$_2$		xxiii. 92	
xxiv. ECG		xxv. Sinus with ST depression	

Once one cycle is completed correctly then (see Table A12.3).

Event triggers

Initial call for help from ward

Instruction to perform incorrect compression ratio

Administration of atropine for VT

Scenario progression

The ward round has just left the ward. Mr Barlow is having his sheets tucked in by a junior ward nurse. The nurse notices that Mr Barlow is unresponsive, shakes him, and calls for help.

The surgical trainee calls in the two candidates and tells them he is running the cardiac arrest and one must take the airway and one must get the defibrillator.

He does not tell them to put out a cardiac arrest call—the candidates must initiate that.

◆ *Candidate is instructed to do synchronized BVM at ratio 15:2.*

Candidate is given history as they are following these instructions.

Previous MI over ten years ago and he had a bypass then. Since then no chest pain, has stopped smoking, and walks his dog every day. He was admitted for an elective right inguinal hernia repair three days ago. Surgery was uneventful but in recovery he was cold, clammy, hypotensive, and had some chest pain. ECG unchanged but has been kept in for cardiology review and serial troponins. Cardiology due to come round and discharge this morning. The ward round had just left his bed when he became unresponsive.

If candidates do not challenge BVM ratio of 15:2 the nurse says to candidate that when they were at BLS training last week there was talk of new guidelines.

Surgical trainee will continue at 15:2 ratio and give 200/200/360 J shocks and adrenaline every cycle.

After first shock if candidates have still not recognized that surgical trainee does not know new guidelines then rhythm becomes VT and surgical trainee gives atropine to treat it.

Patient details

Past medical history

IHD for 16 years. Presented with acute MI and had single vessel bypass same year. Since then no angina.

Hypercholesterolaemia

Hypertension

Family Hx brother died MI aged 59

Ex-smoker stopped after MI

Drug history

Simvastatin 10 mg

Aspirin 75 mg OD (stopped for surgery)

Losartan 50 mg OD

Enoxaparin 20 mg BD

Temazepam 10 mg nocte

Allergies Nil known

Social Lives at home with wife and dog. Retired undertaker.

Investigations

See Table A12.4 for blood results.

Candidate's information

You are just starting your shift on a general surgical ward. The morning ward round is just finishing.

Faculty characterizations

Nurse instructions

You are friendly to candidate and enthusiastic at chest compressions. You vaguely heard at your BLS training that there were some new guidelines and as the candidate voices concerns you will back them up.

Table A12.4 Blood results

xxvi. Hb	xxvii. 12.2	xxviii. Na	xxix. 136
xxx. WCC	xxxi. 8.0	xxxii. K	xxxiii. 4.7
xxxiv. Platelets	xxxv. 575	xxxvi. Urea	xxxvii. 12
xxxviii. Glucose	xxxix. 4.5	xl. Creat	xli. 50
xlii. ECG	xliii. Old ECG Q-waves	xliv. Troponin	xlv. <0.1

Surgical trainee instructions

You lead the arrest confidently following old protocol.

You initially are dubious about new guidelines having never heard of them but if candidate and nurse are sure you'll ask what you should be doing.

If poster of new guidelines is pointed out to you then you have to accept their word.

After one shock of 200 joules, if candidates have still not recognized that you do not know new guidelines then rhythm will become VT and you give atropine to treat it. As you do this, say loudly: 'One minijet of atropine for the VT.'

Scenario endpoints

Technical skills:

1 Perform simple airway manoeuvres (with adjuncts)

2 Manage cardiac arrest following ALS 2010 guidelines

Non-technical skills:

1 Effective communication

2 Leadership

Debriefing points

2010 ALS guidelines

How does a junior member tell a senior team member they should do things differently?

Chapter 13

Debriefing—theory and techniques

Janice C Palaganas, Brendan Flanagan,
and Robert Simon

Overview

- Debriefing is a conversation held after a real or simulated event aimed at sustaining or improving future performance.
- The debriefing period of structured reflection and feedback is considered to be an essential element of simulation-based education and considered by many to be the most critical phase for learning in healthcare simulation.
- The facilitation skill of the debriefer is arguably the most important element of effective simulation-based education.
- Establishing a safe and supportive learning environment is a fundamental tenet of an effective debriefing.
- Theories underpinning the role of debriefing draw heavily on scholarship in relation to experiential learning and reflective practice.
- There are opportunities for cogent emotional and educational benefits for learners during debriefing.
- Poorly facilitated debriefing may be a source of adverse learning or learning knowledge, skills, or attitudes that lead to degradation of future performance.
- Although the actual style of the debriefing varies, there are recognized sequential phases that provide an effective structure for debriefing.
- Opportunities for formal faculty development with respect to debriefing skills are critical to a successful simulation programme and are increasingly available.

13.1 Introduction to debriefing

In healthcare simulation-based education (SBE), the term 'debriefing' refers to the purposeful, structured period of reflection, discussion, and feedback between learners and educators and is usually held immediately after a case-based simulation event. Video playback may supplement the debriefing through visually guided reflection, illustrating observable actions and results for thought and discussion. For this chapter, we define debriefing as a conversation between two or more people to review a real or simulated event in which participants reflect on outcomes, actions, and thoughts with the intent to assist in developing knowledge, skills and attitudes in clinical judgement, critical thinking, and psychomotor tasks and behaviours for improved future performance and patient safety.

This chapter will outline some of the main theories underpinning debriefing and describe some currently used debriefing techniques to provide assistance to novice and experienced debriefers. There is still a paucity of rigorous research to support much of what occurs during the debriefing process and many promising areas for future research are outlined at the conclusion of this chapter. Given the need for rigorous research around debriefing, the material presented here is the product of proven theories and research programmes from a variety of disciplines including psychology, education, aviation, healthcare, and organizational behaviour; the authors' reflections after almost 20 years of involvement in clinically oriented SBE and debriefing; and developing and conducting a 'train the simulation instructor' course with more than 3,000 educators over the past 12 years. All of this has shaped the material presented in this chapter. Italicized text provides scripting examples that we have found and observed to be useful during a debriefing.

13.2 **The theory**

13.2.1 **Purpose**

In a simulation experience, debriefing fosters the deepest potential for learning. The primary purpose for debriefing is educational: to provide an opportunity for the learners to explore their own and others' practice with respect to knowledge (e.g. task- or event-focused, team management), skills (e.g. technical and non-technical), and frames (e.g. thoughts, emotions, past experiences, or attitudes that drive actions) depending on the goals of the session.

Well-planned debriefings 'can allow for reflection-on-action and planning for different ways of handling a similar event next time'.[1] High-quality debriefings can stimulate participants to continue reflecting upon the experience after the formal debriefing period has ended. This informal reflection may occur individually or with others afterwards.

13.2.2 **Educational theories**

The theory underpinning the role of debriefing is supported by many sources. These theories describe the fundamental purposes in debriefing and its critical role in the learning process using simulation. The five significant theories include: adult learning,[2] experiential learning,[3, 4] reflective practice,[5, 6] deliberate practice,[7, 8] and situated learning.[9] These theories are briefly summarized below. Morrison and Deckers[10] succinctly describe the major learning theories in relation to SBE.

13.2.2.1 **Adult learning theory**

Adult learning theory is based on findings in andragogy, or the study of adult learning. Malcolm Knowles states six assumptions under this theory that motivates adults to learn.

These assumptions include: (i) adults need to know the reason why they are learning what they are learning; (ii) adults need to be involved in their plan and decisions around education (be self-directing); (iii) adults bring vast experiences to the discussion; (iv) adults are most interested in material that is relevant to their lives; (v) adults learn best when the activity is problem-centred; and (vi) adults are internally driven.[2]

13.2.2.2 Experiential learning theory

Experiential learning theory is a learning perspective that conceptualizes learning as a process through the transformation of experience. David Kolb and Roger Fry developed a model of learning from the work of Dewey, Lewin, and Piaget.[4] The model posits that learning is facilitated through cycles of experience (e.g. work, 'real-world' experience, simulations), reflection (e.g. reflecting on a specific action), conceptualization (e.g. analysing and understanding what drove the action and effect), and experimentation (e.g. planning and executing a course of action).[3] This widely adopted and studied perspective on experiential education highlights the crucial role of debriefing in SBE.

13.2.2.3 Reflective practice

Reflective practice aims to create new meaning through the analysis and understanding of actions and values. Donald Schön's work in reflective practice describes two types of reflection: reflection-in-action (i.e. during the simulation) and reflection-on-action (i.e. after the simulation) during debriefing.[5] Debriefing should also allow for a third type of reflective practice identified by Thompson and Pascal[6]: reflection-for-action (i.e. how to apply new meaning for new action in practice or for the next simulation).

13.2.2.4 Deliberate practice

Deliberate practice is to intentionally engage in an activity with the purpose of improving performance. K Anders Ericsson outlines essential components of deliberate practice that optimizes learning and performance, including: internal motivation to engage in a task to improve; building on previous experience, skill, and knowledge; immediate feedback on the performance; and repetition of the task.[7] Ericsson underscores the point that healthcare students need representations that can support planning and practice of the actual performance to allow for adjustments toward mastery and there is a need where feedback can be immediate.[8] With careful planning and skilled facilitation, simulation with debriefing helps to fill this need.

13.2.2.5 Situated learning theory

Situated learning theory defines learning as a social process where knowledge is co-created within the context of how that skill or knowledge is applied.[9] Like experiential learning theory, situated learning theory embraces a concrete experience and reflective observation on the experience. Learning is constructed in a way where knowledge is married to context as defined by all aspects of a particular moment. This deep understanding of the context becomes the means for understanding that situation and the meaning made by the learner. This dynamic perspective adds a larger context to debriefing a particular case and suggests that learning is supported through a social process where beliefs and behaviours are acquired, reinforced, or altered through the exchange and interaction of individuals.

By incorporating these foundational elements into SBE, debriefing is seen as a powerful process to enhance clinical performance and improve patient safety.

13.2.3 Challenges

13.2.3.1 Confusion in terminology

The term 'debriefing' may also elicit another understanding for clinicians. All too often in the clinical environment, a structured debriefing session only happens after an adverse outcome and is often associated with a long discussion of a negative and emotionally charged incident with a tendency to attribute blame or process negative emotions. Despite how the process of debriefing often plays out in the clinical setting, the debriefing process in simulation is structured and aimed at reflection to promote a positive culture.

13.2.3.2 Simulation anxiety

Asking learners to engage in a simulated event that may be video-recorded, followed by a debriefing in the company of others, increases the pressure for good performance which may cause learner anxiety. There are techniques a facilitator can use to acknowledge and ease some of this anxiety. In our experience, we have found that utilization of these techniques to set the stage for learning is one of the most powerful foundations to creating learner engagement, reflection, and deep learning (see section 13.3.3.3).

13.2.3.3 Simulation glitches

Despite vetted plans and dry runs, a simulation scenario may incur technical glitches or proceed down an unplanned path. This may affect the debriefing, since the facilitator likely needs to approach the debriefing differently. When a glitch occurs, the debriefer may be tempted to spend time defending the original intent of the simulation, and too often simulation failures motivate learners to use debriefing time to vent about lack of realism. Learning in the debriefing is still salvageable following a simulation fraught with problems. This requires skilful weaving of learning topics throughout the discussion. Our approach is that even if an objective of the case doesn't play well in the simulation, as long as the idea is introduced in the simulation or debriefing, the objective can be discussed. A simulation failure may even result in abandoning the original objectives of the scenario and discussing other interesting things that occurred.

13.2.3.4 Lack of faculty training

Debriefing significantly enhances the powerful learning opportunity provided by simulation in healthcare and continues to be considered one of the most complex skills of SBE for clinician educators to master. This is not surprising, since the skills required are neither clearly defined nor part of the typical training of healthcare practitioners.[11] Moreover, simulation creates an emotion-laden environment, laden mindfully by the instructor and the environment of simulation that is outside most clinician's repertoire. Debriefers have the challenge of teaching in this emotional context. There are multiple formal training programmes worldwide for debriefing training.[12] While there are multiple approaches to debriefing, the key advantages of formal training programmes in debriefing are the opportunities for practice and direct feedback. Without experience or training, the facilitator is unlikely to reach the potential that SBE affords and runs the risk of jeopardizing relationships with the learner and creating negative learning.

13.2.3.5 The habits of traditional teaching

We teach the way we have been taught.[13] We've found that this statement is all too true. Most clinician educators learn how to teach by following the examples of their clinical educators; who also usually don't have much or any training in the teaching-learning process. Traditional classroom methodologies promote unidirectional teaching (e.g. faculty lectures in a lecture hall to students with the aim that the students will receive the knowledge being lectured). Even during clinical learning sessions, much of the dialogue is based on what the learners have to know. As outlined in section 13.2.2, SBE follows the principles of adult, experiential, reflective, deliberate, and situated learning concepts. The methodologies used in debriefing, under these concepts, require a learner-centred approach based on what the students 'do' much more than what the students 'know'. Solely knowledge-focused SBE is a gross underutilization of the potential learning possibilities; what's usually most interesting and transformative for the learner is to analyse what they did and why. While there are opportunities for 'lecturettes' and knowledge review during a debriefing, learner needs should first be explored and identified to ensure the appropriate teaching is occurring.

In the following sections, we suggest concepts and techniques that can support faculty to overcome the challenges outlined above.

13.3 The practice before the debriefing: a suggested structure

Debriefings usually follow immediately after a corresponding simulation scenario. Several scenario and debriefing iterations may occur in the context of a single simulation-based course. Many of the important issues for successful debriefing are similar to those for any experiential learning activity or small group exercise. A structure for setting a foundation for a high-quality debriefing session is outlined here.

13.3.1 Developing objectives

Prior to the development and running of a simulation course, objectives must be developed to appropriately meet the demands of the curriculum and the needs of the learners. Objectives guide the development of the simulated case and debriefing. Objectives should be written in a way in which they can be observed; e.g. not focusing on learner ability to know or understand facts, but to see how the learner demonstrates observable skills and behaviours. Objectives often stem from a learning needs assessment.[14] A needs assessment typically addresses questions such as: Who are the learners? What are the learning needs of this group? What are the specific training needs of the group and the individuals in the group? How much training is needed? Is simulation the ideal platform for meeting these needs? Which of these learning needs is/are best met using simulation and how?

There are frameworks that provide competencies that could be used as objectives (e.g. student curriculum, published clinical competencies, certification or accreditation programme criteria, etc.).[14] A now, well-established framework in the context of team-based simulation and debriefing is crisis resource management (CRM), which refers to the management of teamwork in a crisis situation (see Chapter 26).

13.3.2 Planning

Healthcare simulation is an exciting platform with the ability to creatively simulate real events. In excitement, faculty often become enthralled with the technology and equipment, with a desire to utilize as many impressive simulator capabilities as possible. As with any educational activity, adequate planning is essential to ensure that the session, the chosen case, the case progression, and the equipment achieve the predetermined objectives. Important practical considerations for the simulation session as a whole and for the debriefings are: is simulation the best platform to meet these needs? Who is the best educator to guide this learning and can they be involved? Who are the learners? Is there one or more than one discipline involved (e.g. medical, nursing, teamwork specialists, perfusionists, etc.)? What level of difficulty is appropriate? What are the learners'—and the teachers'—expectations of the session? What is the group size? Is the purpose of the debriefing predominantly for the participants to explore, discuss, and learn about clinical/ technical issues, behavioural (or non-technical) issues, or both? What are the roles of the respective debriefers, if there is more than one?

When developing the simulation scenario around these considerations, it is key to create a simulation that will highlight actions around the objectives to generate topics for the debriefing. To ensure this, ask: what opportunities need to be embedded into the simulation to allow demonstration, or lack of, these skills and behaviours? Effective debriefing requires time to explore the objectives, so part of the planning is to ensure that adequate debriefing time is available. As a general rule, the length of time for debriefing should not be less than the time taken for the scenario itself and is usually 30–40 minutes or 2–3 times the length of the simulation is ideal.

13.3.3 Establishing a safe and supportive learning environment: setting the stage

Much of the success of the debriefing process is determined well before the start of the debriefing. It is essential that every effort be made throughout the course as a whole to establish and maintain the notion of the learning environment as a 'safe container' in which the participants can and do feel psychologically safe to engage in the simulation and can openly disclose and discuss their true thoughts.[16]

Rudolph, Raemer, and Simon (2014) suggest four practices to establish a psychologically safe environment: declaring and enacting a commitment to respecting learners and concern for their psychological safety; attending to logistic details; clarifying expectations; and establishing a 'fiction contract' with participants. These four practices are presented here with a one additional consideration: set the stage for the clinical case.

13.3.3.1 Declaring and enacting a commitment to respecting learners and concern for their psychological safety

Successful experiential learning activities require a learner-centred approach. A learner-centred approach focuses on the experience and level of comfort of the participants, what topics they would most like or need to cover, with faculty interest in their understanding of the topic. This perspective occasionally means changing the simulation or debriefing plans in real time. When faculty explicitly declare the importance of teaching based on observed behaviour in the simulation and the thoughts of the participants, a tone is set based on teaching and learning in a collaborative manner. Soliciting and being open to addressing questions or concerns demonstrates a commitment to the instructor's goal to respect participants and to remain concerned for their psychological safety.

13.3.3.2 Attending to logistic details

Prior to participant arrival, it is important to ensure the environment is conducive to learning as follows:

+ The simulation has been dry-run with similar participants to ensure it is at the right learning level; will likely meet the objectives with a focus; and that the simulation will run smoothly and without glitches.

+ The room is fully prepared at least 15 minutes prior to their arrival.

+ The educational support equipment is functioning: monitors, computer, etc.

+ If using video playback, a horseshoe or circle arrangement of seating works well with the facilitators at a location where they can control the playback.

+ A whiteboard should be available for illustrating and documenting discussion points and is ready for writing.

+ Relevant cognitive aids are at hand or on the wall in hardcopy or via a data projector; e.g. algorithms, behavioural skills frameworks.

+ Observers and staff are aware of avoiding entering the room during the debriefing. Avoid the presence of 'over the shoulder' observers in the debriefing—their presence can be distracting to the participants and may be a source of disruption by unsolicited comments from outside the learner group.

Upon arrival, an introduction to the environment is helpful. This includes:

+ Orientation to the location, including where the restrooms are, when are good times to use the restroom.

+ If faculty feel it is necessary, orientation to the simulation environment—where to obtain supplies, simulator requirements (e.g. virtual simulator supplies and on-screen directions), etc. Many programmes allow participants to meet the simulators, however other programmes feel as though such an orientation potentially decreases participant ability to act as if the mannequin is a patient and engage in the simulation. Many programmes use an embedded simulated person (sometimes called an actor or confederate) to facilitate the issues that would be met by orientation to the simulation environment (e.g. obtaining the supplies for the group, guiding learners as to where to feel a pulse during the simulation event, etc.). Other programmes have had success using a mannequin that is animated vis-à-vis a realistic voice, demonstrating a likable personality, generation of vital signs, and other mannequin features such as chest excursions, eyes blinking, etc.

◆ Orientation to the schedule, including physical movement of the course (e.g. at the conclusion of each simulation, the participants will return directly to the debriefing room, etc.).

Beyond logistical orientation, the pre-briefing includes clarifying expectations, establishing a fiction contract, and setting up the clinical case.

13.3.3.3 Clarifying expectations

Participant expectations often vary enormously. It is for this reason that their expectations are worth exploring during the introduction to the course. Following the principles of adult learning theory (see section 13.2.2), participants need to understand what, why, and how they are learning. Because adult participants self-direct their own learning, it is important that the facilitator present the learning path of the day so that the faculty and participants come to basic agreement on the learning goals. Some of these matters can be accomplished via provision of pre-course material (e.g. information on the simulation centre, what to expect, the agenda for the day, clinical content or knowledge, etc.).

When using the simulation environment for high-stakes assessment (i.e. summative assessments, using simulation for grading/passing/failing purposes), the goals and expectations should be clearly articulated. High-stakes assessment simulations are very different than simulations structured as a learning exercise; i.e. formative assessment. High-stakes assessment requires detailed clarity around the performance expectations and any planned consequences (e.g. advancement or remediation) as a result of performance (see Chapter 21).

Since simulation exercises often involve observers, participants might experience anxiety around peer evaluation, faculty or supervisor evaluation, or feel some threat to protection of their reputation and privacy. This anxiety may impede their learning, performance, and engagement. Assuring participants that this a normal concern and providing clarity around confidentiality and exactly how video may be used helps to address this anxiety. Equally important, participants—whether trainees or practising clinicians—have the right to be informed of the planned confidentiality of the sessions. Participants should be given answers to the following questions: what can we agree to talk about and not talk about outside this simulation experience and why? What can the faculty running this simulation share with others including my supervisor and why? What will happen with my videos and will they ever be used outside the course and, if so, under what circumstances? Will my supervisor have knowledge about my performance?

13.3.3.4 Establishing a fiction contract

While faculty have worked hard and creatively to engineer a realistic environment and case to allow for situated learning (see section 13.2.2), the simulation is not the same as caring for real patients. Despite simulation's advantages, there are limitations in that the resources (e.g. simulators, actors) and environment may appear to the participant as unrealistic. Success of the simulation-based learning must come from both parties: the faculty/facilitators and the participant learners. Dieckmann, Gaba, and Rall (2007) promote the use of an explicit agreement from both parties.[17] This usually presents as a verbal agreement from the faculty (e.g. 'Within the resources and technology available to us, we have done everything we can to make this simulation seem real. I will continue throughout the exercise to do my best to give you realistic interactive experience. But the fact is that it is simulated and certain things may not seem real to you. To help make our time together successful, I'm asking you to meet me half way. I hope you will agree to act as though things are real, as if you are truly in this clinical event. If we both work at it, then I think we'll have a much better experience. Can you agree to that?').

13.3.3.5 Setting the stage for the clinical case

Faculty who developed the case should determine, depending on the objectives of the session, what information is needed and appropriate for the learners to know prior to the simulation. Faculty must consider the participant role. We've learned from the field of improvisation ('improv') theatre, that participants must know four things: who they are; where they are; who the team is (e.g. surgeon, nurse); and what is the issue; e.g. 'we have an intoxicated patient in the emergency room (department), his girlfriend is at the registration area and the nurse is currently at his bedside'. Many simulation programmes believe that simulation is most powerful for the learner when they are exactly who they are and that they not try to be someone else; e.g. a physician pretending to be a nurse. This school of thought believes that it subtracts from necessary learning for that individual; tends to make the simulation environment more confusing for participants; and may reinforce stereotypes that interprofessional education seeks to break down—stereotypes that have been shown to negatively impact patient care. These programmes will give a general assignment to the participants that allows freedom for them to be who they are clinically in their profession (e.g. 'you are at a nursing station during your clinical shift' or 'you are the on-call team'). Some simulation programmes predetermine the roles of the learners to provide variety and realistic composition of involved teams in the simulation case and under the belief that playing a role other than one's clinical role may provide insight into this other role.[18] Based on our interprofessional experience, the authors recommend against the predetermination of individual roles unless role exposure is one of the main objectives—and if that's the case, the simulation debriefing should be carefully facilitated to address role issues.

13.4 The practice of debriefing: a suggested structure

Although the finer points of the structure of the debriefing may vary somewhat, it is generally agreed that there are three main phases to the process.[15, 19–21] The Institute for Medical Simulation (2014) suggests a three-phase structure:

1 A **reactions phase** that attempts to elicit the participants' feelings, as well as providing the facts of the case in which they have been involved. The facilitator may

preview his/her plan for the debriefing time. Group discussion then elicits the main issues for subsequent reflection, which can be stimulated by video playback if available.

2 An **understanding phase** in which the participants' perspectives around the simulated case are explored to determine performance gaps,[22] discussed to help understand underlying perspectives or other learner perspectives, teaching to help move participants to new understandings, and generalization to the participants' real settings.

3 A **summary phase** in which the learning from the scenario and debriefing is reviewed and extrapolated into a real-world context with consideration of how the participants can implement any new learning into their daily practice.

13.4.1 The reactions phase

Emotion before cognition. One of the aims of the scenario is to get the participants into a heightened state of emotional arousal that may closely represent the physiological state in which clinicians provide care. Creating psychological challenges that trigger emotional engagement gets to the affective component of learning,[2] and, provided it is managed appropriately, sets the scene for a more meaningful debriefing.

Participants need to discharge some of this emotion before they are able to more objectively debrief the scenario. This process begins as soon as the scenario ends. Therefore, getting the participants out of the simulation room and into the debriefing room needs to be managed as thoughtfully and quickly as possible. There should be no break in proceedings at this stage—the important thing is to capture the learners' immediate feelings to gain an insight into their emotional state and comments about the case, even if it means walking behind them down the hallway to the debriefing room. The general level of conversation may be an indicator of the collective mood of the group who have just been in the scenario. A lot of chatter is typical and reflects normal emotional release. A quiet ambiance may indicate a general perception that the situation wasn't handled well.

A useful opening question at this stage is: *How did that feel for you?* Or *How are you feeling at this moment?* Ask this as a general question, and allow each participant to answer if time allows. The question should be aimed toward their emotion in the moment and avoid immediate discussion of their detailed performance. Discussion of specific performance is reserved for the understanding phase. Impress upon the participants that this question is distinct from how they felt during the scenario and is not about the technical aspects of the scenario (e.g. it is not 'How do you think you managed the situation?'). In that vein, debriefers should avoid opening the reactions phase with questions like 'How do you think that went?' or 'What do you think about your performance during the case?' Recognize that identifying and raising vulnerable feelings may be difficult for participants—most won't answer the question, or will, indeed, answer the question as though it was 'How do you think you managed the situation?' It is a good idea to mentally or actually record responses to this question to capture the participants' emotions—it may help assist future discussion. The use of a whiteboard may act as a transparent visual reminder for points of exploration. It is important once you have asked this question to acknowledge the range of emotions—stress, relief, embarrassment, frustration, anger—that this is normal and that it is actually helpful to have an element of high emotion to maximize the learning potential of the debriefing.

Hearing the emotions of the participants also indicates what is most relevant to them from the scenario and what they would most like to discuss. Building on the principles of adult learning theory, this provides insight for the facilitator to weave in learner topics into the faculty-chosen debriefing topics or substitute a faculty-chosen topic with a learner topic.

This short action, usually lasting 2–5 minutes, allows emotional release. Human cognition can be undermined by emotion because it can distract the participant from listening or understanding a discussion and reflecting on his/her thoughts.[23, 24] Therefore, emotion should be released and sanctioned prior to delving into cognition, understanding, and discussion.

Be aware that some participants will cite a lack of realism, and some learners will genuinely struggle to achieve the level of immersion in the scenario because certain variables of the simulation prevents them from holding the fiction contract.[17] While this is not ideal, it is easier to address having been discussed explicitly during the pre-briefing. When this occurs, faculty should not use precious debriefing time defending the simulation since the participant's perspective is valid: the simulation is no more or less real than the participant perceives it to be. Instead, faculty should validate this perspective and stay focused on the objectives. One technique is to redirect to previous real experiences; e.g. *Yes, it is not real. I agree it can be confusing. So let's not talk about simulation artefacts. Instead, let me ask you if you have ever, in your experience, tried to feel a pulse on a patient and wasn't sure if you felt it or not or read it correctly or not?*

Following this short assessment of emotions, a proactive helpful technique is to give the facts of the case (e.g. 'This was a 76-year-old female admitted to the ICU for myocardial infarction who progressed into pulseless electrical activity'). The facts do not include the performance of the participants, but the facts of the clinical case as though one was giving a transfer-of-care report. If facts are not clarified early in the debriefing, it places the debriefing at risk of not having a shared understanding of the event and questions clarifying the nature of the case may continue to be asked throughout the entire debriefing. Clarifying the facts of the case most often saves discussion time so that precious time can be used effectively for understanding and teaching.

13.4.2 **The understanding phase**

After the reactions phase, a good transitional action into the understanding phase is to preview the debriefing. A preview is a short description that orients participants about the conversational topics in the debriefing. While this is sometimes done before the reactions phase, it tends to dampen the potential for emotional release and immediately focuses participants to think about their performance in relation to the topics. An example of a preview is: *We have about 30 minutes to talk about what happened in the context of current best practice. I have two things that I'd like to discuss and, from your reactions just now, I think it will be interesting for us. First, I'd like to talk about how the team handled deciding and implementing a plan for the patient's asthma and then I'd like to change direction and talk about how the upset mother was handled.* The topics mentioned should be general headline topics, since added detail and judgement may stimulate detailed discussion in response to a preview, throwing the agenda off track. The topics chosen should tie into some of the emotions or topics that arose during the reactions phase and an explicit statement that their identified topics will be covered can help the participants feel at ease and create engagement in the discussion. If time permits, another option is to ask the participants if there are any additional topics that they would like to discuss and openly negotiate how to work any additional topics into the timeframe allotted.

At this time, to maintain psychological safety, it might be helpful to remind the participants (or debriefees) that:

♦ Everyone should feel free to contribute, though it is usual for the discussion to start with those who were actually in the scenario, moving on later to the observations of those who were watching.

♦ For some of the things that are discussed there will be quite clear guidelines for what is supposed to happen in such clinical situations.

♦ For some there will be no right or wrong answer or scripted solution.

♦ Criticisms should be constructive and specific and be sensitive to the feelings of others: one way to manage this is to remember to critique the perform**ance** not the perform**er**.

The understanding phase consists of three sub-phases: exploring, discussion and teaching, and generalizing and applying. The sub-phases may be repeated with each topic that is debriefed.

13.4.2.1 Exploring

During the simulation, faculty may note some actions or inactions and judge them to be right or wrong actions. The problem with this is that learner thoughts cannot be observed and the observed actions may not be for the reasons faculty assume. Rather than assuming that the actions or inactions reflect competency or missing knowledge of the observation, faculty judgements and assumptions should first be tested by exploring the trainee's perspective. Exploring the trainee's perspective effectively and directly is a something of an art and takes practice to do well. The most effective explorations include what was observed and transparency of the faculty's judgements and assumptions. Using this art of transparency is called 'debriefing with good judgement'.[25]

Rudolph[25] has outlined the theory and method for 'debriefing with good judgement'. This approach helps debriefers manage on the one hand the need for critical inquiry without being overly confrontational with learners, and on the other the temptation to avoid or 'sugar-coat' errors so as to avoid being non-judgemental. The method has three elements. Rudolph et al. first propose a conceptual model whereby people's (participants') actions are shaped by how they interpret the situation they are in—that is their 'mental model' or 'cognitive frame' of the situation. Second, is that an important role of the debriefer is, therefore, to uncover the learners' underlying frames that determined their actions through a process of genuine inquiry. Finally, the debriefer reveals (advocates) their own view of the situation as a means to explore the learners' views in more depth. This process promotes an environment in which the debriefer can work with the learners to develop alternative frames and actions for the future. Rudolph's group has extensive experience both using and teaching this technique. Readers are strongly encouraged to read Rudolph's and other Institute for Medical Simulation faculty's approach to gain a clearer understanding of this method.

The use of video in the debriefing session provides a powerful trigger for reflection and discussion as it allows replay of the actual sequence of events in the scenario. Video depicts an objective reflection to merge or contrast with participants' recollections/perceptions, which are sometimes flawed. In addition, using video can help participants recall more precisely what they were thinking and trying to accomplish at that moment in time.

The use of video can be expensive; the system available may not be entirely user-friendly; and the technology can be fragile leading to failures at inopportune times. Using video can be anxiety-provoking and even threatening for the participants, especially if they are unclear about the purpose of the video. Thus, it is important to know which clips to review (whether by marking the video in real time or writing down the time of the clip) and 'previewing' what they are about to watch prior to playing the video. Previewing provides a preface to the segment through a description of where it takes place in the chronology of the scenario and what issues you the debriefer want participants to think about in the context of this particular video clip. This act of previewing helps prevent the 'gotcha' approach where the video is played to show that participants' recollection of the case may be faulty. Making participants feel inadequate undermines trust between the facilitator and the participants and generates defensiveness. A preview focuses all the participants on one aspect of the video and leads to more meaningful, focused discussion. If the video illustrates aspects of management of the scenario that were problematic, it can be reassuring for the participants to have them also acknowledge things that went well in that time frame before moving on. Try to avoid showing a large number of segments or very long segments. If any discussion starts up while you are showing the video, pause the tape and pursue the discussion. A useful sequence for video review is:

1 Preface the video (e.g. *'Let's have a look at this piece of video. It's at the point in the scenario when the patient starts to complain about chest pain. I'd like you to pay particular attention to how the team's communication pattern changed.'*)

2 Show the video clip.

3 Discuss the issue in question in relation to the video (e.g. 'I noticed that Albert started to speak louder and, it seemed to me in a confident way. I'd like to discuss what was going on for Albert at that time and how others felt about it. Albert, what were you

thinking at the time?. . . Juan, when Albert appeared to be the leader, what were your thoughts? *What aspects of the communication were effective? Why? Ineffective? Why?*')

4 Discuss the issue in question in a broader context (e.g. '*What are the features of effective communication?*')

13.4.2.2 Discussion and teaching

Once performance and knowledge gaps are identified from the exploring sub-phase, the faculty now knows what to further discuss and can insert short teaching moments or 'lecturettes' to assist participants in filling these gaps.

During the understanding phase, a challenge for the faculty is to facilitate the agenda of the debriefing toward rich learning within a time frame, but not with too rigid a plan that may stifle participant perspectives. Other challenges include:

◆ Keeping everyone engaged/involved, not just the outspoken participants. 'Cold calling' or redirecting of conversation to the objectives or to the quiet participants can help with this challenge.

◆ Raising important medical/technical or behavioural issues not covered by participants in their discussion. Failing to address an oversight or misconception is too likely to be interpreted as validation of a particular form of medical management by the participants. For this reason, patient safety or poor practices must be brought up. Participants need to be made aware of inappropriate decisions and actions or inactions and be made aware of the consequences of such if translated into the workplace. This may involve periods of instruction within the debriefing that aims to enhance the knowledge base of the group and highlight issues the group may have overlooked. The debriefer is not obligated to spend a lot of precious time on mistakes, but they must be noted. Having fact sheets on the medical management of the simulation cases available for participants to take home is a good way to save time and ensure the learners can brush up on any knowledge gaps afterwards.

◆ Stressing that inappropriate actions (or inaction) does not necessarily imply that the participants would have handled the situation the same way if the situation was actually real—or that they are 'below standard'. But it is important to question them as to why they did what they did and to ensure they realize such management would be inappropriate in a real situation.

13.4.2.3 Generalize and apply

The interest in this sub-phase is to meet adult learning criteria and allow the participants to conceptualize how the topics just discussed and the lecturette just provided are relevant to their practice. The facilitator can ask the participants about their real-life experiences in this type of situation: '*Has anyone been in this situation in real life? Would the things we just discussed work for you in that situation or in a future situation similar to this?*'

Some things to do during the understanding phase:

◆ Be familiar with the event you will debrief and, if you missed something during the running of the simulation, be transparent that you missed that part and may need the participants to help recall what happened.

- Use open-ended questions (e.g. What were you thinking? What's your take on that? What was going on for you at the time? I'm curious about your perspective?) to initiate discussion. Once participants have finished discussing a topic, use follow-up questions to acknowledge the importance of group ideas and encourage deeper discussion.

- Reflect questions to you by participants back to the group to get their thinking on the question, rather than giving your own opinion too prematurely (if at all).

- Get used to using silence as a technique to encourage participant input to the discussion. It can be really hard to avoid answering your own questions when no one responds. However, if you don't speak, someone else almost always will. Try counting to 20 after you ask a question if necessary before speaking again. And then, if you think the question is an important one, ask the participants if they need you to rephrase the question.

- Body language is important. Leaning forward with open hands facing outwards and an interested, enthusiastic facial expression is far more engaging than gestures that indicate boredom, frustration, or negativity (such as folded arms or not looking at the speaker).

Some things to avoid during the understanding phase:

- Instructor-centred discussions.
- Long lecturing.
- Giving the impression that only your opinion is important.
- Interrupting participants.
- Interrogation and asking many questions that only the debriefer knows the answer. A good principle: the debriefer can see what happened but cannot know what participants were thinking.
- An overly rigid agenda: you need to have an agenda, but be prepared to be flexible.
- Patient death, unless issues surrounding death and dying form part of the objectives of the session, it's probably better to avoid having 'patients' die during a simulation.

13.4.2.3 The summary phase

One important reason for staying on schedule is to ensure adequate time is available to close out the debriefing appropriately. Make it clear that the debriefing session is ending; e.g. *'It's time to wrap up the debriefing session.'* This involves summarizing the topics covered and lessons learned, emphasizing their importance in relation to the workplace. Ask the participants to state the important things they learned from the discussion and how this will influence their future practice. *'What will you take away to your daily practice? How will you do it?'* Remind the participants that the system in which they work is likely to tacitly support their current behaviour. If they have learnt something today that needs to change, how are they going to make it happen?

At the end of the course, make sure to provide the participants with options for further discussion/counselling should they so desire, including a method of contact.

13.5 **Debriefing instructor training**

Debriefing varies from programme to programme, session to session. Because these topics are beyond the intent of this chapter, we provide here resources for some of these variables:

- one or more debriefers
- the use of a 'content expert'—someone who understands the topic being taught more so than the debriefers and participants
- group size
- experience level of the participants:
  - novice or experienced?
- single specialty or professional group versus an interprofessional group
- participants' prior experience with simulation-based education:
  - is it the same or is the extent of previous exposures mixed?

Following the phases and steps of debriefing presented above can still guide effective debriefings despite the presence of these variables.

Formal debriefing instructor training is strongly recommended to allow for reflective practice, guidance, and feedback of debriefing skills. Debriefing exposes the debriefer at times to challenging questions, to uncontrolled emotions, and to divergent and even irrelevant ideas and viewpoints. Debriefers need to have organizing skills, group process skills, communication skills, conflict resolution skills, and counselling skills.[26] A common finding is that debriefers initially seek and need control over the debriefing process, often related to their own anxiety about loss of control, reflecting a lack of confidence in their debriefing skills. However, true learner-centredness requires the debriefer to have respect for the participants by allowing them to share control of the process—the participants' needs and expectations are extremely important factors in any debriefing. The ideal is an open and flexible style, based on mutual negotiation and collaborative learning—meaning that the needs and expectations of all members of the group can be made explicit and shared. Openness, warmth, and flexibility are likely to be important characteristics for debriefers.

Many established centres around the world, recognizing the challenge of developing and maintaining accomplished simulation faculty, provide training opportunities.[12] These programmes devote a portion of time to debriefing training in the form of interactive workshops outlining the theory underpinning simulation debriefing as well as generous opportunities to practice and get feedback on their debriefing. While these courses provide a useful introduction to the debriefing, as with any valued and complex skill, a lengthy apprenticeship with generous coaching is required to develop a degree of mastery.[27]

The principles involved in optimizing the effectiveness of simulation-based training apply also to the process of instructor debriefing training; in particular, the need for systematic and repetitive practice with timely feedback on performance. As a minimum this should involve routine discussion about the conduct of practice debriefings, with peer-to-peer and expert-to-peer feedback for the debriefer. Just as video is a powerful tool to stimulate reflection after a simulation scenario for course participants, so too is video of the debriefing to assist in honing the skills of the instructor. Use of video enables feedback on a number of important debriefing skills, such as: body language; amount of talking by the debriefer rather than the participants; the debriefer/s questioning style; the use of silence; attention to group dynamics, etc.

The Debriefing Assessment for Simulation in Healthcare (DASH) is a generalized instrument designed to assist in evaluating the quality of a debriefing and developing debriefing skills. The DASH provides criteria that indicates what a good or poor debriefing looks like.[28, 29]

13.6 **Debriefing research**

The debriefing process during SBE is increasingly studied and continues to have areas for future research. Some of the areas in need of rigorous research include the following:

- How important is the use of video? What is the return on investment? What are the downsides?
- What is the optimum number of instructors? How does this relate to the group size?
- Is professional group equity important in relation to debriefing? Do interprofessional participant groups benefit more from interprofessional debriefers?
- What is the place of humour in debriefing? Is it helpful or harmful?
- What verbal/non-verbal debriefer techniques optimize or compromise the debriefing process?
- What is the impact of stress on learning? Who learns better by doing and who learns better by observing? How do you best activate observers?
- What type of Kolb's Learning Style Inventory does better or worse in simulation?
- What constitutes optimal instructor training for attainment and maintenance of debriefing competence?
- What are the benefits of being a student observer of a simulated case and what are the best practices for students who are observing;
- What techniques maximize transfer of learning to the real world?
- Does debriefing have a role as a means to learn and develop cognitive decision-making skills?

13.7 **Conclusion**

Most of what individual participants will take away from a simulation session is predicated on their view of their performance in their simulated cases—how the debriefing is conducted will have implications for whether this is a positive or a negative experience. The debriefer's task is to give honest and supportive feedback to guide participants to new perspectives by turning a challenging, albeit artificial, clinical situation into a rich learning experience. There are tried-and-true steps and phases before, during, and after a debriefing to help guide a debriefer toward providing learners with a rich debriefing and a beneficial learning experience. These steps and phases have been discussed in this chapter.

Debriefing requires a lot of practice to develop expertise. The good news is that increasing attention is being paid to the development of models and theories of debriefing and the skill set required of expert debriefers. Clinician-educators who dedicate themselves to maximize the learning power of simulation and debriefing can make a significant difference in relation to enhancing the education of clinicians, and by extension, to patient safety.

Acknowledgement

Material in this chapter is from the Simulation Instructor Training Course developed and taught by Harvard Medical School faculty and adjunct faculty from the Center for Medical Simulation.

References

1 **Dannefer EF, Henson LC.** Refocusing the role of simulation in medical education: training reflective practitioners. In: Dunn WF (ed). Simulators in critical care and beyond. Des Plaines, IL: Society of Critical Care Medicine; 2004, 25–28.

2 **Knowles M.** The modern practice of adult education: from pedagogy to andragogy. Wilton, CT: Association Press, 1980.

3 **Kolb D.** Experiential learning. Experience as the source of learning and development. Englewood Cliffs, NJ: Prentice-Hall, 1984.

4 **Kolb D, Fry R.** Toward an applied theory of experiential learning. In: Cooper C (ed.). Theories of group process. London: John Wiley, 1975.

5 **Schon D.** The reflective practitioner. New York, NY: Basic Books, 1983.

6 **Thompson N, Pascal J.** Developing critically reflective practice. Reflective Practice: International and Multidisciplinary Perspectives 2012;**13**(2):311–325.

7 **Ericsson A, Krampe RT, Tesch-Romer C.** The role of deliberate practice in the acquisition of expert performance. Psychological Review 1993;**100**(3):363–406.

8 **Ericsson KA.** Deliberate practice and the acquisition and maintenance of expert performance in medicine and related domains. Academic Medicine 2004;**79**(10):S70–81.

9 **Lave D, Wenger E.** Situated learning: legitimate peripheral participation. New York, NY: Cambridge University Press, 2008.

10 **Morrison JB.** Deckers C. Common theories in healthcare simulation. In: Palaganas JC, Maxworthy J, Epps C, Mancini MB. Defining excellence in simulation programs. Philadelphia, PA: Wolters Kluwer Lippincott Williams & Wilkins, 2014.

11 **Littlewood KE, Szyld D.** Debriefing. In: Palaganas JC, Maxworthy J, Epps C, Mancini MB. Defining excellence in simulation programs. Philadelphia, PA: Wolters Kluwer Lippincott Williams & Wilkins, 2014.

12 **Navedo D, Simon R.** Specialized courses in simulation. In: Levine A, DeMaria S, Schwartz A, Sim A. Comprehensive textbook of healthcare simulation. New York, NY: Springer, 2013.

13 **Hess FM.** The same thing over and over: How school reformers get stuck in yesterday's ideas. Cambridge, MA: Harvard University Press, 2010.

14 **Goldstein IL.** Training in organizations: needs assessment, development, and evaluation (3rd edn). Belmont, CA: Thomson Brooks/Cole Publishing Co., 1993.

15 Gaba D, Howard S, Fish K, et al. Simulation-based training in anesthesia crisis resource management (ACRM): a decade of experience. Simulat Gaming 2001;**32**:175–193.

16 Rudolph JW, Raemer DB, Simon R. Establishing a safe container for learning in simulation: the role of the presimulation debriefing. Simulation in Healthcare 2014.

17 Dieckmann P, Gaba D, Rall M. Deepening the theoretical foundations of patient simulation as a social practice. Simulation in Healthcare 2007;**2**(3):183–193.

18 Salas E, Cannon-Bowers JA. The science of training: a decade of progress. Annu Rev Psychol 2001;**52**:471–499.

19 Lederman LC. Debriefing: toward a systematic assessment of theory and practice. Simulat Gaming 1992;**23**:145–160.

20 Cheng A, Eppich W. PEARLS: a mixed method approach to debriefing. Pre-conference workshop to the International Meeting for Simulation in Healthcare 2013, Orlando, FL (January 2013).

21 Zigmont J, Kappus L, Sudikoff S. The 3D model of debriefing: defusing, discovering, and deepening. Seminars in Perinatology 2011;**35**(2):52–58.

22 Rudolph JW, Simon R, Raemer D, Eppich W. Debriefing as formative assessment: closing performance gaps in medical education. Academic Emergency Medicine 2008;**15**:1010–1016.

23 Kindler CH, Szirt L, Sommer D, Häusler R, Langewitz W. A quantitative analysis of anaesthetist-patient communication during the pre-operative visit. Anaesthesia 2005;**60**(1):53–59.

24 Eysenck MW, Derakshan N, Santos R, Calvo MG. Anxiety and cognitive performance: attentional control theory. Emotion 2007;**7**(2):336–353.

25 Rudolph JW. There's no such thing as 'nonjudgmental' debriefing: a theory and method for debriefing with good judgment. Simul Healthcare 2006;**1**:49–55.

26 Pearson M, Smith D. Debriefing in experience-based learning. Simulat Gaming 1986;**16**(4):155–171.

27 Mort TC, Donahue SP. Debriefing: the basics. In: Dunn WF (ed). Simulators in critical care and beyond. Des Plaines, IL: Society of Critical Care Medicine; 2004, 76–83.

28 Center for Medical Simulation. Debriefing Assessment for Simulation in Healthcare, available at: <https://harvardmedsim.org/debriefing-assesment-simulation-healthcare.php>

29 Brett-Fleegler M, Rudolph J, Eppich W, Monuteaux M, Fleegler E, Cheng A, et al. Debriefing assessment for simulation in healthcare: development and psychometric properties. Simulation in Healthcare 2012;**7**(5):288–294.

Chapter 14

Training and assessment with standardized patients

John R Boulet and Anthony Errichetti

Overview

- The use of standardized patients, lay people trained to model the medical conditions of and mannerisms of 'real' patients, for training and assessing medical and allied health professionals is widespread.

- Although standardized patients are used primarily for formative assessment purposes, they have been in high-stakes certification and licensure examinations.

- Developing standardized patient programmes can be complex and special attention should be paid to centre design, case development, and standardized patient recruitment and training.

- Based on four decades of research, standardized patient assessments can yield valid and reproducible scores as long as there are sufficient numbers of encounters, the evaluation rubrics are properly designed and the assessors and standardized patients are well trained.

- The lessons learned from administering and validating standardized patient assessments can be used to help develop and improve other healthcare simulation modalities, including those employing part-task trainers and full-body mannequins.

- For all healthcare simulations, including those that use standardized patients, additional research efforts focused on refining the scoring models, developing integrated assessments, and identifying potential threats to the validity of score interpretations are warranted.

14.1 Introduction to training and assessment with standardized patients

Although simulation in healthcare can take many forms, the use of standardized patients (SPs), lay people trained to model the mannerisms and complaints of real patients, is prevalent throughout the world.[1-6] Starting with their employment for medical student training,[7] SP-based evaluation methods have evolved to be of sufficient quality to become part of high-stakes certification and licensure examinations.[8] SPs have also been used in many disciplines outside medicine, including dentistry, nursing, audiology, and pharmacy.[9–14] Along the way, numerous research studies have published covering diverse topics ranging from case development to training methods to equating performance scores.[15–17] These research endeavours, while extremely valuable for the advancement of SP-based evaluation and training activities, also provide some lessons for all performance-based simulation activities in all healthcare disciplines. As a result, it will be informative for those individuals involved in simulation activities, not necessarily only those that are SP-based, to have some understanding of how SPs have been used to train and evaluate healthcare practitioners. Moreover, knowing how SP-based training and evaluation programmes are set up, including the development of case materials and the layout of the physical assessment facility, can help guide future, potentially more complex and integrated, simulation activities.

The purpose of this chapter is to provide a wide-ranging overview of the use of SPs in health professions' education and assessment. General information will be provided on setting up SP programmes, the basic layout of the physical facility, administering assessments, using the evaluation data, and judging the quality of the assessments and assessment scores. In addition, the role of SP-based methods in other simulation venues will be briefly discussed. Not only can SP methodology (e.g. scoring mechanisms, validation research) be exported to other simulation environments, but, from a practitioner competence perspective, integrating the knowledge that currently exists with the plethora of other emerging simulation-based evaluation methods should lead to better, more valid, and defensible assessments.

14.2 **Typical structure of SP-based simulations**

Although much more detailed information on SPs and SP-based assessments will be provided later in this chapter, it is important to first be familiar with the general structure of simulations that employ SPs. While there can be much variation in the way that SP encounters are configured, some commonalities exist, especially for those assessments designed to educate and assess medical students, residents, practising physicians, and other healthcare professionals. Typically, those being evaluated receive a brief orientation covering assessment protocols (e.g. the use of equipment, restricted physical examination manoeuvres, timing) prior to beginning any simulated clinical encounters. On the door outside the examination room, the person being evaluated may be provided with some background information about the SP, including vital signs and the reason, or reasons, for the visit. Once this information is reviewed, the person being evaluated enters the examination room and proceeds to take a relevant history and/or perform a focused physical examination. Depending on the nature of the assessment, these encounters normally last from 15 to 45 minutes. The SP, having been trained to model the mannerisms and affect of a 'real' patient, provides semi-scripted answers to the evaluated person's queries and reacts appropriately to any physical examination manoeuvres. In some encounters, SPs can be trained to simulate physical findings (e.g. absent breath sounds on one side) or display, via *moulage*, faux injuries; in others, SPs with stable physical findings (e.g. heart murmur, chronic arthritis) are employed. Once the allocated time is spent, or the interview/examination is finished, the evaluated person leaves the room. Most often, re-entry is not allowed, since the SP is typically involved in scoring activities such as rating communication skills or documenting history-taking questions asked. For some assessment designs, the person being evaluated will complete a timed post-encounter exercise after the SP encounter (e.g. writing a progress note or completing a multiple-choice quiz based on the potential disease mechanism associated with the SP's presenting complaint). If the assessment includes multiple encounters, the person being evaluated then rotates to the next encounter, starting again with a review of the background (doorway) information for the upcoming SP interaction.

14.3 **History**

The use of SPs goes back almost 40 years.[7, 18] Initially, their use was directed primarily at formative educational activities. In most instances, a medical student would interact with one or more trained patients and then be provided with qualitative feedback concerning his/her performance. This feedback was generally unstructured, and often did not reference any quantitative measure of performance. Over time, these SP-based encounters became more formalized; SPs were provided with more training, objective scoring systems were developed, multiple-station assessments were created, administration conditions were standardized, relevant post-encounter exercises were added (e.g. reading an electrocardiogram, composing a clinical note), feedback techniques were enhanced, and so forth. Nevertheless, for the most part, the SP-based assessments, commonly referred to as Objective Structured Clinical Examinations (OSCEs), were primarily used for formative purposes—providing medical students with feedback so that they could improve their clinical skills.

Regarding terminology, the term 'standardized patient' is more widely used in North America. Elsewhere, 'simulated patient' is more prevalent. For our purposes we will define SPs as individuals who have been trained to simulate health problems and conditions in a standardized examination or learning environment.

Beginning in the 1980s, there was general recognition that SP-based evaluation methods might well be used for summative purposes, including credentialing and certification.[19, 20] Numerous studies, conducted by both medical school personnel and licensing/certification bodies, suggested that if there are sufficient numbers of simulated encounters, and they are sampled appropriately from the practice domain, reliable and valid assessment decisions could be made.[21] In 1992, the Medical Council of Canada (MCC) initiated the Qualifying Examination Part II, a licensure requirement for Canadian medical school graduates.[22] This examination, which continues to be offered at various sites throughout Canada, utilizes a series of SP encounters to evaluate clinical skills. Since the start of the MCC exam, other certification and licensure organizations have developed and administered 'high-stakes' multi-station OSCEs.[23] Most notably, these include the General Medical Council (GMC) of the United Kingdom,[24] the Educational Commission for Foreign Medical Graduates (ECFMG),[25] the National Board of Osteopathic Medical Examiners (NBOME),[26, 27] and the United States Medical Licensing Examination (USMLE).[8, 28] In addition, many medical schools now demand successful completion of an SP-based clinical skills assessment in order to graduate.[29] Although the movement of SPs from the formative to the summative arena has taken place rather quickly, it has been supported by a large number of studies, many of which provide guidance in the areas of assessment programme development, SP training, scoring, quality assurance, rater calibration, and psychometrics.[30–32] Going forward, the lessons learned and information gained in the SP arena over the past 40 years will certainly provide some much needed direction for other simulation-based assessment activities.

14.4 Setting up a standardized patient programme

Setting up an SP programme involves many steps, including designing the physical facility, developing simulation content and measurement tools, faculty development, and recruiting and training staff and SPs.[33–36] While this process will vary as a function of the purpose of the programme and the available resources, there are a number of important and interrelated factors that should be considered. In the following sections, we provide a general overview of some of the issues that should be addressed when setting up an SP programme. This is not, however, meant to be a 'how to' manual. The interested reader should consult some of the available references for more detail on programme implementation, architecture, logistics, and costs.[15, 36–43]

14.4.1 Physical facility

Historically, SP-based training and evaluation centres were modelled after real clinics. Typically, there were a few rooms, sometimes only one, constructed and equipped to look like a 'real' patient examination venue. In many instances, existing hospital or clinic facilities were used, after hours, to host evaluation activities. As the Northern American SP medical licensing examinations took hold, medical schools began to model their facilities after high-stakes testing centres (e.g. by equipping exam rooms with digital cameras and PCs to collect performance data). As a result, SP programmes have gradually evolved into multifaceted simulation centres, specifically designed and constructed to host an array of simulation activities.[44–48] These centres can incorporate many simulation technologies, including SPs, mannequins (e.g. full-size electromechanical models, part-task/body trainers, surgical trainers), and virtual reality programmes. However, regardless of the scope of simulation activities, the simulation centre should be built, or modelled, to allow for a smooth integration of SP and patient simulator exercises and for the training of allied health professionals, both individually and together. The following section will focus specifically on the basic set-up and use of the SP facility, highlighting some recent technological advances that can simplify various administrative and logistical tasks.

14.4.1.1 Training/assessment area

The typical SP facility contains a number of identical examination rooms and some peripheral office space for training and teaching, computer and video resources, staff offices, and storage. The SP training and assessment area must be reasonably realistic (simulating a multidisciplinary clinical working environment) and versatile (able to provide experiential and didactic sessions for student, faculty, and SPs). When considering a site, one must weigh the cost of new construction versus the logistical constraints of retrofitting existing space. There are obvious advantages to building a new centre. The ability, for example, to wire, plumb, and design hallways and corridors to better accommodate student-SP traffic flow, on the surface, makes this the preferred option. Locating SP training labs in hospital or clinic environments, when in close proximity to a medical school or health sciences facility, will certainly appeal to students who want to learn in a more realistic environment. In general, simulations, regardless of fidelity, seem to have more relevance when they take place within an actual working environment populated by actual patients and family members, physicians, nurses, and other allied health professionals.

Exam rooms are commonly equipped with basic diagnostic equipment (sphygmomanometer, otoscope, ophthalmoscope, etc.), a working sink, and other peripheral equipment normally found in 'real' exam rooms. Where possible, it is advisable to have separate entrance and exit for those being evaluated (examinees) and SPs. This will help facilitate traffic flow, especially when numerous people are being assessed at the same time in different exam rooms. Outside the exam rooms, equipping stations (carousels or pull-down desks) with wireless Internet connectivity will allow for both pre-encounter (e.g. viewing lab results or reviewing patient information) and post-encounter exercises (e.g. to complete a progress notes or answer a quiz based on the patient's complaint).

In North America, SP programmes, at least those associated with medical programmes, most often concentrate on the education of first- and second-year medical students, preparing them for the clinical clerkship years through a series of training exercises and formative evaluations.[29] Training programmes often include case-based encounters (e.g. a student encountering a simulated patient presenting with an identified illness or condition such as asthma or headache). In some special programmes designed to teach and evaluate communication skills, the student may also encounter an SP and his or her family member.[49] Often, in the role of physical examination teaching associates, SPs are used to train students in select physical examination manoeuvres.[50] In these exercises, the teaching associates typically work with one to three students, reviewing physical examination techniques. For these types of educational activities, the training/exam rooms must often be large enough to accommodate several people.

If multiple simulation platforms are being used (SPs and mannequin-based patient simulators), they should be located in close proximity. For example, in a 'breaking bad news' practice scenario, a medical team works with a dying patient (patient simulator) and then counsels family members (SPs) in a simulated waiting area about possible treatment options.[51] Realism can be enhanced with an audio system playing ambient hospital or emergency room sounds. The general point is that the training/assessment area must be as realistic and as flexible as possible. Although the layouts of centres used for high-stakes credentialing purposes often serve as templates for other programmes, their 'one use' assessment function makes them less desirable as models for the more dynamic, educationally oriented, medical school or residency training programmes.

14.4.1.2 Other functional space

Ideally, the SP centre or laboratory includes a reception area for those who are being evaluated; this provides space for a pre-encounter orientation or post-encounter debriefing sessions. If it includes a personal computer and a large flat screen to view various media, this area can serve as a general purpose classroom. Also, by furnishing this area with moveable tables and chairs, and basic diagnostic equipment, training sessions can be held there. Trainers can conduct didactic sessions, demonstrate physical examination manoeuvres, and role play with patients in front of the entire group. Individual SP training can also occur in the trainer's office or any of the available exam rooms. If exam video technology is available, exam room training allows for recording and reviewing of practice sessions.

14.4.2 Simulation connectivity systems

Today's state-of-the-art centres are typically equipped with advanced simulation connectivity systems. These systems include hardware and software for managing and distributing simulation activities. They tie together the various simulations activities through digital audiovideo systems, performance data collection capabilities, scoring and reporting modules, and programme-management algorithms.

If possible, exam rooms should be equipped with two digital pan-tilt-zoom cameras managed by a technician in a control room. All training and assessment sessions can be recorded and stored on a server and access given according to defined security protocols. Live or previously recorded videos can be used by students and clinical faculty to review students' performances, by SPs and trainers to conduct quality assurance activities, and by SPs to review their own work or to learn how to portray a case more accurately.[52-54] For certain types of assessments, including research projects, clinical faculty may want to rate individuals, or teams, using live or recorded video.[55] Faculty, or any other evaluators, can view work live or recorded at the training site or, provided the web-based infrastructure is adequate, remotely from other locations. This 'anytime, anywhere' feature of web-based digital systems effectively solves many logistical issues associated with training and scoring. Training videos can be produced as needed or culled from existing video recorded during teaching sessions.

To generate scores, provide feedback, or assign outcomes (e.g. pass/fail), the SP-based performance assessment requires a system to gather, analyse, and report data. Historically, this was accomplished with paper-based forms. Today, the preferred approach is a personal computer (PC) or tablet placed in an exam room, or other area, for the SP, or any other evaluator, to assess each performance. If external raters are used (e.g. faculty, senior students, residents), they can view recorded performances and enter ratings wherever there is an available computer. To produce individual or group score reports, 'canned' statistical programs, designed to analyse and summarize the performance data, are usually included as part of the connectivity software.

Simulation centres are busy operations that can be made more efficient and cost effective through the use of programme-management software and hardware. Examples include automated announcements that time programmes and move those being evaluated between rooms, automated video-recording that switches cameras on and off, e-mail notification system for scheduling trainees and SPs, room-scheduling software, and an inventory control system for allocating and tracking simulation equipment.

14.5 **Developing the simulation content**

SP cases and performance checklists, or rating scales, are typically developed by case development committees or teams.[15, 56] For medical programmes, the committees are typically composed of clinical faculty and SP trainers. Within the group, it is preferable to have a mix of specialties and some first-hand knowledge of the skill level of those individuals who are going to be educated or evaluated using the simulated cases.

14.5.1 **Case development**

The basis of SP encounters is the case. The case is not a medical record but rather a training document used by SPs to learn how to simulate, or present, a clinical problem. The case is normally generated from a template that lists the important scenario facets, including clinical classification (e.g. setting for the encounter, SP hiring criteria, differential diagnosis, etc.) and the patient characteristics (e.g. chief complaint, past medical history, psychosocial information, body mass, ethnicity, etc.). Template information is generated and discussed by clinical faculty, and then edited into a training document by the SP trainer. A web-based case template enables committee members to develop the content on the 'paperless' scenario efficiently; edits can be made instantaneously and SPs can also give input regarding the case over the web. In medical schools, where meeting frequently is not possible, web-based tools can greatly facilitate the case-writing process.

After completing the case, the development team (or committee) typically reviews the subject matter before it becomes part of any educational or assessment activities. As a step toward content validation, discussed later in the chapter, a faculty member or student surrogate can examine a SP trained to the case. The development team can then critique the case as well as the verisimilitude of the patient simulation with respect to demeanour, symptoms, affect, and response to the physical examination.

14.5.2 **Constructing performance measures**

Currently, most SP-based assessment and evaluation activities involve some sort of data-collection activity.[57] Historically, analytic tools (e.g. checklists) have been used to gather data related to history-taking and physical examination (i.e. data gathering). The checklist items are usually developed by expert committees and can be weighted to reflect clinical importance.[58–60] Most often, the checklists are constructed with the SP's specific medical condition in mind. For example, a modelled encounter that covers 'atypical pneumonia' may incorporate history-taking checklist items such as 'asks about muscle or body aches' or 'pain when taking a deep breath'. Similarly, in terms of physical examination, the person being evaluated might be expected to 'examine the throat' or 'palpate the anterior cervical lymph nodes'. The creation of case checklists should also take into account the expected skill level of the person to be evaluated. For example, a history checklist constructed for a first-year medical student may include basic mastery questions (i.e. basic data the student must gather from all patients). More advanced history checklists should include discriminatory questions: ones that test for advanced clinical judgement or problem-solving.

Although checklist scoring is common, at least for data-gathering activities, holistic, or global, rating scales are also incorporated in many SP-based assessments.[61, 62] For some traits such as doctor–patient communication, rating scales provide a means to assess multifaceted behaviours that may not be amenable to checklist-type decomposition. Although these types of rating scales can be difficult to construct, and have often been criticized as being 'subjective', there is ample psychometric evidence to support their use.[63–65] Furthermore, cases can be constructed to foster certain types of interactions (e.g. interplay between patient physician when breaking bad news), providing more opportunities to measure relevant constructs.[66] Overall, provided the rubrics are defined, the raters are well chosen (e.g. are intimately familiar with the trait being assessed), and their training is appropriate, reliable and valid ratings can be procured.[67–70] Ultimately, the choice of scoring modality (analytic—checklists; holistic—rating scales) will be dependent on a number of factors, including what is being measured, the expertise level of those who are being assessed, the availability of 'experts' to serve as raters, logistics, and cost.[71]

14.6 SP recruiting and training

SPs are lay people trained to simulate patient problems, document skills, and, in some instances, give feedback. Although SPs can be trained to simulate various physical conditions, there are many clinical abnormalities that cannot be imitated, at least realistically. For these situations, it is sometimes possible to recruit SPs with stable physical findings. Regrettably, while this may be an effective strategy for low-stakes formative assessments, questions concerning the constancy of the 'real' physical findings, comorbidity, and potential patient harm from repeated physical assessments usually dissuade credentialing organizations from employing these types of SPs. Fortunately, technology has improved over the past decade, and other simulation modalities (e.g. full-body mannequins, virtual reality) can be used to fill some of the gaps in the assessment practice domain.[72, 73]

14.6.1 Recruitment

The SP recruitment challenge is finding individuals who are intelligent, literate, who exhibit good will toward the learner and enjoy learning themselves, and who have basic acting skills.[36] Screening of individuals can involve basic tests of literacy and memory. For example, potential SPs can be asked to review selected patient encounters and complete rudimentary checklists. Viewing videos also informs them what to expect when a doctor, or other health professional, takes a history and performs a physical examination.

14.6.2 Training

In case-based encounters, where individuals demonstrate or practise patient examination skills, the SP training process usually involves learning to simulate medical illnesses and conditions, documenting abilities, rating certain skills such as doctor–patient communication, and debriefing those who are being evaluated.[37, 74] This instruction is typically done by SP trainers using a variety of educational strategies.[75–78] Since the encounters typically last from 15 to 45 minutes, SPs are often taught memory-enhancing techniques. A new innovation in SP training involves the use of computers to deliver case content. In this self-training model, SPs work through a series of modules alone in which they learn how to portray a case and document skills using a checklist. Such training uses text, graphics, and recorded performances to deliver the content, and has been shown to be efficient and effective.[79] When these computer-based modules are delivered over the web, training can take place anywhere the SP has access to a high-speed Internet connection.

14.6.3 Debriefing candidate performance

For many formative assessments, in addition to portraying the case and documenting what transpired in the encounter, SPs provide those being evaluated with feedback concerning their performance.[36] Here, SPs are best utilized for giving information about interpersonal communication and physical examination technique. Feedback on history-taking should be confined to quality of questioning and to specific topics; for example, discussing psychosocial issues or health maintenance/risk factors that are pertinent to the case. For communication debriefing, SPs can complete a rating scale after the encounter and then discuss those ratings with the person being evaluated. This is best accomplished through an observation-comment approach whereby the SP offers an observation about a communication issue and asks the person being assessed to comment. Normally, SPs are trained to avoid a didactic approach during this debriefing process and those being evaluated are encouraged to reflect upon SP observations. Debriefing and feedback is greatly enhanced through a video review process; for example, where a recording of the encounter is viewed and the person being evaluated is asked to self-reflect on their performance. Giving feedback about the physical examination is more straightforward; using a physical examination checklist as a guide, SPs can ask individuals to perform the skills done incorrectly or incompletely and then correct errors (e.g. demonstrating how to place a blood pressure cuff correctly). Debriefing and giving feedback is a specialized skill, and may be one of the most difficult tasks for SPs. Screening SPs for this pedagogical responsibility is essential.

14.6.4 Performance fidelity

One method of working toward patient accuracy and consistency in performance and documentation (checklist completion) is to involve SPs in quality-assurance activities.[80] Variations on this method include getting patients to observe each other and give feedback or to observe and self-reflect on their own performance. In both cases they can observe either live or recorded sessions and complete a performance fidelity or accuracy checklist in which salient performance points are listed, such as delivering the correct opening line, giving correct information, and not volunteering information that wasn't asked for.

14.7 **Using the evaluation data**

As mentioned in previous sections, various clinical skills can be measured via SP-based evaluations, including data gathering (history-taking and physical examination), doctor–patient communication, interpersonal skills, clinical reasoning, and patient management. These skills can be measured via both analytic (e.g. checklist) and holistic (e.g. rating scale) tools.[81, 82] For some elements, the scoring/rating can be completed by the SP (after the clinical encounter) or by an observer (e.g. faculty) who can be inside or outside the room. Where the technology is available, scoring digital recordings can also be accomplished. If a post-encounter exercise is included in the assessment, ratings, or scores, can be procured from individuals who are specifically trained to evaluate the particular performance domain that is being assessed.[83, 84]

For history-taking and physical examination, case-specific checklists are the norm for documenting performance. More often than not, the performances for each checklist item (completed, not completed) are simply added together to generate an encounter or case score. This can be done separately for history-taking and physical examination, or combined. While individual items can be weighted, there is some debate in the literature as to whether this yields more valid scores.[60] If the SP-based assessment has multiple stations, the data-gathering scores can be averaged. Although the use of checklists is rather simplistic, and they have been criticized for rewarding thoroughness as opposed to efficiency,[85, 86] they provide a reasonably reliable documentation of what the candidate did and did not do.[87] From a formative assessment viewpoint, they can serve as a reference point for providing meaningful performance feedback.

When an SP-based assessment is being used for summative purposes, and not all students/candidates encounter the same cases or SPs, it is often necessary to equate individual scores. Fairness issues arise if one set of candidates sees less (or more) challenging test content (mixes of cases), or is evaluated by less (or more) stringent raters. Although the process of equating can be technically complex, it involves collecting data to be able to establish the difficulty of specific cases and leniency/stringency of particular raters.[16, 88] These data are then used to adjust individual scores based on particular test form (SPs, cases, raters) that the examinee encountered. Basically, if a candidate encounters a particularly difficult set of cases, or more stringent evaluators, a few points are added to his/her score. The converse would be true for someone who has a less challenging assessment form. Regrettably, score equating, even for high-stakes assessments, is often ignored, potentially compromising the validity of the assessment scores.

Whenever numerical scores are gathered as part of an SP assessment, especially if the stakes are high (e.g. certification and licensure examinations), it is important to gather quantitative quality-assurance data. This usually takes the form of double scoring based on some sampling of performances. If these secondary scores can be obtained, various statistical measures can be used to identify discrepant scorers or raters.[80] Even if only the 'live' scores are available, potential scoring problems can be identified fairly easily by looking at basic statistical summaries. For example, if clinical skills domains such as doctor–patient communication are being evaluated, one would expect that an examinee's ability would not vary considerably from one encounter to the next. Therefore, within a given test session, where all examinees see the same SPs, the mean of each SP's ratings, calculated for all encounters, should be close. For larger-scale operations, where there may be more than one SP for a given clinical encounter, it can also be useful to look at mean scores. If all SPs are consistently trained, both for scoring and portrayal, and they encounter examinees of approximately equivalent ability, then one would anticipate that their mean scores (e.g. checklist documentation of history-taking and physical examination) would be comparable.

14.8 **Assessing the quality of the evaluation**

Regardless of whether the purpose of the SP-based evaluation is formative or summative, some attention needs to be paid to the psychometric properties of the scores. Ultimately, it is important to know how the assessment results can be extrapolated to other situations and whether the results generalize to similar evaluations.[89–91] The answers to these queries can be obtained by gathering evidence to support the validity and reliability of the assessment scores.[92, 93]

14.8.1 **Validity**

For SP-based assessments, numerous studies have been conducted in an attempt to provide evidence that the scores are valid; i.e. they provide a sound scientific basis for the proposed score interpretations.[42, 94–96] While there are many potential sources of validity evidence, they can be categorized into five general areas: test content, response processes, internal structure, relations to other variables, and consequences of testing.[97] For test content on SP assessments, one wants to make sure that the types of cases are reflective of the practice domain and that the skills being measured are important to the healthcare field. For case content, this is often accomplished by referencing local or national databases to see what types of patients healthcare workers normally see.[98] Cases can then be developed with reference to the 'true' practice domain. In terms of determining the important skills, efforts are usually made to solicit the opinions of experts and to explore the curricular materials that are used to train practitioners. By crossing the skill domain with the practice domain, and constructing the SP assessment with this in mind, content validity is assured.[99]

Validity evidence from response processes can take many forms, including the documentation of how examinees proceed through the examination,[100] the investigation of whether the evaluators use the score scale as intended,[55, 101] questioning test-takers about their performance strategies,[102] and looking at score gains over time.[103] For example, if checklists are used for scoring, and there is no penalty for irrelevant inquiries, it would be useful to know whether examinees are purposefully asking more history-taking questions and performing additional physical examination manoeuvres, even though the patient's condition does not necessarily warrant them. If so, this could be a threat to the validity of the test scores. The realism of the clinical scenarios, and how those being evaluated interact with the SPs in the simulated environment, can also raise some validity concerns. To the extent that individuals who are being evaluated cannot 'suspend disbelief', their interaction with the SP may be somewhat artificial. Here, it is important to gather evidence to support the verisimilitude of the simulated clinical scenarios and the fidelity of the SP portrayals. This can be accomplished through normal quality-assurance activities and/ or targeted surveys of trainees who have participated in the assessment. One would also expect that SPs would rate physicians, or other healthcare workers, in the simulated environment, at least for some skills such as communication, similarly to how 'real' patients would evaluate them in actual clinical situations. To the extent that this is not true, validity could be compromised.[104]

Investigating the internal structure of assessment can also yield validity evidence. If the SP assessment includes both history-taking and physical examination elements, it would be reasonable to hypothesize that performance in one of these domains would be related to the other. Likewise, individuals with better communication skills should be able to gather more relevant data from the SP. More important, it is essential to know whether particular items function differently for identifiable subgroups of examinees.[105] On SP assessments, the item could be the case, the SP, or the associated combination. For example, where communication ratings are used in the evaluation, one would not expect that examinee scores would differ meaningfully as a function of gender of the SP or the type of case.[68] If they do, this may indicate some form of bias or, equivalently, threat to the interpretation of the test scores.

Analysing the relationship between the SP assessment scores and other variables is another way of procuring validity evidence.[106, 107] External variables can be other test scores (e.g. knowledge examination) or even group membership (e.g. experts, novices). For example, one would expect that, in terms of clinical skills, practising physicians would outperform medical students. Here, it also useful to investigate whether coached and uncoached groups perform differently. If clinical skills performance can be elevated substantially via short-term coaching, this may be a threat to validity. Finally, from a test–criterion relationship viewpoint, one would anticipate that scores obtained in the simulated environment will, to some extent, predict performance with 'real' patients.[108, 109] Unfortunately, these types of investigations often yield only moderate associations. Like a driver's test, the SP assessment provides information on what a candidate can do at the time of testing, not necessarily what he or she will do in the future. Nevertheless, it is still very important to gather data to help establish that performance with simulated patients translates to real-world situations.[110] Without this evidence, some of which can be difficult to procure, the value of simulation-based education and assessment can be questioned.[111]

The final, frequently ignored, source of validity evidence is based on the consequences of testing. Often, there are both intended and unintended consequences of test use; these should be investigated and acknowledged. Based on the historical use of SPs, especially for assessment-related purposes, many benefits appear, including, among others, the fact that the students get better clinical training, there is an increased emphasis on doctor–patient communication and, because of standardization, the perceived fairness of the assessment is enhanced.[112, 113] Ultimately, albeit difficult to establish cause and effect, one would expect, for example, practising doctors to be better trained, patient satisfaction to increase, and there to be fewer malpractice claims or referrals to licensing boards. For countries with national SP-based clinical examinations, the validation process would involve gathering evidence to support the fact that these potential benefits of testing are actually happening.[114, 115]

14.8.2 Reliability

To establish the quality of SP-based assessment, one also needs to provide some evidence that the scores are consistent and relatively free of error.[89] Traditionally, this has been accomplished by providing measures of internal consistency (how well performance on one case is related to the next) and inter/intra rater reliability (how consistent are evaluators in their provision of ratings or scores). These reliability estimates can be provided for the whole exam, if total scores are calculated, or individual parts (e.g. history-taking). While this strategy is effective, it may be conceptually easier to think about reliability in terms of specific error sources.

For SP-based examinations, the decomposition of sources of error has been reported in numerous studies.[16, 21, 116] In general, regardless of the scoring methodology employed, task-sampling variability is the key facet that impacts the reproducibility of scores.[117] For multi-station performance assessments in general, and SP-based models in particular, the content of individual exercises tends to drive performance, at least to some degree.[118] That is, even though specific skills are being measured across cases, individuals will perform better, or worse, as a function of their familiarity/experience with the content. As a result, if the content (mix of cases) is different from one test form to another, an individual's score may not be generalizable, especially if the number of cases is small. Therefore, if score reproducibility is an issue, it is usually advisable to increase testing time (number of cases). This will help ensure that estimates of an examinee's ability will not be overly dependent on the choice of particular cases.

Although other sources of score variability exist for SP assessments, namely those associated with the rater, they usually do not play a significant role if proper training is provided.[70, 83, 119] Here, whether SPs or external observers are scoring, it is important to establish specific criteria that pertain to the assignment of ratings or the crediting of checklist items. Furthermore, as part of the training regime, it is useful to provide benchmarked performances so that individual scorers will know why their ratings are discrepant and make appropriate corrections. By doing this, variability attributable to the raters can be reduced.

14.9 **Applicability of SP-based methodology to mannequin-based simulation**

Although SP-based methods have been around for over three decades, their use in high-stakes certification and licensure examinations has come only recently. This movement from primarily formative teaching to summative assessment spurred numerous research efforts, many of which were designed to address methodological shortcomings and psychometric concerns.[49, 72] The resultant literature can be of much assistance to those individuals who are, or are considering, employing simulations as part of the training, evaluation, or credentialing of healthcare workers.

While there are some notable exceptions, and development work is underway for some healthcare disciplines and specialties, part-task trainers and electromechanical mannequins are rarely employed as part of certification and licensure examinations. However, given the practice domains that must be covered, and the clinical skills that need to be measured, it would seem useful to integrate these models, where possible, into the assessments.[120, 121] For many SP-based clinical scenarios, it is difficult to simulate abnormal physical findings. Furthermore, certain physical examination manoeuvres are often banned (e.g. pelvic examination, breast examination) because it would be too difficult, and expensive, to recruit willing SPs. Therefore, provided the logistical and measurement considerations can be worked out, it would seem prudent to embrace integrated models—those that employ both SPs and mannequins in the evaluation framework. Recently, this has been accomplished in a number of clinical areas, albeit most often within the context of low-stakes formative assessments.[122–124]

Even though SP-based research has been extensive, and has provided many answers concerning logistics, training, and measurement, there are certainly some issues that will still need to be addressed as simulation technology expands. Some of these issues are briefly outlined below.

14.9.1 **New scoring models**

As noted in a previous section, SP-based assessments often employ checklists and/or rating scales. These rubrics have also been used for mannequin-based scenarios.[82, 125] However, unlike basic clinical abilities (e.g. interviewing), measured most efficiently via SPs, mannequins allow for the assessment of more complex procedural skills (e.g. airway management) under more acute and stressful conditions. As a result, issues such as sequencing and timing come into play. Although some success in scoring has been achieved with holistic and key action methods, additional work is certainly needed.[126–128] Going forward, provided that the physiological reactions of the mannequin accurately model those of a real patient, it may be possible to derive a valid score based on how the simulated patient (mannequin) reacts to management strategies that are employed.

14.9.2 **Validation work**

Much has been written concerning the characteristics, qualities, and utility of SP-based assessment methods. More recently, the feasibility, educational importance, and validity of assessments that employ mannequins and part-task trainers has been highlighted.[129–132] Like SPs, it is important to know whether performance in the simulated environment (i.e. with a mannequin) extends to the real world, with real patients. Moreover, as different simulation models are introduced, research efforts should be focused on determining which methods, or combinations, work best and under what specific conditions.[111] Finally, like SP-based scenarios, the focus of evaluations utilizing mannequins generally concerns the interaction between the patient and the provider. In this type of model, many important facets of effective healthcare delivery go unmeasured. Simulations scenarios, whether they employ SPs, mannequins, part-tasks trainers, or some combination, need to be developed to effectively tap other domains such as teamwork, professionalism, and patient safety.[133]

14.9.3 **Task specificity**

In general, SP-based assessments are used to measure basic clinical skills such as history-taking, physical examination, and doctor–patient communication. Therefore, it is possible to generate a reasonably reproducible measure of someone's ability as long as multiple scenarios (usually ten or more) are employed and effective training methods, both for the SPs and any evaluators, are employed.[134] As the cases become more specific, perhaps demanding higher-level skills (e.g. breaking bad news), the overall reliability of the skill scores in a multi-station evaluation tends to diminish.[135] An examinee may do extremely well on one scenario yet, because of lack of familiarity with the medical content, perform poorly on the next.

The problem of content specificity is even more pervasive when mannequins or part-task trainers are employed in the assessment. Here, the modelled scenarios tend to be more content-driven. For example, mannequins can be used to simulate a wide range of clinical conditions, including acute haemorrhage, anaphylaxis, and myocardial ischemia. If an assessment was designed to measure patient-management skills, an individual's performance may fluctuate quite dramatically as a function of specific experience with these types of conditions. Therefore, to get a reasonably precise measure of patient-management ability, several scenarios, purposefully sampled from the practice domain, are required. While the reproducibility of SP-based clinical skills scores has been studied in depth, and documented in numerous articles, similar work for evaluations that employ part-task trainers or mannequins is relatively sparse in comparison.[136] Here, as has been done for SP-based assessments, generalizability studies should be employed to determine the optimal measurement designs.[137, 138] These studies can inform test length (number of stations or cases), timing, the selection of content (scenarios to be modelled), and choice and number of raters.

14.10 **Conclusion**

Employing SPs to educate and evaluate healthcare workers, although often expensive and logistically challenging to implement, is commonplace. From an assessment perspective, unlike other modalities (e.g. observation of interactions with real patients), individuals can be exposed to the same clinical content, ensuring fairness, and allowing for valid comparisons of performance. Advancements in the field are coming in many areas; namely, computer-based SP training modules, more sophisticated scoring models, better-designed physical facilities, standard-setting protocols, and more efficient and effective feedback methods. As a result, there is likely to be a further expansion of the use of SPs, especially as part of summative assessment activities.

The experience gained over the past four decades of SP use will be invaluable to those who are embracing other forms of healthcare simulation. Whether part-task trainers, full-body mannequins, or computer-based case simulations are being employed, knowledge of centre design, case development, scoring, and validation research are all needed to establish effective training and/or evaluation programmes.

References

1 Reznick RK, Blackmore D, Dauphinee WD, Rothman AI, Smee S. Large-scale high-stakes testing with an OSCE: report from the Medical Council of Canada. Acad Med 1996 Jan;**71**(1 Suppl):S19–S21.

2 Barrows HS. An overview of the uses of standardized patients for teaching and evaluating clinical skills. Acad Med 1993 Jun;**68**(6):443–451.

3 Glassman PA, Luck J, O'Gara EM, Peabody JW. Using standardized patients to measure quality: evidence from the literature and a prospective study. Jt Comm J Qual Improv 2000 Nov;**26**(11):644–653.

4 Levine AI, Swartz MH. Standardized patients: the 'other' simulation. J Crit Care 2008 Jun;**23**(2):179–184.

5 May W, Park JH, Lee JP. A ten-year review of the literature on the use of standardized patients in teaching and learning: 1996–2005. Med Teach 2009 Jun;**31**(6):487–492.

6 Cantillon P, Stewart B, Haeck K, Bills J, Ker J, Rethans JJ. Simulated patient programmes in Europe: collegiality or separate development? Med Teach 2010;**32**(3):e106–e110.

7 Harden RM, Gleeson FA. Assessment of clinical competence using an objective structured clinical examination (OSCE). Med Educ 1979 Jan;**13**(1):41–54.

8 Dillon GF, Boulet JR, Hawkins RE, Swanson DB. Simulations in the United States Medical Licensing Examination (USMLE). Qual Saf Health Care 2004 Oct;**13** Suppl 1:i41–i45.

9 Broder HL, Janal M. Promoting interpersonal skills and cultural sensitivity among dental students. J Dent Educ 2006 Apr;**70**(4):409–416.

10 Wilson L, Gallagher Gordon M, Cornelius F, Smith Glasgow ME, Dunphy Suplee P, Vasso M, et al. The standardized patient experience in undergraduate nursing education. Stud Health Technol Inform 2006;**122**:830.

11 Rushforth HE. Objective structured clinical examination (OSCE): review of literature and implications for nursing education. Nurse Educ Today 2007 Jul;**27**(5):481–490.

12 Horton N, Payne KD, Jernigan M, Frost J, Wise S, Klein M, et al. A standardized patient counseling rubric for a pharmaceutical care and communications course. Am J Pharm Educ 2013 Sep 12;**77**(7):152.

13 Hofer SH, Schuebel F, Sader R, Landes C. Development and implementation of an objective structured clinical examination (OSCE) in CMF-surgery for dental students. J Craniomaxillofac Surg 2013 Jul;**41**(5):412–416.

14 Dinsmore BF, Bohnert C, Preminger JE. Standardized patients in audiology: a proposal for a new method of evaluating clinical competence. J Am Acad Audiol 2013 May;**24**(5):372–392.

15 King AM, Pohl H, Perkowski-Rogers LC. Planning standardized patient programs: case development, patient training, and costs. Teach Learn Med 1994;**6**(1):6–14.

16 Swanson DB, Clauser BE, Case SM. Clinical skills assessment with standardized patients in high-stakes tests: a framework for thinking about score precision, equating, and security. Adv Health Sci Educ Theory Pract 1999;**4**(1):67–106.

17 Hoppe RB, King AM, Mazor KM, Furman GE, Wick-Garcia P, Corcoran-Ponisciak H, et al. Enhancement of the assessment of physician-patient communication skills in the United States Medical Licensing Examination. Acad Med 2013 Nov;**88**(11):1670–1675.

18 Harden RM, Stevenson M, Downie WW, Wilson GU. Assessment of clinical competence using objective structured examination. BMJ 1975;**1**:447–451.

19 Norman GR, Barrows HS, Gliva G, Woodward CA. Simulated patients. In: Neufeld VR, Norman GR, editors. Assessing clinical competence. New York, NY: Springer Publishing Company; 1985, 219–229.

20 Swanson DB, Stillman PL. Use of standardized patients for teaching and assessing clinical skills. Eval Health Prof 1990;**13**(1):79–103.

21 Newble DI, Swanson DB. Psychometric characteristics of the objective structured clinical examination. Med Educ 1988 Jul;**22**(4):325–334.

22 Medical Council of Canada. Qualifying Examination Part II, Information Pamphlet. 2012. Ottawa, Ontario, Canada, Medical Council of Canada.

23 Kim KS. Introduction and administration of the clinical skill test of the medical licensing examination, republic of Korea (2009). J Educ Eval Health Prof 2010;**7**:4.

24 Tombleson P, Fox RA, Dacre JA. Defining the content for the objective structured clinical examination component of the professional and linguistic assessments board examination: development of a blueprint. Med Educ 2000 Jul;**34**(7):566–572.

25 Whelan G. High-stakes medical performance testing: the Clinical Skills Assessment program. JAMA 2000 Apr 5;**283**(13):1748.

26 Boulet JR, Smee SM, Dillon GF, Gimpel JR. The use of standardized patient assessments for certification and licensure decisions. Simul Healthc 2009;**4**(1):35–42.

27 Gimpel JR, Boulet JR, Errichetti AM. Evaluating the clinical skills of osteopathic medical students. J Am Osteopath Assoc 2003 Jun;**103**(6):267–279.

28 Federation of State Medical Boards I, National Board of Medical Examiners. 2013 USMLE Step 2 CS Content Description and General Information Booklet. Philadelphia, PA: FSMB and NBME; 2013.

29 Hauer KE, Hodgson CS, Kerr KM, Teherani A, Irby DM. A national study of medical student clinical skills assessment. Acad Med 2005 Oct;**80**(10 Suppl):S25–S29.

30 Whelan GP, Boulet JR, McKinley DW, Norcini JJ, van Zanten M, Hambleton RK, et al. Scoring standardized patient examinations: lessons learned from the development and administration of the ECFMG Clinical Skills Assessment (CSA). Med Teach 2005 May;**27**(3):200–206.

31 Stillman PL, Swanson DB, Smee S, Stillman AE, Ebert TH, Emmel VS, et al. Assessing clinical skills of residents with standardized patients. Ann Intern Med 1986 Nov;**105**(5):762–771.

32 Vu NV, Baroffio A, Huber P, Layat C, Gerbase M, Nendaz M. Assessing clinical competence: a pilot project to evaluate the feasibility of a standardized patient—based practical examination as a component of the Swiss certification process. Swiss Med Wkly 2006 Jun 24;**136**(25–26):392–399.

33 Boursicot K, Roberts T. How to set up an OSCE. Clin Teach 2005;**2**(1):16–20.

34 Jain SS, Nadler S, Eyles M, Kirshblum S, DeLisa JA, Smith A. Development of an objective structured clinical examination (OSCE) for physical medicine and rehabilitation residents. Am J Phys Med Rehabil 1997 Mar;**76**(2):102–106.

35 Selby C, Osman L, Davis M, Lee M. Set up and run an objective structured clinical exam. BMJ 1995 May 6;**310**(6988):1187–1190.

36 Adamo G. Simulated and standardized patients in OSCEs: achievements and challenges 1992–2003. Med Teach 2003 May;**25**(3):262–270.

37 Ainsworth MA, Rogers LP, Markus JF, Dorsey NK, Blackwell TA, Petrusa ER. Standardized patient encounters. A method for teaching and evaluation. JAMA 1991 Sep 11;**266**(10):1390–1396.

38 Reznick RK, Smee S, Baumber JS, Cohen R, Rothman A, Blackmore D, et al. Guidelines for estimating the real cost of an objective structured clinical examination. Acad Med 1993 Jul;**68**(7):513–517.

39 Stillman PL. Technical issues: logistics. Acad Med 1993 Jun;**68**(6):464–468.

40 Kelly M, Murphy A. An evaluation of the cost of designing, delivering and assessing an undergraduate communication skills module. Med Teach 2004 Nov;**26**(7):610–614.

41 Wilkinson TJ, Newble DI, Wilson PD, Carter JM, Helms RM. Development of a three-centre simultaneous objective structured clinical examination. Med Educ 2000 Oct;**34**(10):798–807.

42 Motola I, Devine LA, Chung HS, Sullivan JE, Issenberg SB. Simulation in healthcare education: a best evidence practical guide. AMEE Guide No. 82. Med Teach 2013 Oct;**35**(10):e1511–e1530.

43 Casey PM, Goepfert AR, Espey EL, Hammoud MM, Kaczmarczyk JM, Katz NT, et al. To the point: reviews in medical education—the Objective Structured Clinical Examination. Am J Obstet Gynecol 2009 Jan;**200**(1):25–34.

44 Parr MB, Sweeney NM. Use of human patient simulation in an undergraduate critical care course. Crit Care Nurs Q 2006 Jul;**29**(3):188–198.

45 Earle D. Surgical training and simulation laboratory at Baystate Medical Center. Surg Innov 2006 Mar;**13**(1):53–60.

46 Magee JH. Validation of medical modeling & simulation training devices and systems. Stud Health Technol Inform 2003;**94**:196–198.

47 Kurrek MM, Devitt JH. The cost for construction and operation of a simulation centre. Can J Anaesth 1997 Nov;**44**(11):1191–1195.

48 Ross K. Practice makes perfect: Planning considerations for medical simulation centers. HFMMAGAZINE [Internet]. 2012 Nov [cited 14 Nov 2014]; available from <http://www.hfmmagazine.com>

49 Petrusa ER. Taking standardized patient-based examinations to the next level. Teach Learn Med 2004;**16**(1):98–110.

50 Davidson R, Duerson M, Rathe R, Pauly R, Watson RT. Using standardized patients as teachers: a concurrent controlled trial. Acad Med 2001 Aug;**76**(8):840–843.

51 Bowyer MW, Rawn L, Hanson J, Pimentel EA, Flanagan A, Ritter EM, et al. Combining high-fidelity human patient simulators with a standardized family member: a novel approach to teaching breaking bad news. Stud Health Technol Inform 2006;**119**:67–72.

52 Furman GE, Smee S, Wilson C. Quality assurance best practices for simulation-based examinations. Simul Healthc 2010 Aug;**5**(4):226–231.

53 Furman GE. The role of standardized patient and trainer training in quality assurance for a high-stakes clinical skills examination. Kaohsiung J Med Sci 2008 Dec;**24**(12):651–655.

54 Erby LA, Roter DL, Biesecker BB. Examination of standardized patient performance: accuracy and consistency of six standardized patients over time. Patient Educ Couns 2011 Nov;**85**(2):194–200.

55 Boulet JR, McKinley DW, Norcini JJ, Whelan GP. Assessing the comparability of standardized patient and physician evaluations of clinical skills. Adv Health Sci Educ Theory Pract 2002;**7**(2):85–97.

56 Gorter S, Rethans JJ, Scherpbier A, van der Heijde D, Houben H, Van d, V, et al. Developing case-specific checklists for standardized-patient-based assessments in internal medicine: a review of the literature. Acad Med 2000 Nov;**75**(11):1130–1137.

57 O'Connor HM, McGraw RC. Clinical skills training: developing objective assessment instruments. Med Educ 1997 Sep;**31**(5):359–363.

58 Gorter S, Rethans JJ, Scherpbier A, van der Heijde D, Houben H, van der Vleuten C, et al. Developing case-specific checklists for standardized-patient-based assessments in internal medicine: a review of the literature. Acad Med 2000 Nov;**75**(11):1130–1137.

59 Boulet JR, van Zanten M, De Champlain A, Hawkins RE, Peitzman SJ. Checklist content on a standardized patient assessment: an *ex post facto* review. Adv Health Sci Educ Theory Pract 2008 Mar;**13**(1):59–69.

60 Sandilands DD, Gotzmann A, Roy M, Zumbo BD, De CA. Weighting checklist items and station components on a large-scale OSCE: is it worth the effort? Med Teach 2014 Jul;**36**(7):585–590.

61 Solomon DJ, Szauter K, Rosebraugh CJ, Callaway MR. Global ratings of student performance in a standardized patient examination: is the whole more than the sum of the parts? Adv Health Sci Educ Theory Pract 2000 May;**5**(2):131–140.

62 Cohen DS, Colliver JA, Marcy MS, Fried ED, Swartz MH. Psychometric properties of a standardized-patient checklist and rating-scale form used to assess interpersonal and communication skills. Acad Med 1996 Jan;**71**(1 Suppl):S87–S89.

63 Guiton G, Hodgson CS, Delandshere G, Wilkerson L. Communication skills in standardized-patient assessment of final-year medical students: a psychometric study. Adv Health Sci Educ Theory Pract 2004;**9**(3):179–187.

64 Hobgood CD, Riviello RJ, Jouriles N, Hamilton G. Assessment of communication and interpersonal skills competencies. Acad Emerg Med 2002 Nov;**9**(11):1257–1269.

65 Jonsson A, Svingby G. The use of scoring rubrics: reliability, validity and educational consequences. Educ Res Rev 2007;(**2**):130–144.

66 Kiluk JV, Dessureault S, Quinn G. Teaching medical students how to break bad news with standardized patients. J Cancer Educ 2012 Jun;**27**(2):277–280.

67 Hodges B, Turnbull J, Cohen R, Bienenstock A, Norman G. Evaluating communication skills in the OSCE format: reliability and generalizability. Med Educ 1996 Jan;**30**(1):38–43.

68 Chambers KA, Boulet JR, Furman GE. Are interpersonal skills ratings influenced by gender in a clinical skills assessment using standardized patients? Adv Health Sci Educ Theory Pract 2001;**6**(3):231–241.

69 Boulet JR, Ben-David MF, Ziv A, Burdick WP, Curtis M, Peitzman S, et al. Using standardized patients to assess the interpersonal skills of physicians. Acad Med 1998 Oct;**73**(10 Suppl):S94–S96.

70 Blum RH, Boulet JR, Cooper JB, Muret-Wagstaff SL. Simulation-based assessment to identify critical gaps in safe anesthesia resident performance. Anesthesiology 2014;**120**(1).

71 Hodges B, McNaughton N, Regehr G, Tiberius R, Hanson M. The challenge of creating new OSCE measures to capture the characteristics of expertise. Med Educ 2002 Aug;**36**(8):742–748.

72 Boulet JR. Summative assessment in medicine: the promise of simulation for high-stakes evaluation. Acad Emerg Med 2008;**15**(11):1017–1024.

73 Crosby E. The role of simulator-based assessments in physician competency evaluations. Can J Anaesth 2010 Jul;**57**(7):627–635.

74 May W. Training standardized patients for a high-stakes Clinical Performance Examination in the California Consortium for the Assessment of Clinical Competence. Kaohsiung J Med Sci 2008 Dec;**24**(12):640–645.

75 Amano H, Sano T, Gotoh K, Kakuta S, Suganuma T, Kimura Y, et al. Strategies for training standardized patient instructors for a competency exam. J Dent Educ 2004 Oct;**68**(10):1104–1111.

76 Foley KL, George G, Crandall SJ, Walker KH, Marion GS, Spangler JG. Training and evaluating tobacco-specific standardized patient instructors. Fam Med 2006 Jan;**38**(1):28–37.

77 Schlegel C, Bonvin R, Rethans JJ, Van d V. The use of video in standardized patient training to improve portrayal accuracy: a randomized post-test control group study. Med Teach 2014 Oct 14;1–8.

78 Ju M, Berman AT, Vapiwala N. Standardized patient training programs: an efficient solution to the call for quality improvement in oncologist communication skills. J Cancer Educ 2014 Sep 5.

79 Errichetti A, Boulet JR. Comparing traditional and computer-based training methods for standardized patients. Acad Med 2006 Oct;**81**(10 Suppl):S91–S94.

80 Boulet JR, McKinley DW, Whelan GP, Hambleton RK. Quality assurance methods for performance-based assessments. Adv Health Sci Educ Theory Pract 2003;**8**(1):27–47.

81 Norcini J, Boulet J. Methodological issues in the use of standardized patients for assessment. Teach Learn Med 2003;**15**(4):293–297.

82 Boulet JR, Murray D. Review article: assessment in anesthesiology education. Can J Anaesth 2012;**59**(2):182–192.

83 Boulet JR, Rebbecchi TA, Denton EC, McKinley DW, Whelan GP. Assessing the written communication skills of medical school graduates. Adv Health Sci Educ Theory Pract 2004;**9**(1):47–60.

84 Durning SJ, Artino A, Boulet J, La Rochelle J, van der Vleuten C, Arze B, et al. The feasibility, reliability, and validity of a post-encounter form for evaluating clinical reasoning. Med Teach 2012;**34**(1):30–37.

85 Cunnington JPW, Neville AJ, Norman GR. The risks of thoroughness: reliability and validity of global ratings and checklists in an OSCE. Adv Health Sci Educ Theory Pract 1996 Jan;**1**(3):227–233.

86 Day RP, Hewson MG, Kindy P, Van Kirk J. Evaluation of resident performance in an outpatient internal medicine clinic using standardized patients. J Gen Intern Med 1993 Apr;**8**(4):193–198.

87 Regehr G, MacRae H, Reznick RK, Szalay D. Comparing the psychometric properties of checklists and global rating scales for assessing performance on an OSCE-format examination. Acad Med 1998 Sep;**73**(9):993–997.

88 Boulet JR, Swanson DB. Psychometric challenges of using simulations for high-stakes assessment. In: Dunn WF, editor. Simulations in critical care education and beyond. Des Plains, IL: Society of Critical Care Medicine; 2004, 119–130.

89 Boulet J, McKinley D. Criteria for a good assessment. In: McGaghie WC, editor. International best practices for evaluation in the health professions. 1st edn. New York, NY: Radcliffe Publishing; 2013, 19–43.

90 Schuwirth LW, van der Vleuten CP. The use of clinical simulations in assessment. Med Educ 2003 Nov;**37**(Suppl 1):65–71.

91 Roberts C, Newble D, Jolly B, Reed M, Hampton K. Assuring the quality of high-stakes undergraduate assessments of clinical competence. Med Teach 2006 Sep;**28**(6):535–543.

92 Weller J, Henderson R, Webster CS, Shulruf B, Torrie J, Davies E, et al. Building the evidence on simulation validity: comparison of anesthesiologists' communication patterns in real and simulated cases. Anesthesiology 2014 Jan;**120**(1):142–148.

93 Cizek GJ. Defining and distinguishing validity: interpretations of score meaning and justifications of test use. Psychol Methods 2012;**17**(1):31–43.

94 Brailovsky CA, Grand'Maison P, Lescop J. Construct validity of the Quebec licensing examination SP-based OSCE. Teach Learn Med 1997;**9**(1):44–50.

95 Pangaro LN, Worth-Dickstein H, MacMillan MK, Klass DJ, Shatzer JH. Performance of 'standardized examinees' in a standardized-patient examination of clinical skills. Acad Med 1997 Nov;**72**(11):1008–1011.

96 Tamblyn R, Abrahamowicz M, Dauphinee D, Wenghofer E, Jacques A, Klass D, et al. Physician scores on a national clinical skills examination as predictors of complaints to medical regulatory authorities. JAMA 2007 Sep 5;**298**(9):993–1001.

97 American Educational Research Association, American Psychological Association, National Council on Measurement in Education. Standards for Educational and Psychological Testing. Washington, DC: American Educational Research Association; 2014.

98 **Boulet JR, Gimpel JR, Errichetti AM, Meoli FG.** Using National Medical Care Survey data to validate examination content on a performance-based clinical skills assessment for osteopathic physicians. J Am Osteopath Assoc 2003 May;**103**(5):225–231.

99 **Mookherjee S, Chang A, Boscardin CK, Hauer KE.** How to develop a competency-based examination blueprint for longitudinal standardized patient clinical skills assessments. Med Teach 2013 Nov;**35**(11):883–890.

100 **Chambers KA, Boulet JR, Gary NE.** The management of patient encounter time in a high-stakes assessment using standardized patients. Med Educ 2000 Oct;**34**(10):813–817.

101 **McKinley DW, Boulet JR.** The effects of task sequence on examinee performance. Teach Learn Med 2004;**16**(1):18–22.

102 **Arbuckle MR, Weinberg M, Harding KJ, Isaacs AJ, Covell NH, Cabaniss DL, et al.** The feasibility of standardized patient assessments as a best practice in an academic training program. Psychiatr Serv 2013 Mar 1;**64**(3):209–211.

103 **Raymond MR, Kahraman N, Swygert KA, Balog KP.** Evaluating construct equivalence and criterion-related validity for repeat examinees on a standardized patient examination. Acad Med 2011 Oct;**86**(10):1253–1259.

104 **Fiscella K, Franks P, Srinivasan M, Kravitz RL, Epstein R.** Ratings of physician communication by real and standardized patients. Ann Fam Med 2007 Mar;**5**(2):151–158.

105 **Bienstock JL, Tzou WS, Martin SA, Fox HE.** Effect of student ethnicity on interpersonal skills and objective standardized clinical examination scores. Obstet Gynecol 2000 Dec;**96**(6): 1011–1013.

106 **Hauer KE, Chou CL, Souza KH, Henry D, Loeser H, Burke C, et al.** Impact of an in-person versus web-based practice standardized patient examination on student performance on a subsequent high-stakes standardized patient examination. Teach Learn Med 2009 Oct;**21**(4):284–290.

107 **Boulet JR, McKinley DW, Whelan GP, van Zanten M, Hambleton RK.** Clinical skills deficiencies among first-year residents: utility of the ECFMG clinical skills assessment. Acad Med 2002 Oct;**77**(10 Suppl):S33–S35.

108 **Cadieux G, Abrahamowicz M, Dauphinee D, Tamblyn R.** Are physicians with better clinical skills on licensing examinations less likely to prescribe antibiotics for viral respiratory infections in ambulatory care settings? Med Care 2011 Feb;**49**(2):156–165.

109 **Tamblyn R, Abrahamowicz M, Dauphinee D, Wenghofer E, Jacques A, Klass D, et al.** Physician scores on a national clinical skills examination as predictors of complaints to medical regulatory authorities. JAMA 2007 Sep 5;**298**(9):993–1001.

110 **Schwartz A, Weiner SJ, Binns-Calvey A.** Comparing announced with unannounced standardized patients in performance assessment. Jt Comm J Qual Patient Saf 2013 Feb;**39**(2):83–88.

111 **McGaghie WC, Siddall VJ, Mazmanian PE, Myers J.** Lessons for continuing medical education from simulation research in undergraduate and graduate medical education. Chest 2009 Mar;**135**(3 Suppl):62S–8S.

112 **Errichetti AM, Gimpel JR, Boulet JR.** State of the art in standardized patient programs: a survey of osteopathic medical schools. J Am Osteopath Assoc 2002 Nov;**102**(11):627–631.

113 **Larsen DP, Butler AC, Lawson AL, Roediger HL, III.** The importance of seeing the patient: test-enhanced learning with standardized patients and written tests improves clinical application of knowledge. Adv Health Sci Educ Theory Pract 2013 Aug;**18**(3):409–425.

114 **Cohen AG, Kitai E, David SB, Ziv A.** Standardized patient-based simulation training as a tool to improve the management of chronic disease. Simul Healthc 2014 Feb;**9**(1):40–47.

115 Murdoch NL, Bottorff JL, McCullough D. Simulation education approaches to enhance collaborative healthcare: a best practices review. Int J Nurs Educ Scholarsh 2013;10.

116 Shatzer JH, Wardrop JL, Williams RG, Hatch TF. Generalizability of performance on different-station-length standardized patient cases. Teach Learn Med 1994;6(1):54–58.

117 Swanson DB, Norcini JJ. Factors influencing reproducibility of tests using standardized patients. Teach Learn Med 1989;1(3):158–166.

118 Norman GR, van der Vleuten CP, De Graaff E. Pitfalls in the pursuit of objectivity: issues of validity, efficiency and acceptability. Med Educ 1991 Mar;25(2):119–126.

119 Boulet JR, Gimpel JR, Dowling DJ, Finley M. Assessing the ability of medical students to perform osteopathic manipulative treatment techniques. J Am Osteopath Assoc 2004 May;104(5):203–211.

120 Berkenstadt H, Ziv A, Gafni N, Sidi A. Incorporating simulation-based objective structured clinical examination into the Israeli National Board Examination in Anesthesiology. Anesth Analg 2006 Mar;102(3):853–858.

121 Rathmell JP, Lien C, Harman A. Objective structured clinical examination and board certification in anesthesiology. Anesthesiology 2014 Jan;120(1):4–6.

122 Nestel D, Kneebone R, Black S. Simulated patients and the development of procedural and operative skills. Med Teach 2006 Jun;28(4):390–391.

123 Kneebone RL, Kidd J, Nestel D, Barnet A, Lo B, King R, et al. Blurring the boundaries: scenario-based simulation in a clinical setting. Med Educ 2005 Jun;39(6):580–587.

124 McKenzie FD, Hubbard TW, Ullian JA, Garcia HM, Castelino RJ, Gliva GA. Medical student evaluation using augmented standardized patients: preliminary results. Stud Health Technol Inform 2006;119:379–384.

125 Boulet JR, Murray D, Kras J, Woodhouse J, McAllister J, Ziv A. Reliability and validity of a simulation-based acute care skills assessment for medical students and residents. Anesthesiology 2003 Dec;99(6):1270–1280.

126 Murray D, Boulet J, Ziv A, Woodhouse J, Kras J, McAllister J. An acute care skills evaluation for graduating medical students: a pilot study using clinical simulation. Med Educ 2002 Sep;36(9):833–841.

127 Devitt JH, Rapanos T, Kurrek M, Cohen MM, Shaw M. The anesthetic record: accuracy and completeness. Can J Anaesth 1999 Feb;46(2):122–128.

128 Devitt JH, Kurrek MM, Cohen MM, Fish K, Fish P, Noel AG, et al. Testing internal consistency and construct validity during evaluation of performance in a patient simulator. Anesth Analg 1998 Jun;86(6):1160–1164.

129 Devitt JH, Kurrek MM, Cohen MM, Cleave-Hogg D. The validity of performance assessments using simulation. Anesthesiology 2001 Jul;95(1):36–42.

130 Morgan PJ, Cleave-Hogg DM, Guest CB, Herold J. Validity and reliability of undergraduate performance assessments in an anesthesia simulator. Can J Anaesth 2001 Mar;48(3):225–233.

131 Pugh CM, Youngblood P. Development and validation of assessment measures for a newly developed physical examination simulator. J Am Med Inform Assoc 2002 Sep;9(5):448–460.

132 Cheng A, Auerbach M, Hunt EA, Chang TP, Pusic M, Nadkarni V, et al. Designing and conducting simulation-based research. Pediatrics 2014 Jun;133(6):1091–1101.

133 Salas E, Paige JT, Rosen MA. Creating new realities in healthcare: the status of simulation-based training as a patient safety improvement strategy. BMJ Qual Saf 2013 Jun;22(6):449–452.

134 Wind LA, van Dalen J, Muijtjens AM, Rethans JJ. Assessing simulated patients in an educational setting: the MaSP (Maastricht Assessment of Simulated Patients). Med Educ 2004 Jan;38(1):39–44.

135 van der Vleuten CP, Norman GR, De Graaff E. Pitfalls in the pursuit of objectivity: issues of reliability. Med Educ 1991 Mar;25(2):110–118.

136 **McBride ME, Waldrop WB, Fehr JJ, Boulet JR, Murray DJ.** Simulation in pediatrics: the reliability and validity of a multiscenario assessment. Pediatrics 2011 Jul 11.

137 **Boulet JR.** Generalizability theory: basics. In: Everitt BS, Howell DC, editors. Encyclopedia of statistics in behavioral science. Chichester: John Wiley & Sons, Ltd; 2005, 704–711.

138 **Donoghue A, Ventre K, Boulet J, Brett-Fleegler M, Nishisaki A, Overly F, et al.** Design, implementation, and psychometric analysis of a scoring instrument for simulated pediatric resuscitation: a report from the EXPRESS pediatric investigators. Simul Healthc 2011 Apr;**6**(2):71–77.

Chapter 15

Team-building exercises and simulation

Andrew Anderson

Overview

- Team building and the associated communication skills are now recognized as a vital element in healthcare training.
- Simulated environments are now being used widely to develop team skills and human factors training.
- The use of assessment tools and a move to competency measures provides potential for measuring outcomes of team and communication training.
- We can borrow techniques and training programmes from other industries such as aviation and use them for team building in medicine.
- The use of personality profiling can greatly enhance team building.
- By using icebreakers and non-medical-based team-building games, training can become fun and team building more effective.
- By integrating actors with high-fidelity simulators, very realistic scenarios can be generated to allow combined training in technical and team skills.

15.1 Background and team-building theories

15.1.1 Introduction to team-building theories

The advantages of simulators in enhancing the objectivity and efficiency of training are clear, and the increased emphasis placed on the ability to perform a task (rather than simply having knowledge of it) is now an accepted advantage of such systems. Anaesthesia was one of the first areas of medicine which embraced the use of simulator technology,[1] and a network of high-fidelity simulator centres has been developed in the United Kingdom since 1997. There are now more than 80 such centres across the country and most offer team-building training courses. The higher the fidelity designed into the simulator, the more expensive they are and this remains a barrier to adoption of complex skills-based systems, but the use of simulation in all its forms for team training is now widespread across the United Kingdom.

There is now clear recognition that training healthcare professionals in human factors, including situation awareness, team performance, and communication skills, reduces errors and increases patient safety. The UK Department of Health document 'A Framework for Technology Enhanced Learning'[2] states:

> High environmental and equipment fidelity (sometimes known as full immersion simulation) can be used to explore the influence of human factors in health and social care practice, by examining the impact of the environment, equipment and other system processes on individual and team performance. This aspect of using simulation can be linked to learning important lessons from serious patient harm events, which have been reported nationally. It can also be used to evaluate proposed changes in systems or processes of care within local or wider healthcare organisations.

There is also a recognition that training courses need to deliver outcomes and demonstrate value. In addition, the move from a time-based to competency-based curriculum has driven a need for improved assessment techniques. It has also shifted the measurement of competence from being based on purely technical skills to a more rounded assessment based on specified areas of good medical practice (GMP). In the UK, the GMP Guidance[3] identifies the skills necessary for working with colleagues (see Box 15.1).

Making the assumption that assessment drives learning, interest in the use of simulators for assessment has grown in recent years as their capability has increased and the relative cost of obtaining some of the higher-fidelity systems has fallen. If simulation is to take its proper place in medical training it needs to embrace two things—a broader, more relevant applicability to curriculum and assessment criteria that provide better measures of the effects of simulated training. Team-building training (TBT) offers a potential application

---

Box 15.1 UK guidance for good medical practice—working with colleagues

- respect the skills and contributions of your colleagues
- communicate effectively with colleagues within and outside the team
- make sure that your patients and colleagues understand your role and responsibilities in the team, and who is responsible for each aspect of patient care
- participate in regular reviews and audit of the standards and performance of the team, taking steps to remedy any deficiencies
- support colleagues who have problems with performance, conduct, or health

Source: data from General Medical Council (GMC), 2015, *Good Medical Practice*, http://www.gmc-uk.org/guidance/index.asp, accessed 1 March 2015.

that fulfils both requirements and could enable training and simulation centres the opportunity to widen their appeal to all areas of healthcare.

A team can be defined as:

> a small number of people with complementary skills who are committed to a common purpose, performance goals, and approach for which they are mutually accountable.[4]

Team building can be defined as: a planned effort made in order to improve communications and working relationships by managed change involving a group of people. Team building is most effective when used as a part of a curriculum strategy that identifies the types of teams and their interactions with patients. Simulation has a major role to play in effective team building by offering the opportunity to analyse and practise team skills in realistic patient-based environments and to improve patient care as a result. This chapter explores the reasons why team building is important and offers suggestions about how simulation can be used as a platform for change in the way we train and manage teamworking in healthcare. Good teamwork involves the sharing of ideas, mutual respect, accountability, responsibility, and a clear direction towards a common goal.

By necessity, teamwork requires individuals to manage themselves as well as others and to solve problems together. Teamwork is the sum of all the non-technical skills described in this section, but it **begins with individuals managing themselves** while appreciating that they are part of something bigger.

15.1.2 **Measurement of outcomes**

Before embarking on any training initiative, it is imperative that those attending the courses are going to benefit from them and there is some measure of positive behavioural change. The Foundation programme in the United Kingdom is a two-year general training programme which forms the bridge between medical school and specialist/general practice training. It is pioneering the measurement of competence by using a range of assessment instruments to provide objective measures of skills, knowledge, and attitudes. Early data suggests the most useful of these tools is multi-source feedback (MSF)—a means of assessment based on collated questionnaires that ask co-workers to rate skills and attitudes of colleagues, including communication and teamworking (see Box 15.2). Tools such as case-based discussion (CBD) and direct observation of procedural skills (DOPS) may suggest areas of communication or teamwork where performance is below standards. By conducting these assessments before and after training, some measure of effectiveness can be demonstrated. Team performance is reduced when members fail to share unique information with other members of the team. Stasser[5] showed that team members who have some common and unique information tend to spend time discussing the common information and fail to share enough of the unique information, and therefore make poor decisions. Real-world studies of high-level political decisions and airline crashes demonstrate that groups make poor decisions when members fail to speak assertively. Blum et al.[6] showed that anaesthesiology faculty or residents participating in one-day training programmes in a simulated operating suite did not share vital clinical

---

Box 15.2 Working with colleagues—peer-review factors

- ◆ verbal communications with colleagues
- ◆ written communications with colleagues
- ◆ ability to recognize and value the contribution of others
- ◆ accessibility/reliability
- ◆ leadership skills
- ◆ management skills

---

information due to a variety of factors. Individual team members were given 'probes' or pieces of specific, potentially important information for patient management, and how and when these probes were shared were observed. This study offers another example of the importance of effective communication in medicine and a way of highlighting them in a simulated setting.

15.1.3 Why team building is important and types of teams

West et al.[7] examined the relationship between the people-management practices in hospitals and patient mortality and found the higher percentage of staff working in teams, the lower the patient mortality. On average, in hospitals where more than 60% of staff worked in formal teams, mortality was around 5% lower than expected. Two major studies found that adverse events caused by poor medical management and miscommunication occurred in 2.9% and 3.7% of patients, respectively.[8]

The same report made several notable recommendations that training institutions should adopt with regard to medical education—the main one being for them to: 'Establish interdisciplinary team training programmes, such as simulation, that incorporate proven methods of team management.'

There are many types of teams found within the healthcare environment. These include:

- ◆ primary healthcare teams
- ◆ secondary healthcare teams
- ◆ emergency teams
- ◆ management teams
- ◆ clinical teams
- ◆ operating room teams

For the purpose of planning team training using simulated environments, teams can be divided into two categories—semi-permanent teams, such as clinical firms and operating theatre teams, and ad hoc teams, such as those dealing with emergencies or cardiac arrests. For permanent teams who have to work together on a regular basis, the One Minute

Manager series offers an insight into successful techniques used in large corporations. The One Minute Manager Builds High-Performing Teams[9] has several useful techniques and insights that can be applied to medical training. These include:

◆ the stages of team development—orientation, dissatisfaction, production, and integration

◆ things to observe in teams—participation, decision-making, conflict, problem-solving, etc.

◆ leadership styles—validating, collaborating, resolving, and structuring

For those situations where healthcare workers come together to deal with short-term situations, the requirements for effective team performance (see section 15.1.5) are even more relevant. The aviation industry has managed to build selection and training programmes that allow flight crew members who have never met to perform effectively, eliminating barriers to communication such as status, personality clashes, and hidden agendas. Simulation is critical in providing effective training for pilots and so medical training should copy this paradigm.

15.1.4 **What makes an effective team?**

The basic requirements for a team to be effective are:

Communication and negotiation: team members need the ability to state ideas or questions clearly, listen to others attentively, and to resolve disagreements in a non-confrontational manner. This is a skill that many students may lack.

Analytic and creative skills: team members need to evaluate information and propose creative solutions. Many students have these skills, but may not be able to effectively communicate their views or concerns.

Organization: the team needs to be able to track and complete all of its tasks on time. Tensions can often arise if deadlines are missed.

For a team to function effectively there must be a clarity of purpose for what the team will achieve and the interpersonal relationships of the team must not be hampered by hidden agendas or personality clashes. Members must have a chance to contribute, learn from, and work with others. In medicine, a team can often be made up of members who have never met and the importance of leadership, clear roles, and absence of conflict are even greater in these situations. Simulated exercises are extremely useful in throwing together multidisciplinary groups and observing how they interact.

Team members have a responsibility to become involved in the working of the team and should:

◆ contribute ideas and solutions

◆ recognize and respect differences in others

◆ value the ideas and contributions of others

◆ listen and share information

◆ ask questions and get clarification

◆ care about the team and the outcomes

15.1.5 **Understanding personality types and team dynamics**

Multidisciplinary teamworking has become an in-vogue approach over recent years. The use of simulation to put teams together in semi-realistic situations and film there inter-actions for formative assessment has been one of the major factors in the increased adop-tion of simulated patient systems worldwide. Anecdotal evidence suggests that the success of these courses in making teams more effective is limited. This could be due to two fac-tors: (i) status issues (hierarchical gradients) and clashes between healthcare professionals, especially between doctors and nurses; and (ii) the lack of understanding of personality types and their impact on human interactions.

Only by focusing on the clinical outcomes can we overcome the inherent status issues exacerbated by the differences in medical and nurse training. The use of psychometric profiles such as Myers Briggs® or Belbin® has become more widespread in healthcare but their use in analysing team dynamics is limited. Dr Belbin's work at Henley Management College demonstrated that balanced teams comprising people with different capabilities performed better than teams that are less well balanced.

A simple and easy source of information about how team members will interact is the DISC approach. Dr John Geier brought the DISC system into practical application with substantive research and while this isn't a full 'personality test' in the strict technical sense, it provides an insight into an individual style that is more than adequate to predict the likely trends of their behaviour in the future and, in particular, in team-building situations. It has a major advantage in that it can be completed quickly and can be interpreted easily. The system evaluates four key factors in an individual style, rather than the 16 or more that are often seen in full personality tests (for example, DISC makes no attempt to measure such factors as intelligence).

The tests classify four aspects of personality by testing a person's preferences in word associations. DISC is an acronym for:

♦ **Dominance**: relating to control, power, and assertiveness

♦ **Influence**: relating to social situations and communication

♦ **Steadiness**: relating to patience, persistence, and thoughtfulness

♦ **Compliance** (or conscientiousness or caution): relating to structure and organization

These four dimensions can be grouped in a grid with D and I sharing the top row and representing extroverted aspects of the personality, and C and S below representing intro-verted aspects. D and C then share the left column and represent task-focused aspects, and I and S share the right column and represent social aspects (see Figure 15.1).

	Task Focused	Social Focused
Extrovert	Dominance	Influence
Introvert	Conscientious	Steadiness

Fig. 15.1 DISC-factor relationships

◆ **Dominance**: people who score high in the intensity of the D styles factor are very active in dealing with problems and challenges, while low D scores are people who want to do more research before committing to a decision. High D people are described as demanding, forceful, egocentric, strong willed, driving, determined, ambitious, aggressive, and pioneering. Low D scores describe those who are conservative, low-keyed, cooperative, calculating, undemanding, cautious, mild, agreeable, modest, and peaceful.

◆ **Influence**: people with high I scores influence others through talking and activity and tend to be emotional. They are described as convincing, magnetic, political, enthusiastic, persuasive, warm, demonstrative, trusting, and optimistic. Those with low I scores influence more by data and facts, and not with feelings. They are described as reflective, factual, calculating, sceptical, logical, suspicious, matter of fact, pessimistic, and critical.

◆ **Steadiness**: people with high S styles scores want a steady pace, security, and don't like sudden change. Low S intensity scores are those who like change and variety. High S persons are calm, relaxed, patient, possessive, predictable, deliberate, stable, consistent, and tend to be unemotional and poker-faced. People with low S scores are described as restless, demonstrative, impatient, eager, or even impulsive.

◆ **Conscientious**: persons with high C styles adhere to rules, regulations, and structure. They like to do quality work and do it right the first time. High C people are careful, cautious, exacting, neat, systematic, diplomatic, accurate, and tactful. Those with low C scores challenge the rules and want independence and are described as self-willed, stubborn, opinionated, unsystematic, arbitrary, and careless with details.

Prior to building teams or training a group of people who have never worked together before, it is very helpful for the trainer, but even more important for the team members, to understand their personality types and how they will feel when interacting with other types. For example, a high D personality can find a high S person frustrating because they make slow decisions. The high S or high C personalities are not generally assertive and can, therefore, not contribute what could be vital information to the team if they feel dominated.

The effectiveness of multiprofessional training is greatly enhanced if participants have a basic understanding of their own personality and other types and how each type reacts to others. This also helps break down some of the hierarchal barriers that exist between, for example, doctors and nurses. I would recommend the use of such analysis in any team-building scenario.

15.2 **Practical aspects**

15.2.1 **Running a team-building day**

As for all training, the key to success is in the planning. In preparation, trainers should:

◆ Practise the team-building exercise yourself first to check that it works, check timings, materials, and to ensure you have all the answers. Anticipation and planning are vital.

Box 15.3 Outline of a team-building day

- Objectives: personal and for the day
- Icebreaking exercises
- Team-building games/scenarios
- Discussion on what the team needs to achieve
- Simulated exercises
- Review and de-brief

- Make sure all team-building games instructions are clear and complete—essential for keeping control and credibility.
- Become proficient yourself first with any team-building games or equipment that you use.

For the day itself, an outline plan is shown in Box 15.3. Given time, you can bring many of the techniques described above to make the day more effective including:

1 Distribute Post It™ notes and ask each attendee to write one thing they wish to achieve from the training. Use these notes to review what was achieved at the end of the course.

2 Use icebreaking exercises to open discussion and team dynamics (see below).

3 Either in advance or on the day, conduct psychometric profiles to facilitate understanding of how team members interact.

4 Once these dynamics are understood, review the purpose of the team and what makes teams effective. Ask delegates to engage with each other and expose any hidden agendas or status issues.

5 Utilize video and verbal feedback from the simulator sessions to explore team and communication issues.

15.2.2 Exercises for opening communication and breaking down barriers

15.2.2.1 Interactive team games[10]

If you have time, examples of more interactive exercises that generate a lot of communication and feedback are as follows.

15.2.2.2 Skills knowledge and attitudes exercise

First, using a flip chart, brainstorm with the team their ideas of great managers and leaders—can be real and fictional—famous, celebrity, local business personalities—whatever. Allow a few minutes to collect a selection of names. Tack this sheet to the wall. Then ask the team to call out what they think are the attributes most associated with the various names on the list, that make them good at what they do. In any order, doesn't matter. Write these attributes on the flip chart. Then ask one of the more dominant delegates to come to the front and circle all the 'skills' on the sheet, with the help of the team, and the facilitator if necessary. There will be hardly any. Next ask a quiet team member to come to the front and circle all the 'attitudes' on the sheet. It will be most of them.

The point for discussion is that while a certain **skill** level is necessary to do a job, the fact is that **attitude** determines whether the job is done well, and whether the job holder makes a real difference to their organization, colleagues, and environment. People commonly believe that skills are the most important attributes and the biggest training priorities. Often they are not. Usually, lifting beliefs and changing attitudes have a far greater impact on individual performance and organizational effectiveness. This simple exercise helps to explain the differences between skills and attitude, and why attitude is so much more important than skill. The activity is for groups of any size, although you can split large groups into smaller teams with appointed team leaders to run the exercise in syndicates, and then review the different teams' findings afterwards as a whole group.

15.2.2.3 Personal goal-setting exercise[10]

The exercise is then to ask the team members to think about one aspect of their own personal character (how many is up to the facilitator) that they would like to develop, change, or improve. For example, this might be to develop greater confidence; to manage their time better; to deal with stress more effectively; to be more creative; to be more accurate; to finish tasks on time; to take more exercise; to spend more time with their children; to achieve a qualification; or anything about themselves and their lives, at home or work, that it is reasonable to want to change. Depending on the group, you can give extra guidance as to particular areas to focus on or avoid. Be mindful of the group's comfort zone and keep within it in terms of the personal nature of weaknesses and sensitivities that you expect people to think about, and if appropriate, to divulge to others. If you wish to ask the team members to think of more than one aspect for change, you can guide them to select different types of change; for example, one for work and one for home; or one for now, one for the next month, and one for the next three months. Use your imagination and refine your instructions to fit the situation. Bear in mind that certain changes that people seek to make will contain more than one element, which is relevant to the next stage of the exercise.

When people have thought and decided on their aspect(s) for change, you can ask them to discuss their ideas and feelings in pairs, so as to validate, confirm, and reassess their thoughts. Alternatively, you can ask people to keep their thoughts to themselves. It depends on the group as to whether you make the exercise 'open' or 'secret'. Next, ask the team members to translate each desired change into a **specific positive statement**, which (in keeping with the technique), should be in the **present tense**. If a desired personal change contains more than one behaviour then it can help to break it down into two or more statements. Broadly, the more ambitious and complex the desired change then the more likely it will need breaking down into separate statements, which could be different behaviours or steps.

The facilitator should decide and agree with the delegates whether they wish to share their aims and statements with others. It is helpful to share, because people can then work in pairs to give and receive feedback as to the changes and positive statements which represent the changes desired. There are various ways to review the exercise, the process, feelings, and the outputs, and various ways to agree follow-up actions and commitments if appropriate, all of which depend on the group and the situation, and especially the wishes of the individuals involved. This activity can be varied to suit the situation. It is a simple and yet potent exercise to encourage and help team members to think about and hopefully commit to personal change and development, especially if linked to a commitment to take action after the exercise. The exercise will also encourage self-analysis and goal-setting.

15.2.2.4 Mnemonic exercise[10]

This is a simple and very flexible activity to help a team of people (or children) to learn and remember key facts and information—about anything, and certainly relating to the particular theme or subject of the team meeting or training session. The exercise is based on the method of memorizing through association. Examples of mnemonics using association are:

- Richard Of York Gave Battle In Vain (the initial letters match those of the colours of the rainbow, Red Orange Yellow Green Blue Indigo Violet)
- Every Armpit Does Get Body Odour Eventually (Notes of the strings on a guitar)
- SWALK (Sealed With A Loving Kiss)
- The word 'stalagmites' contains an 'M' for mountain (which points up, as opposed to stalactites, which point down)
- The word 'stationery' (relating to paper) contains an 'er', as does 'paper' (as opposed to the word stationary = 'not moving')
- Numbers can be remembered by association with similarly shaped images, for example: 1 = wand, 2 = swan, 3 = flying bird, 4 = yacht, 5 = hook, 6 = elephant (trunk), 7 = cliff, 8 = spectacles, 9 = balloon on a stick, 0 = beach ball, 10 = stick and a hoop. There are many other alternatives. This memory method enables long numbers to be remembered by creating a story linking the respective images.

The exercise itself is simply to ask team members, individually or in pairs, to create their own mnemonic for a given piece of important information, facts, or figures. The information could be related to the theme of the meeting or not, depending on the situation. Examples of types of information that are useful to support with mnemonics are: a process, a theory or model, a formula, technical data, product range, codes and numbers, procedures and policies, document references, etc. Mnemonics should then be presented back to the group and discussed as to their effectiveness. Sharing ideas for memorizing key data helps teams on a number of levels: it improves retention of the particular subject matter used in the exercise; it teaches people how to improve their memory, and it gets people working together in creative way. There is also always the likelihood that some particularly good ideas will come out of the exercise, which can then be conveyed and used to reinforce key information across the wider organization.

15.2.2.5 Life raft scenario[10]

The scenario is that the team is stranded in a life raft which is too small to hold everyone without sinking. Someone (or you could say two or three people—it's flexible) must to be thrown overboard (or eaten, if you prefer the really macabre version)—the group must decide who is/are to be the unfortunate victim(s). First, delegates have the opportunity to present their reasons why they should stay (the facilitator can decide what media is to be used, but watch out for the time—this part needs to be reasonably brief). Delegates can be directed either to base their presentations on their own real selves, or if a less emotive approach is required, to adopt the personality of a character from history, or a TV soap, etc. The facilitator must decide how best to instruct the team on this aspect. After presenting their own cases, the group then debates people's relative values and strengths. Within this debate individuals can continue to argue their own cases if they wish, after which the group makes its decision. Set a time limit for each presentation, the debate, and the decision; for example, two minutes per presentation; 20–30 minutes for the debate; and five minutes for the decision or vote. The facilitator can guide the group as to the decision method; for example, secret ballot, show of hands, or preferably to leave the group to decide the decision process, as this highlights other interesting behaviours and capabilities within the team. This is also an interesting exercise to use in group selection recruitment as an interaction game:

1 decide on who you are—yourself or another personality

2 list qualities about why you should not be thrown overboard

3 one minute for each person to make their case

4 debate each one

5 five minutes to decide voting method (can be secret or open)

6 vote

7 discussion

Points to review if used in other than a group-selection context:

◆ Quality and effect of individual presentations.

◆ How individuals behave and respond to threat and possible rejection.

◆ How different personality types within the group react in different ways to the debating and decision process.

◆ How the group organized itself to manage the difficult discussion process.

◆ The different perceptions among the team of relative strengths, weaknesses, values, etc.

◆ The way the group decided on how to make the decision (unless told how by the facilitator).

◆ The reaction of the team members and colleagues of the victim(s) after the vote—balance between relief and sympathy.

For more ideas and a wealth or business-related ideas about team building I would recommend the following websites:

+ <http://humanresources.about.com/od/icebreakers/>
+ <http://www.businessballs.com/>

15.2.3 Audience engagement and management

Attending simulation centres and associated training programmes can be a stressful exercise for participants. The effectiveness of any team-building exercise can be greatly enhanced by laying some ground rules at the outset. This includes making it clear that teamwork is the focus of the simulated exercise and the participants should not focus on the fidelity of the simulator or situational reality. The use of low-cost simulation, including the use of simulated patients or simple low-fidelity mannequins, can bring team training 'alive' providing the participants accept this is the objective and not to create the real world in detail.

The engagement of a clinical audience in simulation can sometimes be a challenge. The educator can improve engagement by:

+ Telling relevant stories around the situation to be practised.
+ Use of humour allied to personal experience.
+ Patient involvement, either via video or in person.
+ Avoiding lengthy, boring slide presentations.
+ Allowing open feedback from participants to other participants.
+ Applying professional de-briefing techniques.
+ Use of relevant but extreme examples of teamwork breakdown (e.g. Teneriffe Air Disaster).
+ Discussion around serious incidents within the participant institution.

Another issue to be considered is that of 'Generation Y' students. A systematic review[11] confirms the rapid dissemination of technology in the formative years of 'Generation Y' students, with the purported consequence that this group thinks and processes information differently. Consequentially, it is claimed that 'Generation Y' has a relationship with technology that is intuitive and spontaneous. Blended courses, in one comparative study of student nurses,[12] has also been reported as being more effective than traditional formats, finding that students that participated in a blended-learning course received higher grades than those who participated in the same course using traditional delivery.

The use of other technologies to enhance learning (e.g. e-learning and mobile learning via apps) and 'Just in Time' exercises can support the classroom-based education programme and if integrated into a programme can ensure engagement of the Generation Y individual. Use of tablet computers or other digital media within the simulation can also help to create realism and dynamism but technology must never be allowed to get in the way of the training objective—improving human interactions and performance.

15.3 **Conclusion**

The techniques of team-building and communication training are vital to improving patient care and safety. The use of realistic exercises based around new simulator technologies and in controlled environments offers the simulation community the chance to educate a wide variety of healthcare professionals in the benefits of simulated training. By using assessment instruments and follow-up skills evaluation, the investment made in simulation technologies can be justified by demonstrating observable improvements in patient safety.

References

1 **Galvin R**. Simulation and anaesthetic training: a personal viewpoint. Bulletin of the Royal College of Anaesthetists 2006;**35**:1746–1748.

2 A Framework for Technology Enhanced Learning DOH Online 2011: <https://www.gov.uk/government/uploads/system/uploads/attachment_data/file/215316/dh_131061.pdf>

3 General Medical Council (GMC), Good Medical Practice, 2015: <http://www.gmc-uk.org/guidance/index.asp>

4 **Katzenbach JR, Smith DK**. The wisdom of teams: creating the high-performance organization; 1993.

5 **Stasser G**. Pooling of unshared information during group discussion. In: Worchel S, Wood W, Simpson JA, eds. Group process and productivity. Newbury Park, CA: Sage, 1992:48–67.

6 **Blum RH, et al.** A method for measuring the effectiveness of simulation-based team training for improving communication skills. Anesthesia & Analgesia 2005;**100**(5):1375.

7 **West MA, et al.** The link between management of employees and patient mortality in acute hospitals. International Journal of Human Resource Management 2002;**13**(8):1299–1310.

8 Quoted in Institute of Medicine. To err is human: building a safer health system. Washington, DC: National Academy Press; 2000.

9 **Blanchard, Carew and Carew**. The One-Minute Manager Builds High-Performing Teams. Harper Collins; 2004.

10 **Chapman A**. From the free resources website <http://www.businessballs.com>. Not to be sold or published. Alan Chapman accepts no liability for any issues arising; 1995–2006.

11 Preferred teaching and learning approaches of students considered 'Generation Y' in health professions pre registration education: a comprehensive systematic review protocol. In: The JBI Database of Systematic Reviews and Implementation Reports, ISSN 2202–4433, available at <http://www.joannabriggslibrary.org/index.php/jbisrir/article/view/986/1228>

12 **Lancaster J, Wong A, Roberts S**. 'Tech' versus 'talk': a comparison study of two different lecture styles within a Master of Science nurse practitioner course. Nurse Education Today 2012;**32**(5):e14–18.

Chapter 16

Teaching and learning in simulation using the problem-based approach

Russell W Jones

Overview

- Problem-based learning (PBL) is an ideal educational approach to achieve many desirable educational objectives (or outcomes) within simulation in healthcare.

- PBL and simulation seek to equip learners with the ability to solve problems far beyond those encountered within any specific learning experience.

- Most definitions of PBL have four common elements: (i) learning objectives are translated into a problem; (ii) successful solutions require an explanation, with possible diagnosis and treatment; (iii) learners use small group discussions to analyse and understand the problem and potential solutions; and (iv) questions or issues that are not answered within small group discussion form the basis for further learning outside the group.

- The many advantages of PBL include a focus on 'real-life' core information, fostering valuable transferable skills such as leadership, teamwork, communication and problem-solving, encouraging a deep approach to learning, and making curriculum content relevant to healthcare problems.

- PBL provides novice learners with experiences that allow them to develop a memory of a broad range of known cases. It is known that experts draw on their own library of familiar cases from their own experience. Therefore, by deliberately providing novices with a library of cases, PBL allows novices to approach a healthcare problem using a similar strategy to that used by experts.

- Although extremely valuable for teaching many educational objectives (or outcomes), PBL is not the optimal method for teaching all simulation sessions.

- PBL scenarios should be developed by specifying the desired educational objectives to be achieved by the scenario, developing one or more triggers to achieve these objectives, and then writing discussion questions to focus learning relevant to each trigger.

Overview *(continued)*

◆ When multiple triggers are used within the same PBL scenario, they should follow chronologically with each trigger adding information to gradually enhance the detail of the scenario.

◆ Multidisciplinary teams including clinicians and professional educators allow input from a variety of different perspectives and are therefore ideal for developing optimal scenarios.

◆ In order to ensure healthcare professionals appreciate they may encounter the same or similar problems in practice, wherever possible PBL scenarios should be based on de-identified real patients, or composites of real patients.

◆ The facilitatory ability of the teacher is the single greatest factor that influences the success of PBL.

◆ Optimal PBL can only occur if facilitators are well trained in how to facilitate PBL.

16.1 Introduction to teaching and learning in simulation using the problem-based approach

Problem-based learning (PBL) extends the learner far beyond merely providing an opportunity to solve problems. Rather, PBL makes problem-solving the main reason for learning. Herein lies the power of PBL because the learner is required to solve specific problems while acquiring knowledge on how to solve similar problems.[1] PBL originated within educational initiatives more than 50 years ago. Unlike many educational initiatives that have risen and fallen over time, PBL has grown in popularity and expanded to cover an extremely broad range of curricula, including all healthcare professions. PBL was initially developed and applied within a medical education context at McMaster University in Canada by Howard Burrows.[2, 3] The perceived value and popularity of PBL among teachers and learners in healthcare professions has grown to such an extent that at least some component of PBL is currently incorporated into most courses in Western healthcare training. These include professions as varied as surgery, anaesthesia, intensive care, pain medicine, nursing, retrieval medicine, speech pathology, pharmacy, paramedicine, and medical administration. Theoretical advances in behavioural psychology were used by several researchers[4] to successfully argue that people who commence learning by focusing on problems prior to attempting to understand underlying principles had equal or greater educational success than people using a traditional approach whereby underlying principles were presented first and then applied to a specific problem.

16.2 Simulation and PBL

The value of PBL parallels the value of simulation in that both seek to equip learners with the ability to solve problems far beyond those encountered within a specific learning experience. Considering the variety and flexibility of real problems that arise within the broad spectrum of healthcare, it may be argued that it is this ability which becomes of greatest benefit to healthcare professional within their professional life.[5] Simulation within healthcare, by its very nature, is replete with excellent opportunities for the effective use of PBL. When applied appropriately PBL is an invaluable aid to teaching specific simulation-related objectives and for learners to achieve specific simulation-related outcomes. Importantly, whereas PBL is an invaluable asset for those involved in simulation instructional design, PBL is not the optimal method for teaching all simulation activities. Rather, PBL is most suited to teach those objectives best taught when their learning commences with a problem, query, or question that learners need to solve.[6] When this occurs consequences include an increase in the ability of the learner with regard to self-directed learning and problem-solving,[7] as well as increased clinical competency and self-efficacy.[8] Learners have also been shown to favourably view the integration of simulation and PBL.[9]

Whereas a universally accepted definition of PBL has yet to be agreed among health educators,[10] when PBL is applied to simulation in healthcare most definitions have four common elements (see Box 16.1).

The remarkable ability of the human mind to learn from a single problem, encountered in a particular context and at a specific time and place, and then to transfer and apply some or all of the knowledge, skills, and abilities learned to similar problems or analogous contexts or comparable places or related times makes every aspect of a skilfully prepared and taught PBL session an incredibly rich learning opportunity. Few approaches to teaching offer such a high ratio of potentially positive learning from a single teaching event. A key to unlocking the many benefits of PBL is the research that revealed experts within healthcare (or, indeed, within any discipline) have a substantial reservoir of experiences. Within simulation these experiences form a library of real experiences with which the expert is familiar. Research has revealed that experts compare novel scenarios to their library of real scenarios.[11] When applied to reasoning within healthcare it is known this ability occurs naturally within experts, yet novices need to learn this ability. In part, this is because novices lack an extensive library of real experiences. One of the many benefits of

---

Box 16.1 Elements of PBL

1 Learning objectives are translated into a problem.

2 Successful solutions require an explanation, with possible diagnosis and treatment options.

3 Learners use small group discussions to analyse and understand the problem and potential solutions.

4 Questions or issues that are not answered within small group discussion form the basis for further learning outside the group.

Box 16.2 Advantages of PBL

- Making curriculum content relevant by building learning around clinical, community, or scientific problems.

- Focusing learning on core information relevant to real scenarios and reducing information overload.

- Fostering the development of valuable transferable skills useful throughout life-long learning. These include leadership, teamwork, and communication as well as problem-solving.

- Facilitating healthcare professionals to become responsible for their own learning. This is an essential skill for all professionals actively engaged in their own continuing development.

- Increased motivation of healthcare professionals to learn by focusing the learning on 'real-life' scenarios.

- Encouraging a deep, rather than surface, approach to learning by forcing learners to interact with information on multiple levels and to a greater depth than traditional teaching approaches.

- Using a constructional approach to learning whereby learners construct new learning around their existing understanding.

PBL is that it rapidly builds up the library of experiences available to the novice. Therefore, within simulation a scenario is typically used to provide an example from which a learner may extrapolate and apply in later experience. Thus, PBL offers the opportunity to provide healthcare professionals with learning experiences that will be of use throughout their professional life.[1]

16.3 Value of PBL to simulation

Researchers have consistently argued for the benefits of PBL since it was first conceived throughout its history to the present day.[3, 12–14] The popularity of PBL, as well as its rapid widespread adoption by the healthcare community, has arisen from several powerful advantages. Many of these advantages are particularly pertinent to simulation in healthcare and should be optimally exploited by simulation course designers[15] (see Box 16.2).

16.4 PBL, interprofessional learning, and critical thinking

Unlike many educational innovations, PBL has kept pace with contemporary educational needs. To this end, PBL has been embraced by health educators seeking a suitable technique by which to teach new content including both interprofessional learning and critical thinking. Recent years have seen increasing awareness about the value of interprofessional understanding and learning within healthcare teams. Largely pioneered among teams of healthcare professionals working within the operating theatre (where positive and negative outcomes were increasingly obvious with regard to the extent of positive or negative patient outcomes), the development of educational activities that facilitate enhanced interprofessional team performance has gradually spread from the surgical, anaesthetic, and theatre nursing teams to all other clinical and many administrative teams. PBL is well placed to facilitate increased knowledge, skills, and abilities within the individuals who comprise interprofessional teams. Indeed, research has shown the benefits of PBL in creating positive interprofessional learning outcomes include enhanced interpersonal cooperation compared with traditional educational programmes.[16] By virtue of its group approach to learning, PBL is able to facilitate interprofessional learning because it provides numerous opportunities to learn about other professions and members of these professions, to learn from other members of interprofessional teams, and to learn together with interprofessional colleagues.[12]

Another ability that has received considerable attention within health education in recent years is critical thinking. Once again, research has shown the ability of PBL to keep pace with evolving healthcare education and PBL has been found to foster the ability of learners to develop critical thinking.[13, 17, 18] Specifically, PBL enhances information processing, critical appraisal, cognitive questioning, thought clarification, and communication, all of which are essential for effective critical thinking.[19, 20]

16.5 **Difficulties of using PBL within simulation**

Optimal educational outcomes and objectives are best achieved when these are matched to their ideal teaching and learning strategies. In this regard, no single strategy is perfect for achieving the educational goals for all educational situations. Therefore, despite the significant advantages described above, those responsible for teaching and learning should be aware of several significant disadvantages within PBL[15] (see Box 16.3).

Simulation course designers should be aware of the above potential problems when considering the use of PBL for all or part of a simulation-based learning experience. Designers should carefully consider how to mitigate or eliminate any negative impact on learning.

Box 16.3 **Disadvantages of PBL**

+ Teaching faculty being required to facilitate learning rather than to directly impart their knowledge. This may be considered inefficient and, possibly, demotivating to faculty.

+ Knowledge acquired through PBL being less organized than knowledge acquired through traditional learning.

+ The difficulty of training facilitators and the scarcity of teaching faculty with the skills of facilitating rather than the skills of traditional teaching.

Box 16.3 Disadvantages of PBL *(continued)*

- The time required of healthcare professionals to fully engage in PBL. This can be particularly problematic for the typically crowded simulation curriculum where time-poor faculty and learners are asked to teach and learn under significant time pressures.

- The replacement of the traditional teacher role by the facilitator which may make it difficult for learners using PBL to emulate good traditional teachers as role models. However, learners will be better able to emulate good facilitators.

- Additional disadvantages include the significant costs, resources, and time required to train effective facilitators. PBL experts also point to concerns about the costs of implementing PBL programmes, though note that other researchers argue that PBL is not necessarily more expensive than traditional educational approaches[21] and raise the issue of PBL not necessarily covering all areas within a healthcare topic.[15]

16.6 **PBL scenario structure**

Simulation course designers are encouraged to develop their own scenarios and to contribute to the growing worldwide pool of available PBL-based scenarios. The flexibility of PBL is considerable allowing course designers to tailor the scenarios they develop to match the specific needs of those healthcare professionals who form the clientele of their simulation centre. As simulation has grown in popularity, so the number of available scenarios has also grown. Existing PBL scenarios can be used if they match desired educational outcomes, or available scenarios may be modified and adapted as appropriate. Of course, if a scenario is used as part of summative assessment (i.e. used for the purposes of assigning a grade, score, mark, or pass/fail result) then the scenario should not be altered. This is because such a scenario will have been validated for the purposes of summative assessment and any alteration will reduce this validity. The ethos of the simulation community is collegial to the extent that most simulation centres are willing to share their scenarios. Scenario developers who are new to PBL typically find it easier to modify and apply existing scenarios in the teaching environment before attempting to develop and apply their own.

The following scenarios demonstrate the breadth of healthcare that can be successfully taught and learned using a well-crafted PBL scenario. The first scenario has a focus on paediatric febrile convulsion from the perspective of a nurse working within an emergency department. The second has a focus on a difficult delivery and post-partum haemorrhage from the perspective of an aeromedical retrieval doctor.

16.6.1 **Paediatrics, a case of febrile convulsion**

An essential initial step when developing PBL scenarios is to carefully specify the desired educational objectives (or outcomes) to be achieved by the scenario.

16.6.1.1 Objectives

On completion of this PBL, learners should be able to[22]:

+ Describe appropriate management by childcare workers and ambulance paramedics when encountering a child experiencing febrile convulsions.

+ Explain methods for eliciting key information from childcare workers and parents.

+ Comprehend common causes of febrile convulsions and associated pathophysiology.

+ Describe the diagnosis and treatment of febrile convulsions.

+ Show an appreciation of the need for parents to understand diagnoses and treatment of their children.

+ Specify discharge information and resources to be provided to parents prior to patient discharge.

+ Explain the role of the general practitioner or family physician in ensuring appropriate ongoing care.

Once the intended learning outcomes that are to be achieved from the PBL session have been specified, scenario developers should incorporate trigger scenarios designed to fulfil these outcomes. One or more triggers can then be selected by course facilitators for use with a particular group of healthcare professionals.

16.6.1.1.1 Trigger A (pre hospital) Isobel is a 22-month-old toddler with no significant past medical history other than several viruses experienced with increasing frequency since she commenced childcare. She has achieved all normal developmental milestones. Her vaccinations are up to date. Both parents work. Her mother works part time and father full time. Grandparents care her for one day a week at home and she is cared for two days per week in the local childcare facility.

Isobel had an unsettled night and her parents assumed she was teething. They gave her an oral analgesia. She had a low-grade fever (37.9) which resolved following analgesia. She woke early and although slightly sluggish appeared to be fine and her parents sent her to childcare. While at childcare she became irritable.

Within ten minutes, Isobel had a period in which the childcare worker observed her becoming unresponsive, hot to touch, and she commenced a short period of convulsing. An ambulance was called and Isobel was taken to the local emergency department with one of the childcare workers. Her parents were called and her father met the ambulance at the hospital.

Each trigger should be associated with related discussion questions which offer the PBL session facilitator discussion tools to focus PBL learning by the healthcare professionals participating in the session. The following discussion questions were written for the above trigger.

16.6.1.1.2 Discussion questions A

1 What should have been the immediate actions taken by the childcare centre?

2 What appropriate methods could be used to obtain information from both the childcare worker and/or the child (e.g. the paediatric assessment triangle)?

3 What do you think should be the immediate management of Isobel by the ambulance paramedics?

4 What are the common causes of febrile convulsions and associated pathophysiology?

5 Are pharmacological interventions appropriate? If so, discuss.

6 Are non-pharmacological interventions appropriate? If so, discuss.

Ideally, a series of successive triggers should each chronologically build on preceding triggers. Continuing with this paediatric example, the following triggers build on the scenario initially created by the first trigger. Each successive trigger should add further information to the scenario, which gradually increases in detail (and possibly complexity) via successive triggers. Note also how the discussion questions are specifically designed to achieve the PBL objectives specified at the beginning of the scenario.

16.6.1.1.3 **Trigger B (emergency)** You are a nurse working in the emergency department and you perform an initial assessment. The observations for Isobel are:

- weight 14 kg
- temperature 38.3°C
- blood pressure 88/53 mmHg
- heart rate 118 beats per min
- respiration rate 30 breaths per min
- oxygen saturation 98%
- capillary refill <2 seconds
- widespread erythematous rash

16.6.1.1.4 **Discussion questions B**

1 What are your priorities on presentation of Isobel with her father?

2 In what triage category do you think this patient is and why?

3 What are your thoughts on the immediate clinical management of Isobel?

4 How would you involve other healthcare workers in Isobel's treatment?

5 How would you discuss the cause of Isobel's presentation with her father?

6 Why is it important for Isobel's father to understand the findings from the primary assessment?

7 Often, there is a difference between the level of concern exhibited by clinicians for patients with febrile convulsions and that of parents. How could this be better accommodated?

16.6.1.1.5 **Trigger C (advanced care)** Isobel is moved to the observation ward with a plan to discharge in four hours if she remains well. She has been given paracetamol (150 mg) in the emergency department. Approximately three hours later, Isobel has another period of being unresponsive and becomes rigid for approximately 70 seconds. This occurs while her father is getting coffee and her mother, who has recently arrived at the hospital, is sitting quietly with her.

16.6.1.1.6 Discussion questions C

1 What is the immediate clinical management of Isobel?

2 What issues need to be considered in relation to family-centred care?

3 Does this second convulsion warrant further investigations?

4 If so, what investigations and why?

16.6.1.1.7 **Trigger D (discharge)** Isobel was admitted into the short-stay unit. She has been stable without any further indication of febrile convulsion. She has had a low-grade fever overnight which responded well to six-hourly paracetamol and eight-hourly ibuprofen. The plan is for Isobel to be discharged this morning without any further follow-up.

16.6.1.1.8 Discussion questions D

1 What discharge information do you provide to the parents?

2 Are there any resources available for the parents with a focus on febrile convulsions?

3 What advice about symptom management do the parents require?

4 Do you think Isobel requires further follow-up post discharge?

5 How would you convey this to the parents?

6 What is the role of the family GP in ongoing care for Isobel?

16.6.2 Retrieval medicine, shoulder dystocia, and post-partum haemorrhage

16.6.2.1 Objectives

On completion of this PBL, learners should be able to[23]:

♦ Gain an appreciation of the aloneness of a retrieval doctor.

♦ Demonstrate optimal use of available resources.

♦ Recognize and treat shoulder dystocia.

♦ Apply the neonatal resuscitation algorithm.

♦ Demonstrate management of post-partum haemorrhage.

♦ Describe management of haemodynamic shock in a patient with no vascular access.

♦ Demonstrate effective management of invasive monitoring lines.

♦ Prioritize patients for aeromedical retrieval.

16.6.2.1.1 **Trigger A (presentation)** You are the day doctor who has been tasked to retrieve a 31-year-old G6P5 woman from a remote coastal town 350 km from any major teaching hospital. Her last examination conducted by the nurse on site (not a trained midwife) was ten minutes ago and she was fully dilated with membranes intact and head engaged.

She had a complicated obstetric history with gestational diabetes and uncontrolled blood sugars despite exercise, diet, and insulin. Her salbutamol infusion was commenced on presentation but despite this being at full maximal rate, she continues to have moderate contractions.

You accompany the aircraft with the intention of conducting aeromedical retrieval. You arrive at the town's landing strip and are met by a volunteer ambulance officer who tells you 'the patient's waters have just broken'. The ambulance officer drives you to a nursing post where you examine the patient. You notice a head emerging and a slight turtle-necking of the infant and no further emergence. The infant is currently pink but no crying is observed. A foetal Doppler just before head emergence showed moderate foetal tachycardia with a foetal heart rate of 175 beats per minute and you notice meconium-stained liquor oozing.

16.6.2.1.2 Discussion questions A
1 What is your diagnosis?
2 How do you facilitate delivery of the infant?
3 Explain your treatment. What is the rationale for each stage of treatment?

16.6.2.1.3 Trigger B (delivery)
An infant girl is delivered. You observe no crying from her and you notice her colour is changing to blue. You apply the neonatal resuscitation algorithm. The infant's heart rate suddenly drops to 52 beats per minute despite cpap application via T-Piece.

16.6.2.1.4 Discussion questions B
1 Describe the neonatal resuscitation algorithm.
2 Once the foetal heart rate drops, what further measures should you take?

16.6.2.1.5 Trigger C (the mother)
The infant pinks up in response to your measures and starts crying. Given the emergency appears to be over, you determine it appropriate to allow the mother to have contact with the infant. When you turn to the mother she appears pale and is barely rousable. You check airway; appears unblocked and functional. You check breathing; 20 breaths per minute and shallow. You check circulation; heart rate is 120 beats per minute, blood pressure 70/30. You attempt vascular access twice and fail both times. You proceed to intraosseous access. You check for active signs of bleeding and find a large pool of blood in the bed under the sheets.

16.6.2.1.6 Discussion questions C
1 In broad terms, what are the anatomical and physiological differences between the neonate/infant and adult patients?
2 What is your management of post-partum haemorrhage in the mother?
3 How do you manage haemodynamic shock in a patient with no vascular access?
4 What is the availability of blood products for aeromedical retrieval and what are the relevant massive transfusion protocols?

5 Are there any implications for the newborn baby girl?

6 How would you prepare mother and daughter for transport?

7 If transport of only one patient is possible, which patient would you prioritize? Why?

16.7 **Developing PBL scenarios**

The choice of PBL scenario is second only to the value of the instructor in determining the effectiveness of PBL as a learning experience. Fortunately, simulation centres are replete with resources and should be staffed with educators and clinicians with a combined wealth of educational and clinical knowledge. By including professional educators plus a multi-disciplinary team of clinicians within the scenario development process, scenarios will be sound from both an educational and clinical perspective. The experience of these personnel combined with the wealth of resources available within a clinical simulator means the number of potential scenarios approaches the infinite. Carefully structured problems ensure learners comprehensively cover appropriate knowledge, skills, and abilities relevant to the desired educational objectives. Ideally, a simulation course designer should use a PBL approach if the problem scenario exhibits several characteristics[24] (see Box 16.4).

Wherever possible, PBL scenarios should be based on real patients, or composites of real patients, in order to ensure healthcare professionals appreciate that they may encounter the same or similar problems in practice. Fortunately, such scenarios are reasonably easy to create within the healthcare simulation environment. Furthermore, the use of de-identified actual patients allows the designers of PBL scenarios to incorporate de-identified laboratory results, X-rays, scans, and pathological materials.[25] When choosing

---

Box 16.4 **Characteristics of an ideal scenario for PBL**

1 Address one or more learning outcomes relevant to the healthcare professionals to be taught in the simulation course.

2 Facilitate healthcare learners to raise their prior learning and experience to conscious consideration and to build on existing knowledge.

3 Be consistent with the stage of learning at which the healthcare professionals are located.

4 Motivate learners and, ideally, be related to the current or future practice of healthcare professionals.

5 Provide an overall clinical context in which new knowledge is placed.

6 Stimulate thought and discussion, provide guidance, and encourage healthcare professionals to actively seek solutions.

7 Phrase an open-ended problem to facilitate discussion and explanation (i.e. closed problems with limited scope should be avoided).

a scenario, designers should consider what topic area experts believe should be taught relevant to the intended learning objectives as well as the prevalence, severity, magnitude, treatability, and intervention effectiveness.[25] Once a scenario has been developed it should be piloted with an audience of healthcare professionals representative of the intended simulation clients for whom the scenario has been developed.

16.8 Facilitating PBL

Even more important than the use of optimal PBL scenarios is the quality of the PBL teacher.[13, 26] The single greatest factor that influences the success of a PBL programme is the facilitatory skill, knowledge, and ability of the teacher. Such is the importance of facilitation that, within PBL, the teacher is usually referred to as the 'facilitator'. Adequate facilitator training and experience is essential for any PBL session to function optimally.[1, 13, 25–27] Because PBL is a non-traditional approach that differs significantly from traditional teaching, those potential instructors who have been taught using traditional teaching methodology will be unfamiliar with how PBL should be taught. Therefore, of the pool of potential instructors available to a simulation centre it is likely that few will be familiar with a true PBL approach and even fewer will be able to facilitate PBL sessions without additional training and experience. If PBL is used in simulation then it is essential that those instructors who will undertake the facilitation of PBL sessions receive adequate and appropriate training in facilitation.

In true PBL, the facilitator does not direct learning, dominate conversation, or provide direct answers to questions (unless this is necessary for the preservation and progress of the scenario). Instead, the facilitator becomes a learning guide who assists learners to develop their own reasoning and hypothesizing while concomitantly allowing learners to evaluate these hypotheses and assess their own knowledge, skills, and abilities.[1, 27] The facilitator achieves this by continually monitoring and stimulating the PBL process and interpersonal dynamics of the group. Key tools for the facilitator are the phrasing of open questions, guiding of feedback, managing group dynamics, challenging learners' knowledge and understanding, and raising pertinent facts or issues in a timely manner.

Facilitator competence must include[15] the facilitation of small-group learning; a comprehensive understanding of the PBL programme such that the facilitator can relate immediate and future learning opportunities to the PBL scenario and guide healthcare professionals to these opportunities; and a global understanding of the overall educational curriculum so that the facilitator can place discrete problems within the global educational experiences of the learners. The abilities of facilitators to establish effective two-way communication with learners, empathy, and an open and trusting atmosphere have also been shown to be important.[28] Effective use of PBL within healthcare simulation will best occur if instructors who are not experienced in any of the above are provided with the necessary instruction and experience prior to their involvement as a PBL facilitator in simulation. Once this experience has been gained each facilitator should be fully briefed about the problem and related learning[29] as well as the relationship of the problem and intended learning to the scenario.

Research has shown that content area experts may endanger PBL by exerting too great a director role and reducing the effectiveness of collaborative learning[30] as well as directly answering learners questions, devoting greater amounts of time to the development of learning issues than learners devote to solving them, and by talking 'too often and too long'.[31] However, it is likely that a content area expert, who has been correctly taught in the procedures and nature of PBL, should be able to successfully facilitate a PBL session while resisting reverting to a traditional mode of teaching. Such a facilitator would be ideally placed to be able to limit the extent to which they provide solutions to learners, consistent with a PBL approach, yet able to provide the minimal level of clinical structure necessary for learners to obtain optimal benefit from PBL.[32] However, whereas the extent to which a facilitator is required to be a content expert is a matter of some debate within the literature, all PBL specialists agree that adequate training in the role of facilitator is essential for the success of a PBL programme.

References

1 **Jones RW**. Problem-based learning: description, advantages, disadvantages, scenarios and facilitation. Anaesthesia and Intensive Care 2006;**34**:485–488.

2 **Barrows HS, Tamblyn RM**. An evaluation of problem-based learning in small groups utilising a simulated patient. Journal of Medical Education 1976;**51**:52–54.

3 **Neufeld VR, Barrows HS**. The 'McMaster philosophy': an approach to medical education. Journal of Medical Education 1974;**49**:1040–1050.

4 **Foord M**. Inductive versus deductive methods of teaching area by programmed instruction. Educational Review 1964;**16**:130–136.

5 **Jones RW**. Problem-based learning for simulation in healthcare. In: Riley (ed.). A manual of simulation in healthcare. Oxford: Oxford University Press; 2008.

6 **Charlin B, Mann K, Hansen P**. The many faces of problem-based learning: a framework for understanding and comparison. Medical Teacher 1998;**20**:323–330.

7 **Lee WS, Cho KC, Yang SH, Roh YS, Lee GY**. Effects of problem-based learning combined with simulation on the basic competency of nursing students. Journal of Korean Academy of Fundamentals of Nursing 2009;**16**:64–72.

8 **Liaw SY, Chen FG, Klainin P, Brammer J, O'Brien A, Samarasekera D**. Developing clinical competency in crisis event management: an integrated simulation problem-based learning activity. Advances in Health Sciences Education 20101;**5**:403–413.

9 **Roh YS, Kim SS, Kim SH**. Effects of an integrated problem-based learning and simulation course for nursing students. Nursing and Health Sciences 2014;**16**:91–96.

10 **Taylor D, Miflin B**. Problem-based learning: where are we now? Medical Teacher 2008;**30**:742–763.

11 **Bordage G, Lemieux M**. Semantic structures and diagnostic thinking of experts and novices. Academic Medicine 1991;**66**:S70–72.

12 **Dahlgren LO**. Interprofessional and problem-based learning: a marriage made in heaven? Journal of Interprofessional Care 2009;**23**:448–454.

13 **Martyn J, Terwijn R, Kek M, Huijser H**. Exploring the relationships between teaching, approaches to learning and critical thinking in a problem-based learning foundation nursing course. Nurse Education Today 2014;**34**:829–835.

14 Galveo TF, Siva MT, Neiva CS, Ribeiro LM, Pereira MG. Problem-based learning in pharmaceutical education: a systematic review and meta-analysis. The Scientific World Journal 2014; 1–7, article ID 578382 <http://dx.doi.org/10.1155/2014/578382>.

15 Davis MH, Harden RM. AMEE medical education guide no. 15: problem-based learning: a practical guide. Medical Teacher 1999;**21**:130–140.

16 Faresjo T, Wilhelmsson M, Pelling S, Dahlgren LO, Hammar M. Does interprofessional education jeopardise medical skills? Journal of Interprofessional Care 2007;**21**:573–576.

17 Kek MYCA, Huijser H. The power of problem-based learning in developing critical thinking skills: preparing students for tomorrow's digital futures in today's classrooms. Higher Education Research and Development 2011;**30**:329–341.

18 Kong LN, Qin B, Zhou YQ, Mou SY, Gao MH. The effectiveness of problem-based learning on development of nursing students' critical thinking: a systematic review and meta-analysis. International Journal of Nursing Studies 2014;**51**:458–469.

19 Moore J. An exploration of lecturer as facilitator within the context of problem-based learning. Nurse Education Today 2009;**29**:150–156.

20 Kassab S, Abu-Hijleh MF. Student-led tutorials in problem-based learning: educational outcomes and students' perceptions. Medical Teacher 2005;**27**:521–526.

21 Sefton AJ. From a traditional to a problem-based curriculum: estimating staff time and resources. Education for Health 1997;**10**:165–178.

22 O'Brien R, Mould J. A case of febrile convulsion. Edith Cowan University Health Simulation Centre, Perth; 2014.

23 Buck C, Jones RW. Retrieval medicine scenario: shoulder dystocia and post-partum haemorrhage. Royal Flying Doctor Service, Perth; 2014.

24 Dolmans D, Snellen-Balendong H, Wolfhagen I, van der Vleuten C. Seven principles of effective case design for a problem-based curriculum. Medical Teacher 1997;**19**:185–189.

25 Barrows HS. Problem-based learning applied to medical education. Southern Illinois University School of Medicine, Springfield, IL; 2000.

26 Hmelo-Silver CE. Problem-based learning: what and how do students learn? Educational Psychology Review 2004;**16**:235–266.

27 Barrows HS, Tamblyn RM. Problem based learning: an approach to medical education. New York, NY: Springer; 1980.

28 Schmidt HG, Moust JH. What makes a tutor effective? A structural-equations modelling approach to learning in problem based curricula. Academic Medicine 1995;**70**:708–714.

29 Eagle CJ, Harasym PH, Mandin H. Effects of tutors with case expertise on problem-based learning issues. Academic Medicine 1992;**67**:465–469.

30 Silver M, Wilkerson LA. Effects of tutors with subject expertise on the problem-based tutorial. Academic Medicine 1991;**66**:298–300.

31 Crosby J. Learning in small groups. Medical Teacher 1997;**19**:189–202.

32 Davis WK, Nairn R, Paine ME, Anderson RM, Oh MS. Effects of expert and non-expert facilitators on the small group process and on student performance. Academic Medicine 1992;**67**:470–474.

Chapter 17

Patient safety and simulation

Christine L Mai, Rebecca D Minehart,
and Jeffrey B Cooper

Overview

♦ The initiation of the patient safety movement in the 1970s has evolved over many decades to become a well-established healthcare discipline, which has dramatically changed the practice of medicine.

♦ Accidents are not unidimensional, but are the result of a series of unique interactions which combine to result in injury, as illustrated by the Swiss cheese model.

♦ Utilized extensively in other high-risk organizations, simulation has been applied to healthcare in order to address issues of teamwork development, competency assessment, and evaluation of new processes and technologies.

♦ Simulation may be used to promote a culture of patient safety, to reduce human errors, and reduce risks to patients by allowing a safe environment in which learners of all types can practise and expand their skills.

17.1 Introduction to patient safety and simulation

Patient safety is now a well-established discipline that has permeated almost all aspects of healthcare. The prevention of harm resulting from system failures and human error has become a strong focus for healthcare around the world. Making healthcare safer requires a broad spectrum of tactics and actions. Many different forms of simulation can be applied with the aim of preventing errors and improving systems and thus reducing the numbers of healthcare-related preventable deaths and injuries. In this chapter, we give an overview of the development of patient safety and describe the myriad ways that simulation can be used in service of the goal of reducing harm. In fact, simulation can be seen as having its fundamental purpose in patient safety, although it clearly has at least equal importance in the overall field of healthcare education and training. Since the concept, technologies, and various educational applications of simulation are addressed in other chapters in this book, we will not cover those topics except where there are specialized issues in patient safety that are not covered elsewhere.

17.2 **History of patient safety in healthcare**

Patient safety is a healthcare discipline that emphasizes the reporting, analysis, and prevention of medical errors that can potentially lead to adverse events. The central tenant of the Hippocratic Oath pledges *'primum non nocere'* ('first do no harm'), and emphasizes the obligation to beneficences, namely providing safe patient care.[1] However, despite focus on the scientific basis of medical practice and the best intentions to provide patients with the safest care, errors and adverse events occur on a regular basis. The frequency and magnitude of avoidable patient adverse outcomes was not well known until the 1990s when reports from the United States and Europe revealed a staggering number of patients who were harmed, died directly, or died in part by errors in the course of healthcare.

Anaesthesiology is widely credited with having been the first healthcare specialty to target the avoidance of preventable harm. The motivation was based on research published as early as 1978 into the causes of medical error.[2] Substantial increases in malpractice costs and media attention in 1982 contributed to a call for action. Under the leadership of Dr Ellison C. Pierce Jr, the President of the American Society of Anesthesiologists (ASA) in 1984, the Anesthesia Patient Safety Foundation was established in 1985, which was committed to preventing harm from anaesthesia.[3, 4]

In 1999, the Institute of Medicine (IOM) released a widely cited report: 'To Err Is Human: Building a Safer Health System'. The report estimated that 44,000–98,000 deaths occur in the United States annually due to medical errors in hospitals.[5] The IOM report estimated the cost of preventable errors at $US38–50 billion annually. The alarming statistics, which have since been shown to be an underestimate,[6] raised awareness of the substantial impact of medical errors, which were the sixth leading cause of death. The IOM report made many recommendations to attack the problem of harm from healthcare; it was a loud call to action on many fronts.

It is now widely recognized that the complexity of healthcare systems in industrialized countries contributes to the patient-safety challenge. The lack of inherent safety systems and programmes arose from the history of the development of medicine, where practitioners generally work independently in 'silos'. Stressors such as limited manpower, production pressure, lack of communication, and cognitive errors all contribute to breakdowns in quality care and patient safety.

'To Err Is Human' not only focused on physicians and hospitals, but also covered the full scope of healthcare delivery. The report sent a powerful message that the industry was not acceptably safe, and that most errors were preventable or that better systems, training, and other actions could ameliorate the impact of errors that will continue to occur despite the best efforts made. Furthermore, the report pointed out human factors, the lack of teamwork, and the lack of a culture of safety as overarching components that resulted in adverse events (see Table 17.1). The two main recommendations the report made were,

Table 17.1 Causes of healthcare errors

Factors	Examples
1) Human factors	◆ Variation in healthcare provider training and experience ◆ Cognitive errors ◆ Fatigue ◆ Depression ◆ Burnout ◆ Diverse patients ◆ Time pressure ◆ Production pressure
2) Medical complexity	◆ Advance medical technology ◆ Multiple medications ◆ Unfamiliar medical locations ◆ Intensive care medicine
3) System failures	◆ Lack of communication ◆ Unclear delineation of authority ◆ Lack of manpower ◆ Poor hand-off (handover) system ◆ Medications that look alike, sound alike ◆ Reliance on automated systems to prevent error ◆ Equipment failure ◆ Disconnected medical error reporting systems in hospital ◆ Infrastructure failure

first, to 'make patient safety a priority corporate objective', and second, to 'create a learning environment'.[5]

The IOM report catalysed a national and international movement to fundamentally change healthcare systems and practices to raise priorities for the overall delivery of safest care. Today, there are quality-improvement and safety initiatives in all medical subspecialties and most care settings; more in some than others.

17.3 **Defining patient safety and quality of care**

Quality in healthcare can be viewed as an overarching umbrella under which patient safety is a principle discipline. The IOM defined quality of care as 'the degree to which health services for individuals and populations increase the likelihood of desired health outcomes and are consistent with current professional knowledge'.[5] The concepts of patient safety, quality improvement, and risk management are related but have important distinctions (see Table 17.2). One important difference is that quality is measured in terms of success in achieving desired outcomes, whereas safety is measured in failure, particularly catastrophic oversights. Risk management is directed at managing the aftermath of adverse outcomes, especially managing legal issues, malpractice, and avoidance of financial loss for insurers.[9] In today's healthcare system, risk management focuses on proactive patient-safety initiatives to prevent injuries via medical error reduction and quality improvement in order to decrease adverse events from which malpractice arises.

Table 17.2 Key terminology commonly used to discuss quality and patient safety

Patient safety	The avoidance, prevention, and amelioration of adverse outcomes or injuries stemming from the processes of healthcare. Safety emerges from the interactions among components in a system rather than due to the actions of one person, device, or department. Patient safety is a subset of healthcare quality.[7]
Quality improvement	The process used by individuals and organizations to assure that goals are met through a system of constant scrutiny, measurement, review, and revision.[8]
Risk management	The clinical and administrative activities undertaken to identify, evaluate, and reduce the risk or injury to patients, staff, and visitors.[9]
Quality of care	The extent to which health services for individuals and populations increase the likelihood of desired health outcomes and are consistent with current professional knowledge.[10]
Patient-centred care	Qualities of compassion, empathy, open communication, and responsiveness to patients' needs or preferences.[11]
Adverse event	An injury caused by medical management that results in measurable disability.[12]
Accident	An unplanned, unexpected, and undesired event that leads to an adverse result.[13]
Error	A planned sequence of mental or physical activities fails to achieve its intended outcome. These failures cannot be attributed to the intervention of some chance agency.[14]
Near miss	An event or situation that could have resulted in an accident, injury, or illness but did not, either by chance or thoroughly timely intervention.[12]

Source: data from Cooper, JB and Longnecker, DE, 'Safety and quality: the guiding principles of patient-centered care', in D.E. Longnecker, D.L. Brown, M.F. Newman, and W.M. Zapol, eds., *Anesthesiology*, 2nd edn (China: McGraw Hill Companies, Inc., 2012) p. 16.

17.4 **Understanding failures in the healthcare system**

There is a tendency, in and out of the healthcare system, to assign blame to specific individuals for lapse in performance associated with adverse events. Yet, there is evidence to demonstrate that most medical errors or accidents are the result of complex events for which there is no single cause.[16] Accidents are not unidimensional; rather, they are the result of a series of unique interactions which combine to result in injury. 'The Swiss cheese' model[14] (see Figure 17.1) illustrates that accidents are typically the result of a series of interactions that include precursors known as **latent errors**. These exist in the work environment and have the potential to initiate or propagate an accident.[14] Examples include selection of low-quality supplies, failure to maintain equipment or replace obsolete equipment, and scheduling that promotes haste or fatigue. When the chain of events converges symmetrically as to allow the holes of the 'Swiss cheese' to align, these interactions can result in the final adverse event. This concept is now widely accepted in understanding the failures in the healthcare system.

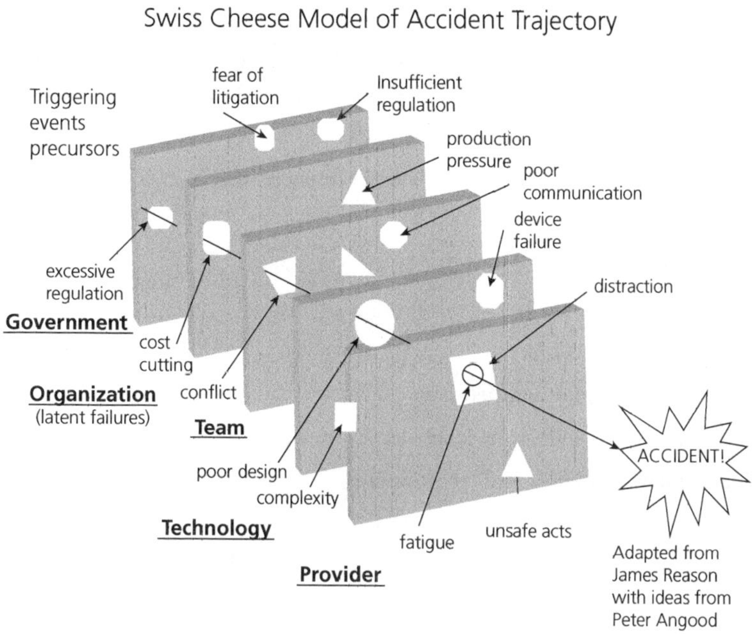

Fig. 17.1 Swiss cheese model of accident evolution.
Adapted from J. Reason, *Human Error*, Figure 7.8, p. 208, Cambridge, UK, Copyright © Cambridge University Press, 1990.

17.5 Simulation-based training in healthcare

Based on the recommendations set forth in 'To Err Is Human', leaders of the healthcare industry looked toward other complex, high-risk industries such as aviation to address their shortcomings. In order to address issues of teamwork development, competency assessment, and evaluation of new processes and technologies, the aviation industry has for years utilized techniques of simulation to train and educate their professionals. Even before the IOM report, simulation was beginning to be used for some patient safety-directed applications, especially in anaesthesiology. As illustrated throughout this book, simulation has a broad array of techniques, technologies, and applications. We now focus on how those applications can be applied to patient-safety problems.

17.6 Simulation applications for patient-safety problems

There are many different ways to catalogue patient-safety issues. Box 17.1 is a set of issues for which simulation applications can be a part of the overall solution. Each is explained in the following sections.

17.6.1 Creating a patient-safety culture

Establishing a culture of safety is one of the most important yet elusive aspects of ensuring safe healthcare. There are different definitions for culture but a common, simple one is 'the

> ## Box 17.1 Patient-safety issues for which simulation is part of the solution set
>
> ◆ Creating a patient-safety culture
> ◆ Education and training in basic skills without exposing patients to risk
> ◆ Training to prevent errors
> ◆ Training to recover from error (CRM)
> ◆ Training for teamwork
> ◆ Improving cognitive skills
> ◆ Assessing clinicians for competency
> ◆ Training and practice in large-scale disaster response
> ◆ Evaluating new processes and technologies
> ◆ Research in human factors
> ◆ Training non-clinicians in patient safety and teamwork

way we do things around here'.[17] Safety culture cannot be measured, but many surveys have been developed to measure safety attitudes, which are best referred to as 'safety climate'. Much has been written about culture in general and specifically in healthcare. Yet, relatively little is said about the role of simulation in creating a safety culture. There are several studies of how simulation has been successful or unsuccessful in improving safety climate.[18] But, doing so is exceptionally challenging because attitudes do not generally change quickly and are not likely to change from the single, team training or similar simulation intervention that is common in most settings. Rather, we expect that the routine use of simulation, as in other high-risk industries, has a positive influence on safety climate by virtue of sending a message that training for emergencies and routinely practising for teamwork are 'the way we do things around here'.

17.6.2 Education and training in basic skills without exposing patients to risk

Medical training has a long history of being an apprenticeship model whereby novice trainees learn skills by practising on patients, under varying degrees of supervision.[19] Over the past decade or more, the practice of learning on patients, especially without adequate supervision, has become less acceptable. The challenge is, how can healthcare providers learn to develop critical medical, nursing, or other allied health professional skills? Simulation clearly provides the most effective possibility and is now increasingly being used in essentially all healthcare specialties and domains within each profession. The chapters in this book illustrate the wide variety of such applications.

Importantly, simulation has been used to replace traditional 'practising' learning skills on patients in a variety of situations, such as advanced airway techniques,[20] central line placement,[21] cardiac surgery,[22] basic surgical skills,[23] intravenous line placement,[24] sterile technique when accessing central venous lines,[25] and accurate blood pressure measurement.[26] In addition to skills attainment, simulation has been used to foster awareness of patient conditions and empathy (e.g. nursing students wearing ostomy bags with simulated faecal material).[27]

Simulation technology is still far from sufficiently realistic or representative of certain aspects of patient care to provide more than superficial training about diagnostic and therapeutic procedures. Furthermore, the economics of payment for education and training, and the reliance on the apprenticeship model do not provide for training of students via simulation (i.e. there are not good incentives for widespread use of simulation to replace practice on patients). Nevertheless, a recent study suggests that simulation can replace clinical exposure for nursing students without decrement in learning what is needed to be prepared to care for patients.[28] There are other challenges; e.g. how much practice is needed in simulation before a clinician is safe to care for patients for each procedure; how realistic must a simulation be to impart the necessary learning? For example, one recent study showed that when medical students underwent CPR training and actually performed chest compressions for full 2-minute cycles, rather than shortened cycles, they were better able to adhere to 2-minute cycles at 12 weeks as compared with controls (shortened cycles).[29]

17.6.3 **Training to prevent errors**

The complexities of the healthcare system create many opportunities for adverse events. While much of simulation training is often seen as generally for educational objectives, in fact, much of that training can incorporate specific and generic approaches to error prevention. Simply providing a safe environment for the student to make mistakes and repeat a procedure allows for training and practising without exposing patients to risk. But, there can be more specific applications, whereby increased opportunities for errors are introduced into the training. These can be distractions or miscues to provide the experience of some types of errors that should be experienced first in simulation to cement the learning (e.g. medication error or communication error). In addition, higher levels of environmental and emotional realism, such as full environment simulation, can create realistic levels of stress under which errors of omission and commission are more likely. This example of realism can introduce failures in interpersonal and team skills (e.g. failure to take a leadership role in a critical event or engage in clear communication).

Many interventions have been developed and introduced to reduce the likelihood of preventable medical errors. Checklists and cognitive aids of various kinds are good examples and, in several cases, have been shown to be effective in reducing harm.[30] Standardized hand-off tools are increasingly being developed to mitigate adverse outcomes related to the increasing numbers of transfer of responsibility in health, due in part to work-hour restrictions and increasing transfers between levels of healthcare facilities. Positive results have been demonstrated.[31, 32] Simulation is perhaps one of the best approaches to training individuals and teams in how to correctly implement emergency procedures and even how to use the various types of cognitive aids effectively. Simulation can also be used to evaluate the usability of any such tools before they are implemented (see section below).

17.6.4 **Training for teamwork**

In the 1980s, via the introduction of anaesthesia crisis resource management (ACRM) into anaesthesia training, Gaba adapted concepts from the aviation industry, such as systematic training, rehearsal, performance assessment, and teamwork.[33] Subsequently, a substantial body of literature demonstrated the value of teamwork for successful prevention of medical errors and management of critical situations.[34, 35] ACRM techniques are now widely applied in healthcare across many healthcare professions and specialties and are usually referred to as CRM. In fact, the original aviation term, crew resource management, is often used in generic teamwork training. Furthermore, there are variations of CRM in healthcare that do not necessarily use simulation to a great extent, if at all (e.g. TeamSTEPPS, which was derived from MedTeams).

The general principles of CRM are based on the observations that an effective team has mutual collegial respect, whereby the members share tasks, goals, and key information to enable all to do their job well. This applies in routine work, which aids in avoiding errors, and in managing critical situations (see next section). Some characteristics of effective high-performance teams include establishing clarity of leadership (which may vary depending on the situation), introduction of team members, closed-loop communication, 'read-back' of verbal orders, perioperative team briefing and debriefing, and the use of communication tools (i.e. SBAR: Situation, Background, Assessment, and Recommendation).[15, 36–38] Today, the importance of teamwork, communication, and resource management is emphasized in nearly all healthcare settings. CRM and other teamwork skills are now widely being taught via simulation.

17.6.5 **Training to manage critical events and recover from error**

Some of the earliest uses of modern mannequin simulators were for training in error recovery via the general methods of CRM. CRM principles emphasize generic skills for team behaviours that optimize the management of critical events, particularly in acute-care situations. CRM behaviours are a subset of general teamwork behaviours noted above. The emphasis is on establishing a clear leader when managing a critical event, communicating clearly (e.g. by stating the name of the person being requested to do something), effectively using resources, and using techniques to maintain situational awareness and avoid fixation errors. There is some evidence that simulation-based training in CRM does improve teamwork behaviours in managing critical events and even can improve outcomes.[39]

7.6.6 **Improving cognitive skills**

Diagnostic errors are increasingly becoming one of the most prevalent contributions to adverse outcomes; however, they are the most challenging to understand and remediate.[40–42] Many diagnostic errors are the result of cognitive lapses of various types. While there are no current established interventions to reduce the incidence and impact of diagnostic errors, simulation-based training and deliberate practice could be implemented to avoid fixations and heuristic-related failures that underlie these kinds of errors. Simulation has been used to teach concepts of metacognition to avoid cognitive errors.[43]

17.6.7 Assessing clinicians for competency

Simulation-based testing is just beginning to be used for some forms of high-stakes assessment. At least one centre in the United States offers assessment and remediation for anaesthesiologists who are referred to them.[44] In addition, simulation may be used to assess and retrain clinicians seeking re-entry into clinical practice.[45] There is evidence that simulation can be used to implement reliable and valid competency testing.[46, 47] There is movement toward competency-based curricula for which simulation can play an important role; however, there is much work to be done to establish reliability and validity of measures.[48] Simulation-based CRM training is a highly weighted option for anesthesiology recertification, although it does not include assessment of competency. Additional points toward the practice-improvement recertification requirement are given to the participant for proposing practice improvements based on the simulation learning and reporting on the success or failure of implementing those changes. Early evidence shows that this form of 'commitment to change' is effective in motivating practice improvements.[49]

17.6.8 Training and practice in large-scale disaster response

The use of simulation has been reported in high-risk industries (such as aviation and the military) to train for more coordinated large-scale disaster response. In healthcare, immersive environments such as Second Life, Advanced Disaster Management Simulator (ADMS), and Multi-User Virtual Environments (MUVE) have been used to teach disaster management using interactive virtual simulation systems.[50–52] Simulations involving large-scale burn disasters,[53] paediatric trauma disasters, and even wide-scale humanitarian crises have been implemented.[54, 55] For example, due to remote, rural areas in Sweden which are variably populated (sparsely in summer, heavily in winter for ski activities), the Swedish National Board of Health and Welfare determined a need for a national burn disaster management plan. Two simulations were held of a rapidly progressing indoor fire in a three-storey building involving 400 affected 'patients' drawn from a database; all 'patients' had unique sets of injuries which needed triaging and attention (ranging from uninjured to non-survivable injuries). Time to evacuate the final 'patient' was five hours in the second simulation, compared with seven hours in the first. In addition, a large number of latent risks were raised which led to further discussion and planning at a national level.[53]

17.6.9 Evaluating and introducing new processes and technologies

Simulation has great potential for evaluation of the safety and efficacy for training prior to introduction of new processes and to test novel technology and medical devices. Yet, it has so far been used only sporadically in healthcare. One of the foremost examples was the introduction of a novel percutaneous carotid stenting technology[56–58] for which simulation-based training was required for certification to use the device. Simulation has been used to assess new anaesthesia technology to identify potential errors before purchase and introduction into use.[59] For example, the introduction of *in situ* magnetic resonance imaging (MRI) in neurosurgery incorporated simulation to evaluate the safety of the process and to train for protecting against the dangers of having a strong magnetic field in the operating environment. At the national level, the US Food and Drug Administration (FDA) is encouraging the use of simulation as part of the process of evaluating new devices.[60] There is evidence that simulation can be used to evaluate ongoing healthcare processes that lead to preventable patient injuries and adverse events; for example, through the use of Failure Modes Effect Analysis.[61]

17.6.10 Research on human performance and human factors

One of the important actions needed to improve overall system safety in healthcare is an understanding of how humans work in their environments of care, and to design systems and technologies that are well suited to avoid errors.[62] Human factors is 'the scientific discipline concerned with the understanding of interactions among humans and other elements of a system, and the profession that applies theory, principles, data and methods to design in order to optimize human well-being and overall system performance'.[63] Simulation has effectively been used to study aspects of human factors in order to aid in the design of systems and technologies to train in prevention of errors. One example is research toward understanding why clinicians do or do not speak up in the presence of a safety hazard during clinical care.[64] The optimal way to learn about potential human-factors issues is to study new designs early in the design process. This can be done in many instances with realistic simulation.

17.6.11 Training non-clinicians in patient safety and teamwork

For patient safety to improve, there must be buy-in and commitment from organizational leaders, administrators, and middle managers about the severity of the issue and the need to allocate resources to solutions, including simulation-based solutions of the type described above. Further, there is good reason to believe that leaders, administrators, and managers must also have good teamwork behaviours in order for the teams in which they work to be safe and effective. For instance, they need to practise crisis-management skills to perform optimally in the types of crises that they experience. Simulation has been used for training these types of teams, both composed solely of non-clinicians or a mix of clinical and non-clinical team members.[65, 66] Simulations of patient-care situations can be created in which non-clinicians can experience the feeling of caring for a patient and being in an acute situation even if the participant has little or no patient-care training or experience. Such exercises can be used as a vehicle to discuss teamwork and leadership skills and to consider how the team can apply them to their normal, non-clinical job functions. From participating in such an exercise, these important organizational players can gain appreciation for patient-safety issues and also for the utility of simulation in helping to solve them.

17.6.12 **Applying simulation for patient safety**

While there are many applications of simulation to make healthcare safer, it is likely still much underutilized directly for this purpose. Most who use simulation likely do so from an education and training perspective rather than thinking in the context of patient safety; i.e. of reducing adverse outcomes. For the sake of reducing preventable harm, it would be wise for educators and leaders to better understand how simulation can be used for this objective. It is also wise for all involved in using simulation to help those who lead patient-safety efforts in healthcare organizations to learn the value of the techniques and technologies of simulation for meeting patient-safety objectives.

17.7 **Conclusions**

Simulation has a wide array of applications for improving patient safety. Perhaps every simulation leader and educator should think of his or her role as being a patient-safety advocate as well as his or her role in healthcare education. And, all who use simulation for educating and training their constituents should consider how simulation could be used more widely towards patient-safety improvement goals.

References

1 Raanan G. 'Primum non nocere' and the principle of non-maleficence. BMJ 1985;**291**:130–131.

2 Cooper JB, Newbower RS, Long CD, McPeek B. Preventable anesthesia mishaps: a study of human factors. Anesthesiology 1978;**49**:399–406.

3 The Anesthesia Patient Safety Foundation: 'The establishment of the APSF' (Pierce, EC, Jr), available at <http://www.apsf.org/about.php>

4 Foundation history, <http://www.apsf.org/about_history.php>, accessed 01 Sep. 2014.

5 Kohn LT, Corrigan JM, Donaldson MS, eds. To err is human—building a safer health system. Washington, DC: National Academies Press; 2000, 312.

6 Leape L. Institute of Medicine's error figures are not exaggerated. JAMA 2000;**284**(1):95–97.

7 Cooper JB, Gaba DM, Liang B, et al. Agenda for research and development in patient safety of the National Patient Safety Foundation. National Patient Safety Foundation, 2000: <http://www.npsf.org/r/npsfrd/>

8 Varkey P, Reller MK, Resar MK. Basics of quality improvement in health care. Mayo Clin Proc. 2007;**82**(6):735–739

9 Joint Commission Resources. Root cause analysis in health care. Chicago, IL. Joint Commission on Accreditation of Healthcare Organizations; 2003.

10 Lohr KNE. Medicare: a strategy for quality assurance. Washington, DC. National Academy Press; 1990.

11 Committee on Quality of Health Care in America. Crossing the quality chasm: a new health system for the 21st century. Washington, DC: National Academy Press; 2001.

12 Quality Interagency Coordination Task Force. Doing what counts for patient safety: federal actions to reduce medical errors and their impact. Washington, DC: Quality Interagency Coordination Task Force; 2000. Report No. 1–58763-000–1.

13 **Senders JW.** Medical devices, medical errors, and medical accidents. In: Bogner MS, ed. Human error in medicine. Hillsdale, NJ: Erlbaum; 1994, 166.

14 **Reason J.** Human error. Cambridge, UK: Cambridge University Press; 1990.

15 **Cooper JB, Longnecker DE.** Safety and quality: the guiding principles of patient-centered care: In: Longnecker DE, Brown DL, Newman MF, Zapol WM, eds. Anesthesiology, 2nd edn. China: McGraw Hill Companies, Inc.; 2012.

16 **Perrow C.** Normal accidents—living with high-risk technologies. New York, NY: Basic Books; 1984.

17 **Weick K, Sutcliffe KM.** Managing the unexpected. San Francisco, CA: Jossey-Bass.

18 **Cooper JB, Blum RH, Carroll JS, et al.** Differences in safety climate among hospital anesthesia departments and the effect of a realistic simulation-based training program. Anesth Analg 2008;**106**(2):574–584, table of contents.

19 **Gawande AA.** Education of a knife. Complications: a surgeon's notes on an imperfect science. New York, NY: Metropolitan Books; 2002, 11–34.

20 **Kennedy CC, Cannon EK, Warner DO, Cook DA.** Advanced airway management simulation training in medical education: a systematic review and meta-analysis. Crit Care Med 2014; **42**:169–178.

21 **Laack TA, Dong Y, Goyal DG, Sadosty AT, Suri HS, Dunn WF.** Short-term and long-term impact of the central line workshop on resident clinical performance during simulated central line placement. Simul Healthc 2014;**9**:228–233.

22 **Macfie RC, Webel AD, Nesbitt JC, Fann JI, Hicks GL, Feins RH.** 'Boot camp' simulator training in open hilar dissection in early cardiothoracic surgical residency. Ann Thorac Surg 2014;**97**:161–166.

23 **Gawad N, Zevin B, Bonrath EM, Dedy NJ, Louridas M, Grantcharov TP.** Introduction of a comprehensive training curriculum in laparoscopic surgery for medical students: a randomized trial. Surgery 2014;**156**:689–706.

24 **Jung EY, Park DK, Lee YH, Jo HS, Lim YS, Park RW.** Evaluation of practical exercises using an intravenous simulator incorporating virtual reality and haptics device technologies. Nurs Educ Today 2012;32:458–463.

25 **Gerolemou L, Fidellaga A, Rose K, Cooper S, Venturanza M, et al.** Simulation-based training for nurses in sterile techniques during central vein catherization. Am J Critical Care 2014;**23**:40–48.

26 **Ballard G.** Effect of simulated learning on blood pressure measurement skill. Nursing Standard 2012;**27**:43–47.

27 **Reed KS.** Bags and blogs: creating an ostomy experience for nursing students. Rehabil Nurs 2012;**37**:62–65.

28 **Hayden JK, Smiley RA, Alexander M, Kardong-Edgren S, Jeffries PR.** The NCSBN national simulation study: a longitudinal, randomized, controlled study replacing clinical hours with simulation in prelicensure nursing education. Journal of Nursing Regulation 2014;**5**:S3–S64.

29 **Krogh KB, Hayer CB, Ostergaard D, Eika B.** Time matters: realism in resuscitation training. Resuscitation 2014;**85**:1093–1098.

30 Stanford Anesthesia Cognitive Aid Group*. Emergency manual: cognitive aids for perioperative critical events: <http://emergencymanual.stanford.edu>

31 **Petrovic MA, Martinez EA, Aboumater H.** Implementing a perioperative handoff tool to improve post-procedural patient transfers. The Joint Commission Journal on Quality and Patient Safety 2012;**83**(3):135–141

32 **Joy BF, Elliot E, Hardy C, Sullivan C, et al.** Standardized multidisciplinary protocol improves handover of cardiac surgery patients to the intensive care unit. Ped Crit Care Med 2011;**12**(3):304–308.

33 **Gaba D, Howard S, Fish K, et al.** Simulation-based training in anesthesia crisis resource management (ACRM): a decade of experience. Simulat Gaming 2001;**32**(2):175–293.

34 Gaba DM, Fish KJ, Howard SK, Burden AR. Crisis Management in Anesthesiology. 2nd ed. Philadelphia, PA: Elsevier Saunders; 2015.

35 Morey JC, Simon R, Jay GD, et al. Error reduction and performance improvement in the emergency department through formal teamwork training: evaluation results of the MedTeams project. Health Serv Res 2002;**37**(6):1553–1581.

36 Leonard M, Graham S, Bonacum D. The human factor: the critical importance of effective teamwork and communication in providing safe care. Qual Saf Health Care 2004;**13**(Suppl 1):i85–i90.

37 Baker DP, Salas E, King H, et al. The role of teamwork in the professional education of physicians: current status and assessment recommendations. Jt Comm J Qual Patient Saf 2005;**31**(4):185–202.

38 Lingard L, Espin S, Rubin B, et al. Getting teams to talk: development and pilot implementation of a checklist to promote interprofessional communication in the OR. Qual Saf Health Care 2005;**14**(5):340–346.

39 Boet S, Bould MD, Fung L, Qosa H, Perrier L, Tavares W, et al. Transfer of learning and patient outcome in simulated crisis resource management: a systematic review. Can J Anesth 2014;**61**:571–582.

40 Croskerry P, Singhal G, Mamede S. Cognitive debiasing 1: origins of bias and theory of debiasing. BMJ Qual Saf 2013;**22**:ii58–ii64.

41 Croskerry P, Singhal G, Mamede S. Cognitive debiasing 2: impediments to and strategies for change. BMJ Qual Saf 2013;**22**:ii65–ii72.

42 Stiegler MP, Tung A. Cognitive processes in anesthesiology decision-making. Anesthesiology 2014;**120**:204–217.

43 Stiegler MP, Neelankavil JP, Canales C, Dhillon A. Cognitive errors detected in anaesthesiology: a literature review and pilot study. Br J Anaesth 2012;**108**:229–235.

44 Levine AI, Bryson EO. The use of multimodality simulation in the evaluation of physicians with suspected lapsed competence. Journal of Critical Care 2008;**23**:197–202.

45 DeMaria S, Samuelson ST, Schwartz AD, Sim AJ, Levin AI. Simulation-based assessment and retraining for the anesthesiologist seeking reentry to clinical practice. Anesthesiology 2013;**119**:206–217.

46 Murray JD, Boulet JR, Kras JF, Woodhouse JA, Cox T, McAllister JD. Acute care skills in anesthesia practice: a simulation-based resident performance assessment. Anesthesiology 2004;**101**:1084–1095.

47 Blum RH, Boulet JR, Cooper JB, Muret-Wagstaff SL. Simulation-based assessment to identify critical gaps in safe anesthesia resident performance. Anesthesiology 2014;**120**:129–141.

48 Mittal MK, Dumon KR, Edelson PK, Acero NM, Hashimoto D, Danzer E, et al. Successful implementation of the American College of Surgeons/Association of Program Directors in Surgery surgical skills curriculum via a 4-week consecutive simulation rotation. Simul Healthc 2012;**7**:147–154.

49 Steadman RH, Burden AR, Huang YM, Gaba DM, Cooper JB. Practice improvements based on participation in simulation for the maintenance of certification in anesthesiology program. Anesthesiology (accepted for publication).

50 Second Life, <http://en.widipedia.org/wiki/Second_Life>, accessed 01 Sep. 2014.

51 Advanced Disaster Management Simulator, <http://trainingfordisastermanagement.com>, accessed 01 Sep. 2014.

52 MUVE, <http://en.wikipedia.org/wiki/MUVE>, accessed 01 Sep. 2014 (Goldhaber-Fiebert et al. Use of emergency manuals).

53 Nilsson H, Jonson CO, Vikström T, Bengtsson E, Thorfinn J, Huss F, et al. Simulation-assisted burn disaster planning. 2013;**39**(6):1122–1130. doi: 10.1016/j.burns.2013.01.018. Epub: 23 Feb 2013.

54 Cicero MX, Brown L, Overly F, Yarzebski J, Meckler G, Fuchs S, et al. Creation and Delphi-method refinement of pediatric disaster triage simulations. Prehosp Emerg Care 2014 Apr–Jun;**18**(2):282–289. doi: 10.3109/10903127.2013.856505. Epub: 8 Jan 2014.

55 Cranmer H, Chan JL, Kayden S, Musani A, Gasquet PE, Walker P, et al. Development of an evaluation framework suitable for assessing humanitarian workforce competencies during crisis simulation exercises. Prehosp Disaster Med 2014;**29**:69–74.

56 Dawson SL, et al. Designing a computer-based simulator for interventional cardiology training. Catheter Cardiovasc Interv 2000;**51**:522–527.

57 Gallagher AG, Cates CU. Approval of virtual reality training for carotid stenting: what this means for procedure-based medicine. JAMA 2004; **292**:3024–3026.

58 Ahmed K, et al. Role of virtual reality simulation in teaching and assessing technical skills in endovascular intervention. J Vasc Interv Radiol 2010;**21**:55–66.

59 Paul Dalley, et al. The use of high-fidelity human patient simulation and the introduction of new anesthesia delivery systems. Anesth Analg 2004;**99**:1737–1741.

60 Feigal DW, Gardner SN, McClellan M. Ensuring safe and effective medical devices. N Engl J Med 2003;**348**:191–192.

61 Nielsen DS, Dieckmann P, Mohr M, Mitchell AU, Østergaard D. Augmenting health care failure modes and effects analysis with simulation (evaluating an ongoing process). Simul Healthc 2014 Feb;**9**(1):48–55. doi: 10.1097/SIH.0b013e3182a3defd

62 Carayon patient safety: the role of human factors and systems engineering. Stud Health Technol Inform 2010;**153**:23–46. Available at <http://www.ncbi.nlm.nih.gov/pmc/articles/PMC3057365/>

63 Clinical Human Factors Group, <http://chfg.org/definition/towards-a-working-definition-of-human-factors-in-healthcare>, accessed 01 Sep. 2014.

64 Pian-Smith MCM, Simon R, Minehart RD, Podraza M, Rudolph J, Walzer T, et al. Teaching residents the two-challenge rule: a simulation-based approach to improve education and patient safety. Simul Healthc 2009;**4**:84–91.

65 Singer SJ, Hayes J, Cooper JB, et al. A case for safety leadership team training of hospital managers. Health Care Manage Rev 2011;**36**(2):188–200.

66 Cooper JB, Singer SJ, Hayes J, et al. Design and evaluation of simulation scenarios for a program introducing patient safety, teamwork, safety leadership, and simulation to healthcare leaders and managers. Simul Healthc 2011;**6**(4):231–238. doi: 210.1097/SIH.1090b1013e31821da31829ec

Chapter 18

Non-technical skills: identifying, training, and assessing safe behaviours

Rhona Flin and Nicola Maran

Overview

- Non-technical skills such as decision-making, situation awareness, teamworking, and leadership are used to underpin the technical skills required for safe and effective practice.

- The aviation industry recognized that many adverse incidents have non-technical failures at their core and responded by providing mandatory non-technical skills (CRM) training for operational staff.

- Despite high numbers of adverse events in healthcare, non-technical skills are not yet widely taught in the medical curriculum.

- Observations and rating of non-technical skills can be carried out using behavioural rating (or marker) systems and these are now used in healthcare.

- Speciality-specific behavioural marker systems for anaesthetists (ANTS), surgeons (NOTSS), scrub practitioners (SPLINTS), and anaesthetic practitioners (ANTS-AP) have been developed for use in both clinical and simulation environments to give feedback for assessment and training.

- Despite their apparent simplicity, in order to use behavioural rating systems accurately and reliably, raters need considerable training.

- Simulation provides the ideal setting in which to examine individual or team skills, especially under stress. Debriefing using video allows individuals to gain insight into their own non-technical skills in such conditions. Repeated exposure to challenging situations allows individuals to develop their skills.

- Behavioural observations are increasingly being incorporated into workplace-based assessment tools.

18.1 **Introduction to non-technical skills**

18.1.1 **What are non-technical skills?**

While adverse events often have organizational and technical causes, many of the errors that contribute to accidents in the workplace could have been avoided if better non-technical skills had been demonstrated by the personnel operating or maintaining the system. In aviation, the term was first used by the European regulator and was defined as 'the cognitive and social skills of flight crew members in the cockpit, not directly related to aircraft control, system management, and standard operating procedures'.[1] These skills include situation awareness, decision-making, leadership, and teamwork. They complement workers' technical skills and should reduce errors, increase the capture of errors, and help to mitigate when an operational problem occurs (see Figure 18.1). Non-technical skills are also called crew resource management (CRM) skills and the civil aviation industry has pioneered the development of CRM training. Focusing on non-technical skills is only one aspect of a human-factors approach to safety management.

In this chapter, the terms non-technical skills (NTS) and CRM skills can be regarded as synonymous. Following an overview of the identification, training, and assessment of NTS in aviation, we describe how this approach has been adopted in healthcare, using simulated as well as real environments. The focus is on individual skills within a team setting rather than on skills at the group level.

18.1.2 **Individual or team skills?**

The issue of whether non-technical skills should be trained and assessed at an individual or a team level is a topic of ongoing debate. In most safety-critical settings, work is carried out by teams of technical specialists and so the work group provides the context for the

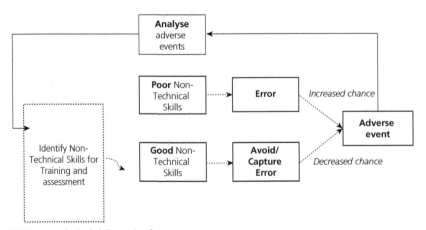

Fig. 18.1 Non-technical skills and safety.

Reprinted by permission of the Publishers from 'Introduction', in *Safety at the Sharp End* by Rhona Flin, Paul O'Connor, and Margaret Crichton (Aldershot: Ashgate, 2008), p. 6. Copyright © 2008, Ashgate, Gower & Lund Humphries Publishing.

individual's behaviour. The main reason for focusing on the individual is because the individual is the basic 'building block' from which teams and larger organizational groupings are formed. Moreover, in many workplaces, the staff do not work in the same team every day. In the larger airlines, the same pilots rarely fly together and for that reason, the focus in European aviation has been on the individual pilot's technical and non-technical competence, rather than on a crew.[2] The introduction of working-time restrictions and the streamlining of medical training forced changes to shift and rotation patterns such that team composition in hospitals is rarely fixed. Although doctors increasingly practise in interdisciplinary teams, they remain individually accountable for their professional conduct and the care they provide.[3]

The counter argument is that the unit of operation is the crew and how the team members interact to accomplish their tasks is the most important issue. Crew members have shared responsibility for the operation and one person's behaviour will be influenced by another's. There are a number of crew rating systems used in aviation, but it should be noted that a flightdeck crew normally consists of only two pilots, both fixed in their seats, operating the same equipment, with one main external communication channel. This is very different from many healthcare teams—an operating theatre or resuscitation room may have ten or more individuals from different professions moving around and engaged in a whole set of interacting tasks, communicating with a range of external sources. It takes considerable skill to observe all these individuals, track their communications, and rate what is happening at a group level of analysis. There are group behaviour rating methods; e.g. for resuscitation teams[4] or operating theatre teams.[5]

It is, therefore, proposed that the initial focus for training and evaluation of non-technical skills should be on the individual. This is especially applicable in healthcare where many professionals are unfamiliar with the basic concepts (e.g. situation awareness) and do not have a shared vocabulary for discussing these within their own profession, never mind across professional boundaries. Single discipline training of non-technical skills is also important in healthcare as most teams will come together on a temporary basis and, therefore, it is important that individuals develop portable team skills which can be used in any 'ad hoc' team. Where groups of staff may come together on a regular basis, individual training can then be followed by training of multidisciplinary teams.

18.2 Background

18.2.1 Non-technical skills in aviation and other industries

In the late 1970s, a series of major aviation accidents, without primary technical causes, forced investigators to turn their attention to the humans in the operational chain.[6] They began to scrutinize the behaviours associated with errors and accidents. Emerging culprits were failures in leadership, poor team coordination, communication breakdowns, lack of assertiveness, lack of attention, and inadequate problem-solving, often exacerbated by stress and fatigue.

The aviation industry realized that the maintenance of high standards of safety was going to require more than efficient technology and proficient technical skills in the system operators (e.g. pilots, engineers, air traffic controllers). It began to take a serious interest in non-technical skills. These were not mysterious or rare behaviours; they were actually normal practices that pilots had always regarded as an essential part of good airmanship. However, these NTS had often been tacitly rather than explicitly addressed and were taught in an informal and inconsistent manner from one generation of pilots to the next.[7] Aviation psychologists and pilots began to run experiments in the flight deck simulators, interview pilots, and analyse accident reports, to discover which skill components either contributed to, or were effective in, preventing adverse events. Once the core NTS had been identified, then the airlines developed training courses to raise awareness of the importance of these skills, to provide the necessary underpinning knowledge and practice for skill development. These were initially called cockpit resource management courses, later amended to crew resource management, as other flight crew members, such as cabin attendants, became involved.[6]

Accidents involving inadequacies in non-technical skills are certainly not unique to the aviation industry. Consequently, many other high-risk industries have introduced CRM training, such as nuclear power, maritime, mining, rail, and the emergency services.[8, 9] Some organizations, for instance the UK nuclear power companies, also assess non-technical skills of staff in safety-critical positions.

18.2.2 **Non-technical skills in healthcare**

Concern about the rates of adverse events to patients caused by medical error grew in the late 1990s and it appeared that many of these could be attributed to failures in non-technical skills.[10, 11] As a result, medical professionals began to look at safety-management techniques used in the high-risk industries. Drawing on the behaviour-based approach adopted by the aviation sector to enhance safety, some of the acute hospital-based specialities began to identify the non-technical skills contributing to safe and efficient performance. Similar to the experience in aviation, skills such as situation awareness, decision-making, and communication have always been regarded as important to good medical practice but have not been explicitly taught in the medical curriculum. The development of behavioural marker systems allows these skills to be more explicitly trained and evaluated. This is vital in an environment of reduced working hours and duration of training, and has led to development and testing of new approaches. Simulated medical environments offer ideal facilities for practising and debriefing healthcare professionals' non-technical skills. More recently, non-technical skills such as situation awareness and teamworking have begun to appear in established workplace-based assessment instruments for both surgery and anaesthesia in the United Kingdom. The rest of this chapter discusses the identification, training, and assessment of non-technical skills in healthcare, with particular reference to the use of simulation facilities.

18.3 **Identifying non-technical skills**

18.3.1 **Introduction**

The specific NTS required for a particular occupation need to be determined by a systematic process of identification based on task analysis.[12] While the main skill categories (e.g.

decision-making or leadership) are similar across professions, the component elements and examples of good and poor behaviours need to be carefully specified for a given profession and task set. These can be distinctive and clearly vary from one technical setting to another. This is why it is inadvisable to use a non-technical skills taxonomy or behavioural marker system devised for one domain (e.g. aviation) in a different work setting (e.g. healthcare).

In essence, a two-stage process should be employed: first, to identify the skills and related behaviours deemed to influence safe and efficient performance; and second, to refine the resulting list and to organize it into a concise, hierarchical structure or taxonomy. This tool then needs to be tested to ascertain usability, reliability, and validity. See Figure 18.2 for an example of the stages in the development of the NOTSS tool to rate surgeons' behaviour in the operating theatre.[13]

The level of detail and scope required will depend on the purpose for which the taxonomy is being developed. A set of behaviours identified for a research tool could be more complex and comprehensive than one being developed for practitioners to use as the basis for training or assessment. The methods that are typically used to develop non-technical skill taxonomies are outlined below.

18.3.2 **Data-collection techniques**

The first place to look for information is the published literature for the job in question. There are research studies examining behaviour in a range of healthcare workplaces and a

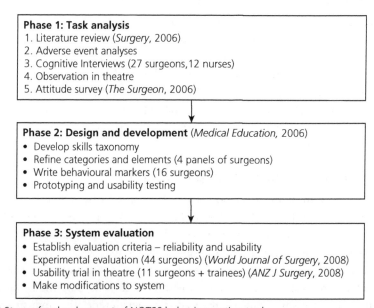

Fig. 18.2 Stages for development of NOTSS behaviour rating tool.
Reproduced from Flin R, Yule S, Maran N, Paterson-Brown S, Rowley D (2005). NOTSS. Non-Technical Skills for Surgeons. Paper presented at European Association of Work Psychology Conference, Istanbul, July.

suitable skill set may already exist. Organizations can hold documents which cover non-technical skills for a particular occupation including job assessments, competence frameworks, training programmes, and appraisal systems.

If no suitable taxonomy is available, there are a number of task-analysis techniques that can be adopted and these methods are normally used in combination to enhance validity. They can be grouped into three main types: (i) questioning techniques—obtaining information directly from practitioners in the relevant job using, for example, an interview,[14], a focus group, or a questionnaire survey; (ii) observational techniques—recording the behaviours of individuals carrying out their tasks[15] can be used but these usually require a coding scheme to organize the information (these first two methods tend to be used with experienced personnel—subject-matter experts); and (iii) event-based analyses—examine accident or near-miss reports to identify patterns of behaviours and related errors. This includes the use of confidential reporting systems,[16] which record safety concerns, as well as actual events. A problem with this method in healthcare is if the reports do not code human factors, being mainly concerned with clinical or technical causes.

18.3.3 Developing a skills taxonomy

The second stage of refining the skill list into a workable taxonomy with skills grouped into categories is normally carried out using panels of subject-matter experts.[17].

18.4 Training non-technical skills

18.4.1 Non-technical skills (CRM) training in aviation

Non-technical skills are trained in aviation and other industries CRM courses. The international aviation regulators generally mandate and monitor CRM courses[2] and they are run by almost all airlines, as both introductory (2–3 days) and refresher courses (e.g. one day annually). Regulators offer guidance on syllabi[2] but airlines design their own courses to suit their operational requirements. In UK aviation, the CRM instructors must be specially trained and formally qualified.[18] Reviews of studies attempting to evaluate the effectiveness of CRM training[19] generally report positive changes in attitudes, knowledge, and sometimes also in behaviour.[20]

18.4.2 Non-technical skills training in healthcare

Anaesthesia has been at the forefront of developments to train non-technical skills in healthcare (see Lighthouse et al., this volume) and there are now a range of courses focusing on one or more non-technical skills.[21] Whichever programme is adopted or designed, the basic principles of training design should be followed.[22] That is, there should be a systematic process of identifying the skills required for the particular profession or team, deciding how best to deliver the instruction and a method of evaluating whether the training was successful. Courses imported from aviation or other industries still require a training-needs analysis and then customization.[23] Baker et al.[24] reviewing medical team-training courses, including CRM, found that, 'not one of the programs was based on a comprehensive pretraining needs analysis and participants had limited opportunities to receive practice and feedback on critical teamwork skills'.

Typically, CRM courses are staged in a classroom setting for two days with about 12 participants and one or two trainers. Ideally, the trainers should be experienced professionals from the relevant domain who have a sufficient understanding of psychology to deliver the material. For those designing their own courses, the methods of training non-technical skills have been outlined in a number of sources on CRM training.[6] Flin et al.[8] outline the basic psychological background, with a range of examples, for seven generic non-technical skills and more material can be found on clinical human-factors websites.[25] Some specialty-specific texts are available; for example, on non-technical skills for surgeons.[26] In our experience, CRM trainers may be willing to allow professionals from other disciplines to sit in and observe their courses.

18.4.3 **Course content and delivery**

Basic CRM or NTS courses provide an introduction to the concept of human error and are designed to raise awareness and convey knowledge of the main non-technical skills, as well as related factors such as stress and fatigue, and how these influence task performance. However, in order to develop these skills, participants must be given an opportunity to put them into practice and to receive feedback and coaching. This can be done to a certain degree in a classroom setting using role play and observed group exercises but scenario-based training using simulators gives trainees the ideal opportunity to take part in real task-based exercises. Video feedback is a particularly powerful way of allowing participants to observe their own behaviours and gain insight into aspects of their performance. Structured debriefing, using a skills framework or taxonomy, allows identification of specific skills with illustration of positive and negative impacts of these actions. The trainers for these sessions must be skilled not only at observing and evaluating non-technical skills but also know how to debrief them in a constructive manner.

It is generally easier to observe the behaviours associated with social skills (such as teamworking, leadership, and task management) than those associated with the cognitive skills of situation awareness and decision-making. Cognitive skills cannot be directly observed and the associated behaviours may be more subtle unless vocalized. Verbalization of observations, thought processes, and rationale for decisions improves ease of observation of cognitive skills and can be prompted by questioning during direct observation (e.g. 'What are you thinking?' or 'Tell me what you are looking at') or during debriefing following a scenario in the simulator. Using observations of specific behaviours lends itself well to the use of the advocacy-inquiry technique of debriefing.[27] Instructors state their observations and disclose their evaluations of behaviour and use questioning to elicit trainees' assumptions about the situation and their reasons for acting as they did. This can allow the facilitator to gain insight into the mental models formed by participants which help to reveal their cognitive frames. Once this understanding is shared between facilitator and learner, supported feedback can help the candidate to identify performance gaps and identify ways in which skills can be improved. Contrasting examples of effective and ineffective behaviours clearly illustrates the skills to be developed and the benefits of doing so. Describing the skills within a structured framework, such as ANTS (Anaesthetists' Non-Technical Skills), allows faculty and learners to focus on distinct categories or elements to build understanding. For this reason, such frameworks are also useful to focus learning objectives for non-technical skills within a scenario. For example, a scenario such as management of anaphylaxis, which may involve few participants but many tasks, may be used to explore skills associated with task management. A scenario involving diagnostic challenges, such as identification of the cause of high airway pressure after induction of anaesthesia, may be used to focus on cognitive skills such as SA and decision-making.

Optimally, further simulator practice with feedback would allow development of these skills; however, few training programmes currently support regular recurrent simulation training such as occurs in the aviation industry. Since simulation training is still relatively infrequent, most scenarios experienced on the simulator currently utilize non-technical skills to recognize and manage emergency situations and are less likely to look at use of these skills in 'everyday' or 'routine' practice. Therefore, it is vital that feedback be given, preferably using the same feedback tools, in the clinical environment on a routine basis. This approach also emphasizes the importance of non-technical skills in the prevention of critical incidents, as well as their use in crisis management.

18.5 Assessing non-technical skills

18.5.1 Assessment of CRM skills in aviation

In UK, it is mandated[2, 18] that an assessment of non-technical (CRM) skills is included in all levels of training and checking of flight crew members' performance. The examination of a pilot's CRM skills must be undertaken by a qualified CRM instructor/examiner (CRMIE) who has been formally assessed as competent for this role.[18] In other countries, there are similar requirements for pilots' CRM skills to be evaluated and there are various systems for rating pilots' non-technical skills. One of these (NOTECHS) is used when evaluating an individual pilot's behaviour during a flight.[1] This system has been recommended by some regulators in Europe as one method of assessing a pilot's non-technical skills and a number of operators have customized it to meet their own fleet requirements.

18.5.2 Behaviour rating systems in healthcare

Behaviour rating systems for healthcare professionals' non-technical skills have been developed using methods derived from aviation and examples are described below.

18.5.2.1 Behaviour rating systems in anaesthesia

A taxonomy of non-technical skills, the ANTS system was developed in Scotland using a similar design and evaluation process to that used in the development of NOTECHS. The content was derived from the research literature on anaesthetists' behaviour, as well as data from observations, interviews, questionnaires, and incident analysis.[28] The system was developed as a tool for giving anaesthesia trainees feedback on non-technical skills, primarily in the clinical environment but also for use in the simulator setting.[29] As can be seen from Figure 18.3, there are four main categories of skill, each subdivided into component elements and for each element a number of positive and negative examples (markers) of behaviour are provided for illustration. Each element and category is rated on a four-point scale: Good, Acceptable, Marginal, Poor. For further details, see the ANTS pages on the Aberdeen of University non-technical skills tools website.[30]

The ANTS behavioural rating system has now been used in a number of settings.[31] The system has been translated into German, Danish, and Hebrew, and has been used to evaluate simulator training for anaesthetists in both Canada[32] and Denmark.[33]

Training courses in identification of anaesthetic non-technical skills are now available.[34, 35] This course presents a brief overview of the underlying psychology on non-technical skills and uses standardized video examples of skills to illustrate a range of behaviours across each of the categories and elements of the ANTS system. A short course such as this is designed only as an introduction to use of the system for those interested in increasing their knowledge of non-technical skills or who are teaching and supervising trainees. It is not possible in such a short time to achieve tight inter-rater reliability or calibration of raters[31] such as would be required in the aviation industry for summative assessment. Some simulation centres run courses specifically focused on developing participants' non-technical skills using scenario-based training with video-assisted feedback based around the ANTS system.[35]

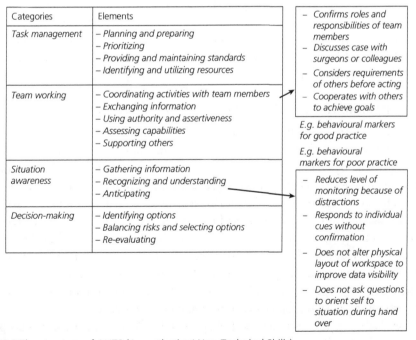

Fig. 18.3 The structure of ANTS (Anaesthetists' Non-Technical Skills).

A new non-technical skills system (ANTS-AP) for the practitioners who assist the anaesthetist has been designed using the same methods as were employed for ANTS.[30, 36] A behavioural rating system describing the skills of anaesthetic nurses has recently been developed in Denmark.[37]

18.5.2.2 Behaviour rating systems in surgery

For rating the non-technical skills of a surgeon conducting an operation, a taxonomy and behavioural rating system has been designed, called the NOTSS system.[30, 38] This uses a method similar to that employed in the development of NOTECHS and ANTS, as shown in Figure 18.2. An example of a NOTSS rating form representing an assessment of a general surgeon's non-technical skills is shown in Figure 18.4.

The NOTSS system has been tested for trainee assessment,[39] has been translated into Japanese, and a Danish version has been independently designed NOTSS-DK.[40] A training course in the use of the NOTSS system has been developed for surgeons.[41] Other rating tools for surgeons are available; some of these have been adapted from the NOTECHS tool for rating airline pilots' non-technical skills.[42] In addition, the SPLINTS system (Scrub Practitioners' List of Intra-operative Non-Technical Skills) is for scrub nurses and other staff who assist the operating surgeon.[30, 43]

18.5.2.3 Behavioural marker systems beyond the operating theatre

The challenges faced by emergency physicians in overseeing activity throughout the emergency department are different from those in the operating theatre, including more regular interruptions and managing multiple patients and tasks at any given time. The development and validation of a tool specifically for use in the emergency department[44] highlights the importance of adapting and testing tools for individual specialties. Another tool describes non-technical skills used by foundation doctors in managing acutely unwell patients and there is recent interest from other specialties, including histopathologists and radiologists.

18.5.3 Implementation of non-technical skills assessment

The process of introducing the ANTS and NOTSS systems has revealed some of the difficulties of bringing a novel type of assessment system into workplace-based assessment. The basic psychological language (e.g. situation awareness) is unfamiliar to most clinicians and, therefore, there is a need for basic awareness training courses in non-technical skills for both ratees and raters before trying to implement the system in training. In aviation, pilots are taught about psychological and physiological factors that influence their performance from the start of their training. As qualified pilots, they undertake CRM courses provided by their airline on a regular basis. Consequently, they are familiar with the cognitive and social skills influencing performance. Teaching on the factors influencing human performance is now being included in the medical curriculum at undergraduate level[45] and some courses are introducing non-technical skills at this stage.

The evaluation of non-technical skills may be undertaken for both training purposes or for a more formal assessment. The latter can be a contentious issue, especially if it

Hospital: Date:		Trainer name: Trainee name:		Operation: Right inguinal hernia repair
Category	Category rating*	Element	Element rating*	Feedback on performance and debriefing notes
Situation Awareness	3	Gathering information	3	Didn't mark side / arrived in theatre late
		Understanding information	4	Aware of INR importance and checked
		Projecting and anticipating future state	3	Take more of a lead in op - i.e. requesting retractions
Decision Making	3	Considering options	3	Be more explicit about relative merits of options
		Selecting and communicating option	2	Not sure about sutures / mesh sizes etc...
		Implementing and reviewing decisions	4	Readily vocalised concerns
Communication and Teamwork	2	Exchanging information	2	Did not relate well to anaesthetist
		Establishing a shared understanding	3	Waited for trainer to take the lead
		Co-ordinating team activities	3	Did not enquire about pt condition from anaesthetist
Leadership	3	Setting and maintaining standards	3	Followed theatre protocol but didn't mark side
		Supporting others	4	Good rapport with trainee OPD and scrub nurse
		Coping with pressure	3	At times seemed to carry on regardless - oblivious to important anatomy - too focused on other things

Fig. 18.4 Completed NOTSS rating form for a trainee general surgeon's performance on a hernia repair.

Reproduced from *Cognition, Technology & Work*, 10(4), pp. 265–274, Debriefing surgeons on non-technical skills (NOTSS), S Yule, R Flin, N Maran, G Youngson, A Mitchell, D Rowley, S Paterson-Brown, Figure 19.1, (c) 2007, Springer Science and Business Media. With kind permission from Springer Science and Business Media.

becomes part of a competence assessment or licensing procedure. For either purpose, the general principles of performance assessment apply,[46] although there are particular considerations to be taken into account when using a behavioural rating system to assess NTS for licensing. In this case, such as in civil aviation in the UK, then specific guidelines need to be developed.[2] In the UK, concern about licensing and revalidation of doctors[47] has introduced competence assurance across the medical specialities. Some of these workplace-based assessment tools, such as Anaesthetic CEX, DOPS, and CBD[33] now include aspects of non-technical skills within the assessments. Most of these tools are currently used in formative assessment of doctors in training grades but some are considered potentially useful in future in summative assessment of doctors who are identified as having concerns in clinical performance.

There are a number of issues concerning behavioural marker systems for summative assessment[48] which should be considered fully before undertaking such high-stakes assessment with these tools in healthcare domains:

- Raters require extensive training (initial and recurrent). They also need to be 'calibrated'— that is, their ratings need to be anchored onto the rating scale in a consistent manner.

- The rating systems do not transfer across domains and cultures without adaptation (e.g. Western behaviours in Eastern cultures, or from aviation to medicine).

- The rating systems need proper implementation into an organization, and need management and workforce support. It is recommended that a phased introduction is required to build confidence and expertise in raters and ratees. Consideration needs to be given to how rating information will be stored and accessed (as with any other performance data held on file).

- Application of the rating system must be sensitive to the stage of professional development of the individual, and to the maturity of the organizational and professional culture (whether used as a diagnostic, training, and/or assessment tool).

- Any use of the system must consider contextual factors when rating behaviour (e.g. crew experience, workload, operating environment, operational complexity).

When using a behaviour rating system for competence assessment, there are additional considerations because the formal assessment of non-technical aspects of performance presents significant challenges. The rating system must capture the context in which that assessment is made (e.g. team dynamics and experience, operating environment, operational complexity, current conditions). For example, the behaviour of one team member can be adversely or positively impacted by another, which could result in a substandard or inflated performance rating. Marker systems should be designed to detect and record such effects.

Most behaviour rating systems consist of a set of observable skills and rating scales on which to record the evaluations. The identification of skill sets was described above and these usually include examples of behaviours that signify whether the skill is being demonstrated. Rating scales come in a range of formats and need to be carefully designed. The behavioural rating method that is used needs to meet a number of psychometric conditions, such as reliability and validity. Flin et al.[8] discuss these, along with the design and use of behavioural rating skills for non-technical skills assessment; see also Hull et al.[49] for suggested guidance and Dietz et al.[50] for a recent review. In order to achieve the optimum quality of ratings, the raters must be properly trained. The training requirements for raters should not be underestimated. The danger is that behaviour rating systems look deceptively simple. Considerable skill is required to make accurate observations and ratings, and to give constructive feedback to those being rated. The following are recommended for a training course in behaviour rating and feedback:

♦ Minimum 2–5 consecutive days training (depending on prior experience).

♦ Ideal group size, 8–12 people.

♦ 1/2 day training follow-up (e.g. meeting, feedback via telephone) after rating practice.

The training for raters should deliver the following:

♦ Make explicit the goals for use of the rating system (e.g. formal assessment, developmental feedback, organizational audit).

♦ Explain the design and content of the rating system, as well as user guidelines.

♦ Review main sources of rater biases (e.g. hindsight, halo, recency, primacy) with techniques to be used for minimization of these influences.

♦ Present the concept of inter-rater reliability and the methods which will be used to maximize it.

♦ Illustrate and define each point of the rating scale and different levels of situational complexity with video examples, discussions, and hands-on exercises.

♦ Provide practical training with multiple examples.

♦ Include calibration with iterative feedback on inter-rater reliability scores.

♦ Teach debriefing skills as appropriate

♦ Conclude with a formal assessment of rater competence.

18.6 **Conclusion**

As simulation facilities have developed in healthcare, there has been an increased recognition that that these offer an ideal opportunity for the development and evaluation of practitioners' non-technical skills. Recent advances in the identification of skill sets, the design of training courses, and the availability of behaviour rating systems are beginning to provide the necessary tools for enhancing the practice of non-technical skills in medicine.

References

1 **Flin R, Martin L, Goeters KM, Hoermann J, Amalberti R, Valot C.** et al. Development of the NOTECHS (Non-Technical Skills) system for assessing pilots' CRM skills. Human Factors and Aerospace Safety 2003;3:95–117.

2 CAA. Crew resource management (CRM) training. Guidance for flight crew, CRM instructors (CRMIs) and CRM instructor-examiners (CRMIEs). CAP 737. Gatwick: Safety Regulation Group, Civil Aviation Authority; 2006. Available at <http://www.caa.co.uk>

3 General Medical Council. Good medical practice. Working with colleagues/working in teams. London: GMC; 2006, paragraphs 41–42.

4 Marsch S, Muller C, Marquardt K, Conrad G, Tscan F, Hunziker P. Human factors affect the quality of cardiopulmonary resuscitation in simulated cardiac arrests. Resuscitation 2004;**60**:51–56.

5 Undre S, Healey A, Darzi A, Vincent C. Observational teamwork assessment in surgery: a feasibility study. World Journal of Surgery 2006;**30**:1774–1783.

6 Kanki B, Helmreich R, Anca J, (eds). Crew resource management. San Diego, CA: Academic Press; 2010.

7 Lodge M. Airline captain. In: Flin R, Arbuthnot K (eds). Incident command. Tales from the hot seat. Aldershot: Ashgate; 2002.

8 Flin R, O'Connor P, Crichton M. Safety at the sharp end. A guide to non-technical skills. Aldershot: Ashgate; 2008.

9 Flin R, Wilkinson. Guidance on crew resource management (CRM) and non-technical skills training programmes. London: Energy Institute; 2014. Available at <http://www.energyinst.org>

10 Bromiley M. Have you ever made a mistake? Bulletin of the Royal College of Anaesthetists 2008;**48**:2442–2445.

11 Reader T, Flin R, Lauche K, Cuthbertson B. Non-technical skills in the intensive care unit. British Journal of Anaesthesia 2006;**96**:551–559.

12 Seamster T, Keampf G. Identifying resource management skills for pilots. In:. Salas E, Bowers C, Edens E (eds). Improving teamwork in organizations. Applications of resource management training. Mahwah, NJ: LEA; 2001.

13 Flin R, Yule S, Maran N, Paterson-Brown S, Rowley D. NOTSS. Non-technical skills for surgeons. Paper presented at European Association of Work Psychology Conference, Istanbul, July 2005.

14 Mitchell L, Flin R, Mitchell J, Coutts K, Youngson G. Thinking ahead of the surgeon. An interview study to identify scrub nurses' non-technical skills. International Journal of Nursing Studies 2011;**48**:818–828.

15 Henrickson-Parker SE, Yule S, Flin R, McKinley A. The Surgeons' Leadership Inventory (SLI): a taxonomy and rating system for surgeons' intraoperative leadership skills. American Journal of Surgery 2013;**205**:745–751.

16 Confidential Reporting System for Surgery, <http://www.coress.org.uk>, accessed 01 Sep. 2014.

17 Yule S, Flin R, Paterson-Brown S, Maran N, Rowley D. Development of a rating system for surgeons' non-technical skills. Medical Education 2006;**40**:1098–1104.

18 CAA. The Crew Resource Management Instructor (CRMI) and Crew Resource Management Instructor Examiner (CRMIE) Accreditation Framework. Standards Doc. 29 Version 5. Gatwick: Civil Aviation Authority;2013.

19 Salas E, Wilson K, Burke S, Wightman D. Does crew resource management training work? An update, an extension and some critical needs. Human Factors 2006;**48**:392–412.

20 Goeters KM. Evaluation of the effects of CRM training by the assessment of non-technical skills under LOFT. Human Factors and Aerospace Safety 2002;**2**:71–86.

21 Van Noord I, Bruijne M, Twisk J, van Dyck C, Wagner C. More explicit communication after classroom-based crew resource management training: results of a pragmatic trial. Journal of Evaluation in Clinical Practice 2015;**21**:137–144.

22 Goldstein I, Ford K. Training in organizations. Belmont, CA: Wadsworth; 2002.

23 **Flin R, Maran N.** Identifying and training non-technical skills for teams in acute medicine. Quality and Safety in Health Care 2004;**13**(Suppl 1):i80–i84.

24 **Baker D, Beaubien M, Holtzman A.** DoD medical team training programs: an independent case study analysis. Publication 06–0001.Washington, DC: AHRQ; 2006.

25 Clinical Human Factors Group, <http://www.chfg.org>, accessed 01 Sep. 2014.

26 **Flin R, Youngson G, Yule S (eds).** Enhancing surgical performance. A primer on non-technical skills. London: CRC Press; 2015 (in press).

27 **Rudolph J, Simon R, Dufresne R, Raemer D.** There's no such thing as 'nonjudgmental' debriefing: a theory and method for good judgment. Simulation in Healthcare 2006;**1**:49–55.

28 **Fletcher G, McGeorge P, Flin R, Glavin R, Maran, N.** Anaesthetists' non-technical skills (ANTS). Evaluation of a behavioural marker system. British Journal of Anaesthesia 2003;**90**:580–588.

29 **Flin R, Glavin R, Patey R, Maran N.** Anaesthetists' non-technical skills. British Journal of Anaesthesia 2010;**105**:38–44.

30 University of Aberdeen, Non-Technical Skills Tools websites: <http://www.abdn.ac.uk/iprc/ANTS www.abdn.ac.uk/iprc/NOTSS>; <http://www.abdn.ac.uk/iprc/SPLINTS www.abdn.ac.uk/iprc/ANTS-AP>

31 **Graham J, Hocking G, Giles E.** Anaesthesia non-technical skills: can anaesthetists be trained to reliably use this behavioural marker system in 1 day? British Journal of Anaesthesia 2010;**104**:440–445.

32 **Yee B, Naik V, Joo H, et al.** Non-technical skills in anesthesia crisis management with repeated exposure to simulation-based education. Anesthesiology 2005;**103**:214–218.

33 **Rosenstock E, Kristensen M, Rasmussen L, Skak C, Ostergaard, D.** Qualitative analysis of difficult airway management. Acta Anaesthesiology Scandinavia 2006;**50**:290–297.

34 Royal College of Anaesthetists, <http://www.rcoa.ac.uk/training-and-the-training-programme/workplace-based-assessments-wpba>, accessed 01 Sep. 2014.

35 Scottish Centre for Clinical Simulation and Human Factors, <http://scschf.org/courses>, accessed 01 Sep. 2014

36 **Rutherford J, et al.** Evaluation of the ANTS-AP system (under review).

37 **Lyk-Jensen H, Jepsen R, Spananger L, Dieckmann P, Ostergaard, D.** Assessing nurse anaesthetists' non-technical skills in the operating room. Acta Anaesthesiologica Scandinavia 2014;**58**:794–801.

38 **Yule S, Flin R, Paterson-Brown S, Maran N, Rowley D, Youngson G.** Surgeons' non-technical skills in the operating room: reliability testing of the NOTSS behaviour rating system. World Journal of Surgery 2008;**32**:548–556. See also <http://www.abdn.ac.uk/iprc/NOTSS>

39 **Crossley J, Marriott J, Purdie H, Beard J.** Prospective observational study to evaluate NOTSS (Non-Technical Skills for Surgeons) for assessing trainees' non-technical performance in the operating theatre. British Journal of Surgery 2011;**98**:1010–1020.

40 **Spanager L, Beier-Holgersen R, Dieckmann P, Konge L, Rosenberg J, Oestergard D.** Reliable assessment of general surgeons' non-technical skills based on video-recordings of patient simulated scenarios. American Journal of Surgery 2013;**206**:810–817.

41 Royal College of Surgeons Edinburgh, <http://www.rcsed.ac.uk/education/patient-safety-and-notss.aspx>, accessed 01 Sep. 2014.

42 **Moorthy K, Munz Y, Forrest D, Pandev V, Undre S, Vincent C, et al.** Surgical crisis management skills. Training and assessment. Annals of Surgery 2006;**244**:139–147.

43 **Mitchell L, Flin R, Mitchell J, Coutts K, Youngson G.** Evaluation of the Scrub Practitioners' List of Intraoperative Non-Technical Skills (SPLINTS) system. International Journal of Nursing Studies 2012;**49**:201–211.

44 **Flowerdew L, Brown R, Vincent C, Woloshynowych M.** Development and validation of a tool to assess emergency physicians' nontechnical skills. Annals of Emergency Medicine 2012;**59**:376–385.

45 Patey R, Flin R, et al. Patient safety: helping medical students understand error in healthcare. Quality and Safety in Health Care 2007;**16**:256–259.

46 Fletcher C. Appraisal, feedback and development. Making performance review work (4th edn). London: Routledge; 2007.

47 Donaldson L. Good doctors, safer patients. London: Department of Health; 2006.

48 Klampfer B, Flin R, Helmreich R, et al. Enhancing performance in high-risk environments: recommendations for the use of behavioural markers. Daimler Benz Foundation; 2001. Available at <http://www.abdn.ac.uk/iprc>

49 Hull L, Arora S, Symons N, Jalil R, Darzi A, Vincent C, et al. Training faculty in nontechnical skill assessment: national guidelines on program requirements. Annals of Surgery 2013;**258**:370–375.

50 Dietz A, Pronovost P, Benson K, et al. A systematic review of behavioural marker systems in healthcare: what do we know about their attributes, validity and application? BMJ Quality and Safety 2014;**23**:1031–1039.

Chapter 19

Current concepts in mannequin-based simulation assessment

Leonie M Watterson and Jennifer M Weller

Overview

- Mannequin-based simulation assessment (MSA) continues to be used for remediation of experienced clinicians and certification of emergency response skills in high-acuity medicine. However, its routine incorporation into assessment programmes has remained limited relative to the rapid growth of workplace assessments and SBA using standardized patients (SPs). Meanwhile, its role is expanding in relation to research, programme evaluation, and quality assurance.

- Clinical performance is now conceptualized in terms of highly integrated, contextually dependent clinical and non-technical competencies which respond to and are influenced by individual human, team, and environmental factors. Teamwork and systems safety are essential components of overall systems performance. These can be assessed with appropriate competency frameworks and test conditions.

- The design and delivery of contextually appropriate scenarios of known complexity is critical to ensure assessments are valid and these should be specified in assessment blueprints. An assessment's blueprint should be individualized and guided by its purpose and consequences. Psychometric specifications aimed to achieve reproducibility should be balanced accordingly with instructional design features aimed at achieving high validity, educational impact, feasibility, and cost-effectiveness.

- As in other forms of assessment, the test should include a broad sample of a clinicians' normal tasks if the results are to be considered reliable and generalizable. Triangulation with other sources of data may offset sampling requirements and improve feasibility and cost.

19.1 Applications of mannequin-based simulation assessment

While assessment using standardized patients (SP)[1] and simulation education without assessment[2] are well established in some certification and recertification programmes, there are only a small number of published accounts of established assessment programmes that incorporate MSA.[3] This is despite its theoretical advantages and its accepted validity and reliability.[4-6] Most recent publications demonstrate its use in research applied to a range of applications, including: validation of assessment instruments,[7] studies of cognitive expertise,[8] identification of performance gaps in training needs exercises,[9] and evaluation of novel educational curricula.[10] MSA continues to have a specified role in certification programmes, specifically in relation to assessment of competencies not easily assessed in the workplace, such as high-acuity emergencies and in recertification and remediation of clinicians with perceived lapsed skills.[11-13] Emerging roles for MSA are team-based assessment and assessment of the workplace[14] and clinical models of care.[15]

19.2 Principles of assessment

All assessment processes should achieve common goals of providing meaningful data that address contextually relevant performance elements; employ defensible methods and standards; and are ethical and procedurally fair.[16, 17] They benefit by being feasible, cost-effective, and by having a positive impact on education.[18] These goals are operationalized for MSA in the elements shown in Box 19.1.[11, 16-19]

Box 19.1 Key features of assessment programmes using MSA

Whole programme administration

- Selection processes are based on established programme guidelines or governance processes.
- Candidates are appropriately recruited and notified and understand the reasons for, purpose and consequences of the assessment, the assessment activities, standards, appeal, and remediation processes. Counselling and support is available.

Competencies and performance elements

- Competencies are relevant to the purpose of the assessment reflecting candidates' normal roles.
- Performance elements and expected standards are supported by competency taxonomies.
- Assessors agree on the range and degree of integration of these and case complexity; including the level of support from acting faculty in scenario design.

Standard-setting

- Scoring standards including minimum acceptable practices are predetermined using evidence-based, benchmarked criteria if possible.

> **Box 19.1 Key features of assessment programmes using MSA** *(continued)*
>
> ♦ Standards are determined relative to case complexity, including expected autonomy, and clinician adaptation to changing clinical complexity, team, and environmental influences.
>
> ### Instructional design features
>
> ♦ Instructional design methods produce testing conditions appropriate to the assessment's purpose.
>
> ♦ Candidates are orientated to the scenario setting, environment, equipment, task, and faculty roles.
>
> ♦ Scenarios are delivered at the predetermined level of complexity including diagnostic cues and prompting that clinicians obtain from teammates, faculty, and assessors.
>
> ### Assessment methods
>
> ♦ Assessors have adequate credentials and undergo prior rater calibration.
>
> ♦ Scenarios sample a wide range of clinical cases unless data are triangulated with other sources.
>
> ♦ Measurement instruments are validated where possible and appropriate to local context. They include behaviourally anchored global scales supported by descriptions or examples of practice.
>
> ♦ Rating methods suit test design. Tests based on direct observation, particularly those with high levels of realism, use global rating scales. These can be supported by criterion-based checklists.[19] Collectively, ratings should incorporate a judicious blend of quantitative and qualitative outcome measures to compensate for the identified limitations of any single test.

19.3 **Recent trends in assessment theory**

Theoretical considerations of clinical-performance assessment have previously focused on the relationship between competencies, scoring standards, and psychometrics. The latter includes the extent to which test results are reproducible (reliability) and the extent to which the test faithfully reflects the tasks and traits it is has the purpose of measuring (validity).[18] As standardization was considered necessary for achieving reliability, early assessment methodology favoured deconstruction of competencies into more discretely measurable components and decontextualization of the setting in which they were measured.[19, 20] The latter involves removal of props, storyline, and cues that identify the domain and situational elements of the setting in which a scenario is presented while retaining the important features of the patient's pathophysiology. This competed with Miller's competence assessment model which proposes that assessment of habitual practice in the workplace ('does') and integrated competency ('shows how') are more valid than assessment of deconstructed competencies.[21] Highly contextualized MSA can achieve test conditions at the 'shows how' and 'does' levels of Miller's model.[22]

This tension has somewhat resolved with studies demonstrating valid and reliable assessment of clinicians' performance achieved with MSA.[4–6] Experts in test psychometrics now agree that test reliability is better achieved by sampling a wide range of clinical tasks and presentations than by achieving highly standardized test conditions.[18, 19] This equates to approximately 12 stations of different subject matter in both the Objective Structured Clinical Examination (OSCE) and context-rich MSA methods.[4, 5] The high cost and reduced feasibility incurred by large samples of assessment scenarios continue to impose constraints on the use of MSA, although these are mitigated by triangulating it with other sources of measurement, particularly when high reliability is required, such as high-stakes certification and recertification.[16]

19.4 Current trends in assessment programmes

An assessment's overall utility is determined not only by its performance against psychometric tests but also other attributes, such as educational impact, feasibility, cost-effectiveness, and acceptability.[18] As mentioned below, instructional design features are crucial in ensuring the assessment is valid in respect to test complexity and alignment with targeted competencies. Hence, assessment blueprints should be individualized against their purpose and consequences. Box 19.2 and Table 19.1 present a series of hypothetical assessments to demonstrate MSA's wide range of applications and describe how an assessment's administration, instructional design, and methodology can be individualized according to its purpose and consequences to achieve the principles presented in Box 19.1.

19.4.1 Competence

Clinical expertise can be viewed in terms of clinical judgements reflecting situation assessment, assimilation of diagnostic information, hypothesis formation, future planning, and decision-making.[4, 8, 17] It is highly context- or topic-dependent and appears intangibly interwoven with somewhat more generic non-technical skills (NTS), such as situation awareness, leadership, communication, general problem-solving, teamwork, and workload management, representing how clinicians interact with, and adapt to, their environment and team.[23] Efforts to understand competency as it relates to individual clinicians have extended to an increased awareness of team assessment. Patient-treatment error represents a major burden of disease,[24] and failures in teamwork and communication are frequently cited as a major factor in these treatment errors.[25] Lingard[26] proposed the concept of 'Collective Competence', where successful patient outcomes depend on the individual competence of each member of the healthcare team involved in care and, critically, the ability of all the members of the team to coordinate their input through effective systems of communication and work as an effective team. In respect to team competence, Salas[27]

Box 19.2 Case examples of assessment activities

Case 1: Assessment within a research study to assess ethical competence (adapted from[10])

The assessment is conducted within a cross sectional observational study investigating ethical competence of clinical teams in an emergency department setting. The study activities are embedded in a routine CRM training course. Institutional Review Board (IRB) approval is provided for the study protocol and recruitment and consent of subjects. Performance elements and standards for five ethical topics are predetermined by an expert group following a review of literature. Validated tools are not available thus a study specific tool is designed with checklists of key actions. Ethical situations are scripted into scenarios and are revealed following resolution of clinical emergencies to control artefact. Ethical authenticity is achieved through script and situational prompts. High-fidelity simulators are available although low to moderate levels of equipment and environmental realism are considered adequate. Feedback is provided as formative assessment after data collections. Subjects complete a sample of five cases accepting this is too small to generalize about individuals' overall ethical competency. Reliability of scores is confirmed for the three trained raters who merge scores and undertake video analysis to manage divergent scores.

Case 2: Programmed certification of medical specialist trainees (adapted from[4])

Assessment is embedded into routine certification examinations of a cohort of individual anaesthesia residents. The assessment examines a sample of five topic domains relevant to emergencies. Results will be triangulated with other assessments to contribute to evidence of attainment of competency prior to completion of their training programme. Reliability has been demonstrated on previous cohorts. Validity is achieved by matching competencies to purpose using modified Delphi method to determine performance elements. Clinical knowledge is integrated with problem solving, decision-making, practical responses, and non-technical competencies of situation awareness. High-fidelity simulators supporting a simple OSCE-style workstation format improves the feasibility of testing this relatively large cohort. Subsequently decontextualized scenarios with one faculty playing a team member is used. The loss of some validity in testing NTS is acknowledged. A validated measurement is used including checklist items and four items with global scores. Standard-setting is achieved via Delphi. A cut score is determined as a 70% pass rate on criteria and consensus of two assessors scoring global items as 'sufficient'.

Case 3: Recertification of clinician with possible lapsed competence (adapted from[11])

A specialist anaesthetist is involuntarily referred by the Medical Accreditation Council to undertake comprehensive performance assessment following a preliminary review

Box 19.2 Case examples of assessment activities *(continued)*

of a serious complaint. The MSA aims to make generalizations regarding routine and emergency response practice in elective and non-elective surgery. A range of integrated competencies are assessed including patient assessment and communication, teamwork, reliance on team support, and adaptive problem solving in high-complexity cases. High-fidelity simulators support highly contextualized scenarios with carefully scripted scenario elements and rehearsed actor faculty. Independent assessors experienced with peer review in the simulation setting are used. The measurement instrument includes global scores for 16 performance elements supported by criterion checklist items. Standards are agreed by assessors using evidence guidelines. Assessors score independently before conferring. No cut scores are predetermined. Quantitative and qualitative data reported to licencing agency for review and determination by a third party. The MSA is incorporated as a component of a broader multifaceted assessment which includes workplace observation, knowledge tests, and medical record review. Hence, results will be triangulated as a means of making generalizations.

Case 4: Formative assessment and quality assurance exercise (adapted from[33])

Twenty experienced operating room teams from one surgical unit volunteer for team-based simulation education as a quality assurance exercise designed to identify opportunities to improve individual team and systems competence. Competencies focus on team information sharing following an initial needs assessment using focus groups. Supported by evidence from a literature review instructional design features include: highly contextualized scenarios reflecting evidence that high contextual realism is required to test competencies which focus on team interaction and the optimization of the work environment; scenarios incorporate events requiring participants to share information and which focus participant reflection during the debrief on strategies to enhance information sharing; explicit reference to the dimensions and underpinning mechanisms of effective teams described by Salas; activities that encourage a structured approach to information sharing between team members, including the use of briefings and checklists such as the World Health Organization Surgical Safety Checklist. Reliability is considered of lower importance given the consequence is formative. The BMRI tool is used to assess team performance for research purposes and formative assessment is achieved with a structured debrief following each simulation.

proposed a model for effective teams, comprising five dimensions: team orientation (focus on the team rather than individual); team leadership (encompassing defining goals and task coordination); mutual performance monitoring (where team members check on, or challenge the actions of others); back-up behaviour (expressed as team members providing assistance or prompts to other team members); and adaptability (recognizing and

Table 19.1 Features of individualized assessment blueprints

	1. Research	2. Certification	3. Recertification	4. Formative
1) WHOLE OF PROGRAMME FEATURES				
a) Selection for assessment				
i) Candidate	Sample of teams	Cohort of individuals	Individual	Cohort of teams
ii) Voluntary selection	Yes	No	No	Yes
a) Consequences	Research data	Certification for stage	Remediation/Re-licensure	Education, quality assurance
b) Preparation, communication, counselling (note i)	IRB consent	Written notification as per training programme guidelines	Notification by licensing agency Medical indemnity insurer and peer support offered	Written invitation
2) COMPETENCIES ASSESSED				
a) Clinical domain	Emergency medicine	Anaesthesia emergencies	Anaesthesia whole of practice	Operating room practices
b) Targeted or generalizable competencies	Targeted	Generalizable	Generalizable	Targeted
c) Competencies (note ii)	EP	CM, ER	CM, CRM, T, P	CM, CRM, T, P
d) Integration of competencies (number of concomitant themes) (note iii)	Moderate (2)	Moderate (2)	High (2 +)	High (2 +)
e) Ability to respond to challenging environmental and or human factors	Not assessed	Not assessed	Assessed	Assessed
f) Degree of reliance on team support assessed? (note iv)	No—faculty are constant	Yes—faculty vary support	Yes—faculty vary support	No—faculty are constant

continued

Table 19.1 (continued) Features of individualized assessment blueprints

	1. Research	2. Certification	3. Recertification	4. Formative
3) ASSESSMENT METHODS				
a) Content sampling (note v)	S (1)	S (12); TT	S (5); TT; MSF; MRR; WO	S (2)
b) Outcome measures (note vi)	C	C, TT	CO, C, E, TS	TT, C, E
c) Data collection (note vi)	Video analysis	Video analysis	DO, PB +/– VA	DO, SAS, TB
d) Scoring tools (note vii)	C,G,Q	L,C,G	C,G,Q	L,C,G
e) Scoring standards—passmarks	Not benchmarked	Benchmarked	Not benchmarked	Not benchmarked
a) Assessor number	2	2	2	1
4) INSTRUCTIONAL DESIGN				
a) Modalities: (note viii)	M	M, SP	M, SP	M
b) Contextual realism				
i) Familiarity of setting	*In situ*	Laboratory	Laboratory	*In situ*
i) Environmental realism	Moderate	Low	High	High
ii) Mannequin realism	Moderate	Moderate	High	Moderate
iii) Faculty actors' role	Scripted	Scripted	Scripted	Scripted
iv) Cueing and prompting from faculty	Moderate	Moderate	Minimal	Minimal
c) Scenario events and complexity				
i) Multilevel events (number of events) (note ix)	CE (1) TI (1)	CE(1)	CE (1); TI (1)	CE (1); TI (1) SE (1)
ii) Scenario progression (linear, branch, looping) (note x)	Looping	Linear	Looping	Branching

iii) Difficulty is scalable within scenario?	No	No	Yes	Yes
iv) Rescue contingencies for unpredicted events	No	No	Yes	Yes
c) Case standardization				
i) Mannequin vital signs and event progression	Operator guided	Software program	Operator guided	Software program
ii) Script parameters	Standardized	Standardized	Guiding	Guiding
j) Interaction between assessor and assese(s)	Modest prompting to support realism	Modest prompting to support realism	Probing used as assessment method	Probing used as assessment method
e) Feedback	Post exercise feedback	Post exercise feedback	Debriefing	Debriefing

Legend

(i) All candidates receive pre-assessment briefing, familiarization on simulator. Candidates and assessors sign confidentiality agreements.

(ii) Ethical practice (EP), clinical practice (CM), emergency response (ER), crisis resource management (CRM), teamwork (T), procedures (P).

(iii) Each affected clinical system, key clinical event or situation is scripted as a discrete story theme. Multiple themes integrate to build authenticity.

(iv) If no, then faculty are briefed to deliver a consistent degree of support/prompting; however, assessment method does not include measures of this competency; if yes, then faculty are briefed to deliver scaled degrees of support/prompting and assessment method specifically includes measures of this competency.

(v) Simulation cases (S), theory test (TT), multisource feedback (MSF), medical record review (MRR), workplace observation (WO).

(vi) Treatment time (TT); case outcomes (CO), competencies (C), errors and adverse events (E), level of team support as a measure of independent practice (TS).

(vii) Computer scored (CS), direct observation (DO), video analysis (VA), interview, probing and debrief (PB), self-assessment survey (SAS), transcription of debrief (TB).

(viii) Computer-generated data and event logs (L), checklists (C), global scales (G), qualitative data (Q).

(viii) Mannequin (M); Standardized patient (SP)

(ix) Clinical events (CE), Situational events (SE); Team-interaction events (T)

(x) Maintaining a scenario's linear progression by overlooking actions and events that would be predicted to take a scenario in a different direction than that scripted may be more appropriate, for instance engineering the stabilization of a patient that is not adequately resuscitated. Alternatively, unplanned events can be allowed to play-out and engineered to resolve satisfactorily before returning or looping back to the main script.

responding to changing circumstances). These dimensions are underpinned by three fundamental requirements for effective teams: shared mental models; mutual trust; and closed-loop communication. While a number of alternative team frameworks have been developed,[28, 29] most published assessment tools reflect these basic principles. Unlike the team as a whole, the ability to make an assessment of an individual's performance within a team is limited, and potentially only reliably measured in a 'standardized team' with faculty playing the roles of other team members.

19.4.2 Instructional design

MSA's capacity to observe individuals and teams under conditions in which contextual elements are scripted and controlled provides considerable benefits over other assessment methods. Consequently, the design and delivery of contextually appropriate scenarios is critical and should be specified in the assessment methodology. Contextual elements include clinical features of the case including time course and clinical complexity. Situational events and cued interactions with acting faculty can be scripted to elicit NTS such as information processing, workload, problem-solving, and team processes mentioned above. Adding or subtracting support and prompting by faculty also changes complexity. Enabling scenarios to branch in response to the quality and timeliness of treatment increases authenticity; however, at the potential cost of unwanted increases in case complexity and reduction in standardization (see Table 19.1). While the controlled environment of a simulation centre has some advantages, *in situ* simulation provides an opportunity to test individuals and, in particular, teams within their workplace. This also tests the environment itself.

19.4.3 Test design

With greater attention given to activities, such as task analysis, designers of assessment programmes are now better able to specify observable performance elements which has led, in turn, to the development of measurement tools that support reliable and valid testing of performance across a range of clinical, non-technical, and team competencies.[3–5, 7, 10, 22] While a single measurement tool for healthcare teams would seem desirable, in general the different contexts and purposes require a tool to be at the very least modified to be fit for purpose. Published team tools include: the Behavioural Marker Risk Index (BMRI),[30] designed to measure information transfer in surgical teams and which is claimed to be predictive of patient outcome; Observational Teamwork Assessment for Surgery,[31] a well-validated instrument that measures teamwork in each of the three sub-teams in the operating theatre (surgery, nursing, anaesthesia); and the Critical Care Teamwork Rating instrument from the University of Auckland,[32] which assesses teamwork of the whole critical care team during a crisis. The latter instrument has been demonstrated to be equally reliable when used by trained external raters and team participants for self-assessment,[33] suggesting the items are relatively intuitive, and may assist teams to reflect on their team processes in the workplace.

19.5 **Conclusion**

MSA's capacity to adjust and control contextual elements makes it a useful alternative or adjunct to other assessment methods. It is particularly suited to assessment focused on management of dynamic events, team processes, and interaction with environment. Programmes should be individualized with careful attention to instructional design elements.

References

1 Dillon GF, Boulet JR, Hawkins RE, Swanson DB. Simulations in the United States Medical Licensing Examination™ (USMLE™). Qual Saf Health Care 2004;**13**(Suppl 1):i41–i45.

2 McIvor W, Burden A, Weinger MB, Steadman R. Simulation for maintenance of certification in anesthesiology: the first two years. J Contin Educ Health Prof 2012;**32**(4):236–242.

3 Berkenstadt H, Ziv A, Gafni N, Sidi A. Incorporating Simulation-Based Objective Structured Clinical Examination into the Israeli National Board Examination in Anesthesiology. Anesth Analg 2006;**102**(3):853–858.

4 Murray DJ, Boulet Kras JF, McAllister JD, Cox TE. A simulation-based acute skills performance assessment for anesthesia training. Anesth Analg 2005;**10**(1):1127–1134.

5 Weller JM, Robinson BJ, Jolly B, et al. Psychometric characteristics of simulation-based assessment in anaesthesia and accuracy of self-assessed scores. Anaesthesia 2005;**60**(3):245–250.

6 Boulet JR, Murray D, Kras J, Woodhouse J, McAllister J, Ziv A. Reliability and validity of a simulation-based acute care skills assessment for medical students and residents. Anesthesiology 2003;**99**:1270–1280.

7 Matos FM, Raemer DB. Mixed-realism simulation of adverse event disclosure: an educational methodology and assessment instrument. Simul Healthc 2013;**8**:84–90.

8 McRobert A, Causer J, Vassialidis J, Watterson L, Kwan J, Williams M. Contextual information influences diagnosis accuracy and decision-making in simulated emergency medicine emergencies. Qual Saf Health Care 2013;**22**:478–484.

9 Hogan MP, Pace DE, Hapgood J, Boone DC. Use of Human Patient Simulation and the Situation Awareness Global Assessment Technique in practical trauma skills assessment. J Trauma 2006;**61**:1047–1052.

10 Gisondi MA, Smith-Coggins R, Horter PM, Soltysik RC, Yornold PR. Assessment of resident professionalism using high-fidelity simulation of ethical dilemmas. Acad Emerg Med 2004;**11**(9):931–937.

11 Watterson LM. High-stakes performance assessment (Chapter 35). In: Riley RH (ed.). A manual of simulation in healthcare. Oxford: Oxford University Press; 2008, 501–518.

12 NSW Medical Council website: Performance Assessment Program <http://www.mcnsw.org.au/page/doctors–performance–conduct–health/professional-performance/performance-assessment/>

13 DeMaria S, Samuelson ST, Schwartz AD, Sim AJ, Levine AI. Simulation-based assessment and retraining for the anesthesiologist seeking reentry to clinical practice: a case series. Anesthesiology 2013;**119**(1):206–213.

14 Schmutz J, Manser T. Do team processes really have an effect on clinical performance? A systematic literature review. Br J Anaesth 2013;**110**(4):529–544.

15 Marshall SD, Mehra R. The effects of a displayed cognitive aid on non-technical skills in a simulated 'Can't Intubate, Can't Oxygenate' crisis. Anaesthesia 2014;**69**(7):669–677.

16 Schuwirth LWT, Southgate L, Page GG, et al. When enough is enough: a conceptual basis for fair and defensible practice performance assessment. Med Educ 2002;**36**:925–930.

17 Stephen R, Lew SR, Page GG, Schuwirth LWT, et al. Procedures for establishing defensible programmes for assessing practice performance. Med Educ 2002;**36**:936–941.

18 Schuwirth LWT, van der Vleuten CPM. Assessing professional competence from methods to programs. Med Educ 2005;**39**:309–317.

19 Boulet J. Summative assessment in medicine: the promise of simulation for high-stakes evaluation. Acad Emerg Med 2008;**15**:1017–1024.

20 Schuwirth LWT, van der Vleuten CPM. Changing education, changing assessment, changing research. Med Educ 2004;**38**:805–812.

21 Miller GE. The assessment of clinical skills/competence performance. Acad Med 1990;**65**(Suppl.): S63–S67.

22 Savoldelli GL, Naik VN, Joo HS, et al. Evaluation of patient simulator performance as an adjunct to the oral examination for senior anesthesia residents. Anesthesiology 2006;**104**:475–481.

23 Flin R, Maran N. Non-technical skills: identifying training, and assessing safe behaviours (Chapter 22). In: Riley RH (ed). A manual of simulation in healthcare. Oxford: Oxford University Press; 2008, 303–320.

24 Jha AK, Larizgoitia I, Audera-Lopez C, Prasopa-Plazier N, Waters H, Bates D. The global burden of unsafe medical care: analytic modelling of observational studies. Qual Saf Health Care 2013;**22**(10):809–815.

25 Rogers SO, Gawande AA, Kwaan M, et al. Analysis of surgical errors in closed malpractice claims at 4 liability insurers. Surgery 2006;**140**(1):25–33.

26 Lingard L. Rethinking competence in the context of teamwork. In: The question of competence: reconsidering medical education in the twenty-first century. Hodges B, Lingard L, editors. New York, NY: Cornell University Press; 2012, 42–69.

27 Salas E, Sims DE, Burke CS. Is there a 'Big Five' in teamwork? Small Group Research 2005;**36**:555–599.

28 Mazzocco K, et al. Surgical team behaviors and patient outcomes. Am J Surg **197**(5):678–685.

29 Passauer-Baierl S, et al. Re-validating the Observational Teamwork Assessment for Surgery tool (OTAS-D): cultural adaptation, refinement, and psychometric evaluation. World J Surg 2014;**38**(2):305–313.

30 Weller J, et al. Evaluation of an instrument to measure teamwork in multidisciplinary critical care teams. Qual Saf Health Care 2011;**20**:216–222.

31 Weller J, et al. Validation of a measurement tool for self-assessment of teamwork in intensive care. B J Anaes 2013;**111**(3):460–467.

32 Weller J, et al. Measuring Team performance in simulation-based training of intensive care teams. In: 15th annual meeting of SESAM. Mainz: Germany; 2009.

33 Cumin D, et al. Creating a multidisciplinary operating room simulation course (MORSIM) for training and research: overcoming barriers. Simul Healthc 2014;**9**(1):73–73.

Chapter 20

Research in simulation

Alexander (Sandy) Garden

Overview

- Good research is based on the application of sound research methods to a worthwhile question, after a thorough literature review.
- The choice of method should be based on the nature of the question.
- Much simulation-based research relates to the investigation of human performance and education to improve the latter.
- The measurement of performance and learning are often complicated by the need to ensure that the measurements are valid and reliable representations of underlying theoretical concepts referred to as constructs.
- Sources of bias and artefact must be adequately controlled, and the experimental design needs to identify and measure covariates, otherwise it will be impossible to exclude alternate explanations for the research findings.
- Because the research may not have any direct benefit to participants, and because of the frequent power imbalance between investigators and participants, there are potentially complex ethical issues.

20.1 Introduction to research in simulation

The methodological considerations in research involving simulation are no different from those in other academic fields, and these are fully discussed in standard textbooks of quantitative[1, 2] and qualitative[3, 4] research methods. This chapter is limited to a discussion about challenges that are commonly encountered while undertaking research in the context of simulation to improve clinician performance and patient safety. Simulation is enticing to researchers because of the potential for a high degree of experimental control. However, in practice it can be difficult to define endpoints for the measurement of experimental effects and there are an enormous number of covariates that can produce biased results. Research in these areas, therefore, draws heavily from the disciplines of applied behavioural research and applied education research using quantitative and qualitative research methods.

From a practical perspective, the key concepts when undertaking research using simulation are the development of worthwhile and feasible research questions, and the use of appropriate research methods to generate trustworthy findings that may be used to change policy and practice.

20.2 **Worthwhile and feasible research**

Any research endeavour is driven by a balance between the interests and aspirations of the investigators, the priorities of those funding the research, and the subsequent 'publishability' of the completed work.

Research involving simulation can be considered in terms of the process of simulation (how it is enacted, including realism), the equipment that is employed, and the subsequent outcomes. In this way it is possible to anticipate the nature of worthwhile questions and the likely difficulties. Early publications included descriptions of simulation technology and addressed relatively simple questions such as the time taken to acquire simple skills such as laryngoscopy.[5, 6] Such studies are straightforward because the performance of technical skill is relatively easy to measure reliably.[7, 8] Numerous studies have described other simple outcomes such as the acceptability of simulation for education and a range of self-reported learning outcomes.[9–11] Because of clinicians' interest in new developments, the latter are likely to continue to be accompanied by relatively simple studies.

In contrast to the numerous and relatively simple types of research described above, evaluations of the technical performance of simulators[12, 13] are uncommon, even though they are important because of the enormous amount of money involved, the manufacturers' conflicts of interest, and the need to spend health budgets wisely. Other important and difficult studies are those that require the measurement of non-technical skills. This is much more difficult because of challenges with the reliability of measurement,[7] and the associated risk that experimental effects may be concealed by 'noise' in the measurement process. Investigations into the validity of generalizing experimental findings from the simulation environment to the clinical environment are just beginning to be reported,[14] and other important knowledge gaps such as the risk of negative transfer (incorrect learning in the simulator being transferred to the clinical arena) are yet to be investigated.

The evaluation of feasibility of a research project includes consideration of the investigators' expertise and track record, the proposed budget (it is easy to underestimate the true cost), the availability and willingness of participants, and the planned time frame. Some questions are thus more feasible within multicentre collaborations[15, 16] and collaborative grant applications are likely to have an advantage.

There are numerous worthwhile research questions and it is easy to fall into the trap of failing to undertake an adequate literature review before undertaking a research project. With easy access to computerized databases, a significant difficulty is limiting the results of a search to a manageable number of potentially relevant publications, and the assistance of a medical librarian can be invaluable.

20.3 **Methods**

The purpose of research methods is to ensure that data are collected in a systematic and ethical manner, and that they are appropriately analysed and interpreted, with conclusions that pay due diligence to competing or alternate explanations. Broadly speaking, research methods can be classified as either quantitative or qualitative. Quantitative research methods typically use statistical tests to analyse numerical data that are obtained through either experimental or observational studies, and to test formal hypotheses. This is the dominant research paradigm in biomedical research, and is frequently contrasted with qualitative research which is widely used in the social sciences, such as anthropology, sociology, and education. Qualitative approaches are particularly useful when attitudes, beliefs, and socially located phenomena, such are those found in teams, are under investigation. Qualitative research has been described as intrinsically exploratory,[17] and it involves making observations that are then analysed using descriptive and interpretive approaches, with hypotheses developed to explain the data. There is increasing acceptance of qualitative research methods within biomedical publications, and the choice of method should be driven by the question. The two approaches are viewed as complementary rather than competing, and can be used in combination.[18]

20.3.1 **Quantitative research**

Notwithstanding the importance of statistical analysis in quantitative research, it is the author's opinion that research training within medical education places excessive emphasis on statistical methods and insufficient attention on other aspects of research methods, such as measurement, experimental control, and sources of bias and artefact. Six consistent flaws have been identified in simulation-based educational research (see Box 20.1) and these should be carefully considered when planning an investigation. Other potential flaws can be avoided by considering the sources of bias as defined in the Cochrane Handbook.[19]

This chapter draws on established research methods from psychology and education[1, 2, 20] to place emphasis on issues related to measurement (including reliability and validity) and experimental control.

20.3.1.1 Measurement

Scientific conclusions regarding the presence or absence of an experimental effect are based on the interpretation of measurements made in relation to an intervention. Valid and reliable measurement is thus at the heart of experimental research, and important early decisions in any research endeavour are what to measure and how to measure it. In addition, because confidence in experimental findings hinges upon their ability to be replicated, experimental control is required, including a clear definition of the circumstances under which the experiment took place.

Research that addresses behaviour, performance, or learning frequently requires the measurement of abstract concepts for which appropriate measurement instruments may not be readily available, in contrast to physical quantities that are readily measured. For example, to measure effectiveness of simulation-based crisis resource management training,

> ## Box 20.1 Consistent flaws in simulation-based educational research[21]
>
> - Poor knowledge of literature beyond the scope of immediate specialty.
> - Lack of awareness of basic research design for education, behavioural science, and clinical discipline.
> - Poor attention to the measurement properties of the educational and clinical research variables, particularly reliability.
> - Properties of educational intervention, such as strength and integrity, rarely described.
> - Inconsistent statistical reporting conventions, with failure to report indices of central tendency (e.g. mean), dispersion (e.g. standard deviation), and effect size.
> - No attention to statistical power.

a tool is needed to measure a theoretical concept called 'competence in crisis resource management'. One solution is to use a pre-existing tool with accepted psychometric properties; alternatively, a new measurement tool could be developed, or a surrogate end-point could be measured (such as time to resuscitate a manikin). Either way, the construct of interest or the 'latent variable'[22] is operationalized into something that can be measured or observed. Typically, a scale or test is created with the assumption that it reveals the level of the underlying theoretical variable (in this case 'competence in crisis resource management'). The difficulty for the researcher is the need to establish that the scale or test actually measures the construct of interest (i.e. is a valid measurement), and that this can be measured in a replicable manner (i.e. that it is reliable).

20.3.1.1.1 **Validity of measurement** Validity in this context refers to the extent to which a measurement tool actually measures what it purports to measure and it is thus a most basic consideration. With theoretical constructs it is important to ensure that the measurement adequately represents the construct of interest and that other constructs are not being measured as well as, or instead of, the construct of interest. The concept of validity can be a source of confusion because numerous definitions have been created to cover different types of validity (see Table 20.1). The underlying idea is quite simple with different types of validity reflecting different dimension of a single concept. An authoritative discussion of these principles can be found in 'Standards For Educational And Psychological Testing'.[23] The Standards place emphasis on the different sources of evidence for validity and do not refer to different types of validity (see Table 20.2). Validity is regarded as a single concept, with no single all-encompassing test of validity. Evidence of validity may be determined by empirical study, theoretical or logical argument, and/or expert opinion. The determination of which aspects of validity are important in any particular situation is based on the

Table 20.1 Types of validity

Type	Description
Construct validity	This is an overarching concept that is supported by the other forms of validity and requires that[24]: i The construct is clearly defined and embedded in a theoretical framework that defines its relationship to other constructs. ii Ways to measure the hypothetical constructs are developed. iii Empirical testing of relationships between constructs and their observable manifestations. For example, discriminant validity where we would expect a high correlation between measures of theoretically related constructs (convergent validity) and low correlation between unrelated constructs (divergent validity).
Criterion-related validity	This refers to the strength of association between the 'new' measurement and an accepted standard measure (a criterion) of the construct of interest. For example, we might expect senior clinicians to perform better than their juniors.[25] Typically, this is calculated as a correlation coefficient. Criterion validity encompasses concurrent validity and predictive validity, where correlations are made with criteria at this point in time (concurrent) or in the future (predictive).

Source: data from Rosenthal R, Rosnow RL. *Essentials of Behavioral Research: Methods and Data Analysis*, 3rd edn. New York, NY: McGraw-Hill. Copyright © 2008 McGraw-Hill Higher Education, New York, NY, USA; Kazdin AE (ed). *Methodologic Issues and Strategies in Clinical Research*, 3rd edn. Washington, DC: American Psychological Association. Copyright © 2003 American Psychological Association; and DeVellis RF. *Scale development theory and application*, 3rd edn. Thousand Oaks, CA: SAGE Publications. Copyright © 2012 SAGE Publications, Inc., Thousand Oaks, CA, USA.

Table 20.2 Sources of evidence of validity

Source	Description
Test content	Does the test content appropriately reflect the construct that it is purporting to measure? This requires empirical analysis, logic, or expert opinion. Important considerations include the potential for construct 'under-representation' when the test fails to capture important aspects of the construct, and 'construct-irrelevance', where matters that are irrelevant to the construct are measured.
Response processes	This refers to the cognitive processes used by both the examinee and the judge. For example do other skills, that are not directly related to the construct, help with performance in a test; and in the case of the judges or raters, are they judging the same thing?
Internal structure of the test	For example, if the internal structure of a test is expected to reflect increasing difficulty, then a novice and an expert would be expected to perform differently on different test items. Internal structure is also used to assess reliability.
Relationship to other variables	This might include performance on related and unrelated constructs, and might involve experimental and correlational evidence.
Consequences of testing	For example if performance is used to determine entrance into a vocational training programme, and the performance is not domain-relevant, then the validity is questionable.

Source: data from American Educational Research Association, American Psychological Association, and National Council on Measurement in Education, Standards for Educational and Psychological Testing, 6th edn. Washington, DC: American Educational Research Association, Copyright © 2014 American Educational Research Association.

purpose for which the test or evaluation is being undertaken, in conjunction with available theory, empirical evidence, and expert judgement.[23] As practical suggestions, Kazdin[20] (p. 200) recommends that the number of theoretical constructs that are measured in any one experiment should be minimized and that more than one index of the construct of interest should be measured (e.g. more than one measure of 'competence in crisis resource management' in the example given above). Most authors are critical of the concept 'face validity', a term which basically means that 'it is reasonable and obvious that the items in a measurement scale assess what they are purported to measure'. However, the underlying assumptions may be wrong, and the name given to a measurement tool frequently reflects the intent of its creators, rather than supporting evidence.

20.3.1.1.2 **Reliability and measurement error** Reliability in this context refers to the consistency or stability of measurement;[20] i.e. the tendency to obtain the same result with repeated measurement. As with validity, this is a fundamentally simple concept that can be confusing because of multiple dimensions with names that suggest different types of reliability. Any form of measurement is subject to a degree of variability, and the difference between the 'true' measurement and a single observation defines measurement error. If the measurement error is randomly distributed, then with sufficient repetitions of the measurement, the error will average to zero and we will have a 'true' measurement. The magnitude of measurement error determines the number of repetitions that are required to determine the 'true' value, and thus defines the value of a single measurement. It is also important to distinguish between random error (which averages to zero) and systematic error, such as some form of offset in a measurement instrument, because the latter constitutes a form of bias that threatens validity.

The sources of measurement error are more complicated than is the case with the measurement of physical quantities. For example, if we administer a 'competence in crisis resource management' tool before and after an educational intervention and we find improved performance, what does this mean? Did the intervention work or did the participant make greater effort on the second administration? Was the participant so anxious on the pre-test that performance was impaired? Was the second rating undertaken using less stringent subjective criteria? Were there significant subject-experimenter effects (see Table 20.3)?

A range of statistical tests are available to evaluate reliability[23] (see Table 20.4). These are based on either correlation or analysis of variance, and the choice of test is determined by the aspect of reliability that is to be quantified. No single test answers all questions, although generalizability coefficients address most. The final decision regarding the degree of reliability that is required in a particular situation is a matter of professional judgement, based on the purpose of the measurement. For example, if an individual's 'competence in crisis resource management' score will be used in a high-stakes decision such as who will graduate from a vocational training programme, then reliability is critical.

20.3.1.2 Experimental design, bias, and artefact

Statistical tests tell us the likelihood or probability that a given experimental finding has occurred due to chance, but do not tell us why an experimental effect was found. The

Table 20.3 Subject-experimenter effects as sources of artefact in behavioural science

Effect	Description
Experimenter expectancy	Experimenter's expectations are conveyed unintentionally to the research subject and influence the results.
Experimenter characteristics	Age, gender, ethnicity, friendliness, attitudes, and status of experimenter may all influence the subject's behaviour. This provides a threat to the generalizability (external validity) of the findings.
Cues from the context of the experiment	This includes aspects of the experiment such as instructions given to the subject; the room where the experiment takes place. These are also called demand characteristics of the experimental situation.
Effect due to roles taken by the subject	Subjects volunteer for research for personal reasons and frequently try to place themselves in a positive light, particularly if there is a power imbalance with the researcher or investigator. For example: Good Subject (tries to please the experimenter) Negativistic subject (tries to disprove research hypothesis) Apprehensive subject (anxiety influences performance)

Source: data from Rosenthal R, Rosnow RL. *Essentials of Behavioral Research: Methods and Data Analysis*, 3rd edn. Boston, MA: McGraw-Hill, 2007 and Kazdin AE, *Research Design in Clinical Psychology*, 4th edn. Boston, MA: Allyn and Bacon; 2003, p. 637.

Table 20.4 Sources of evidence of reliability

Source	Description
Test-retest coefficient	The correlation between scores on an identical test administered at different times. If the test is re-administered soon after the first administration, then the result will be influenced by memory of the test, whereas with a long test-retest interval there may be real change due to uncontrolled confounding influences. The stability of the underlying construct is used to guide the inter-testing interval. If we are testing the effect of an intervention, we will be looking for change.
Internal consistency coefficient	The correlation among items within the test, hence also called the reliability of components. This typically produces an inflated estimate of reliability.
Alternate-form coefficients	Correlation between scores on parallel or equivalent forms of test administered in two independent testing sessions. Split-half correlation uses two halves of a single test rather than two distinct tests.
Rater-reliability	Inter-rater and intra-rater reliability are particularly important when the test score involves a high level of subjective judgement. In clinical psychology testing, a reliability coefficient of ≥ 0.85 is typically regarded as appropriate[20] and this degree of reliability requires appropriate training.
Generalizability coefficient	Based on generalizability theory, analysis of variance is used to estimate the magnitude and source of variability in test results. For example, if differences between raters contribute most of the variance in performance evaluation scores, then generalizability across observers will be reduced.
Test item function	Based on item response theory, enables the investigator to summarize how well the test discriminates among individuals with different levels of the construct being evaluated, i.e. provides a mathematical estimate of precision of measurement.

Source: data from Rosenthal R, Rosnow RL. *Essentials of Behavioral Research: Methods and Data Analysis*. 3rd edn. Boston, MA: McGraw-Hill; 2007, DeVellis RF, *Scale Development: Theory and Application*. 3rd edn. SAGE Publications, Inc.; 2012, p. 217, and *Standards for Educational and Psychological Testing*. 6th edn. Washington, DC: American Educational Research Association; 2014, p. 194.

explanation for experimental findings is inferred from the experimental design and assumptions regarding the control or measurement of covariates. Even with the use of valid and reliable tools, behavioural science is riddled with examples of covariates that must be measured or controlled to avoid erroneous conclusions. For example, in research into the effects of sleep loss on performance, a frequent error has been failure to consider the expected improvement in performance due to practice with the measurement tool, and the latter can be so large that it masks deterioration due to sleep loss. Failure to provide adequate control, with careful consideration of the influence of covariates, results in findings that cannot be adequately explained or cannot be generalized beyond the immediate experiment.

The double-blind, randomized controlled trial (perhaps placebo-controlled) is the gold standard in the evaluation of medical therapy, and the same principles can be applied to behavioural science. However, it may be impossible to blind the subjects regarding the purpose of the experiment or the nature of the treatment. For example, in experiments into the effects of fatigue on performance, the hypothesis is likely to be obvious to anyone with a rudimentary knowledge of the determinants of human performance, and participants are likely to know into which experimental condition they fall.[8] In addition, consideration must be given to the so-called Hawthorne effect, whereby participation in a study may impact upon performance improvement irrespective of the intervention.[1]

In addition to the use of valid and reliable measurement instruments, and management of potential covariates, there must be impeccable experimental technique to avoid or detect errors in data handling and analysis. This includes the use of appropriate techniques of randomization and blinding for those undertaking the data measurements and recordings.[19]

20.3.1.3 Statistical risk

There are two important statistical risks to address. The first is the risk of reporting a statistically significant effect that does not actually exist. This is the 'Type I' error and a probability (known as α) of 0.05 is the traditional threshold for an acceptable level of risk. The Type I error is usually well understood and does not warrant further discussion, except to note that an appropriate value for α in exploratory studies may be 0.1 rather than 0.05.[26] The second risk is of failing to find a statistically significant difference when an effect is really present. This is the 'Type II' error and the probability of this (known as β) is typically expressed in terms of statistical power, the probability of finding an effect if it exists. Power is thus mathematically defined as $1-\beta$ and the traditional value for acceptable power is 0.8, i.e. a 20% chance of failing to detect an experimental effect that is really present.

The importance of power rests in the planning of studies, particularly the calculation of sample sizes, and in the interpretation of negative studies. Statistical power has three determinants[26]: α (the probability of making a Type I error); the effect size (the degree to which the hypothesized phenomenon exists); and N, the sample size. The power of a study will increase if α is reduced, if the actual effect size is large, or if N is increased. Although these are relatively simple concepts, the actual calculation of power is complex and requires the use of an appropriate statistical programme or a nomogram such as those published by Cohen.[27]

20.3.2 **Qualitative research**

The qualitative researcher is typically observing, describing, and using non-numerical analysis, to interpret and explain a phenomenon under investigation. This approach has been widely used to investigate social phenomena, and as such is appropriate when studying phenomena where real, but invisible, social structures are influencing performance during simulation, such as teamwork, communication, decision-making, and conflict management.

Although more than 20 different genres of qualitative research have been described (e.g. ethnography, grounded theory, phenomenology, case-study, content analysis, narrative enquiry), they have common features.[28] These common features include intense and/or prolonged naturalistic contact between the researcher and the participant(s), with the researcher as the main instrument rather than the use of standardized instrumentation. The research typically takes place in a cyclical pattern with data collection followed by analysis and conclusions, followed by more data collection to verify conclusions. Most of the data for analysis are words that are records from observations, interviews, discussions, documents, and reflective notes. These words can amount to hundreds of pages of text, and they need to be condensed into patterns, frequently using some form of thematic analysis, such as 'grounded theory'.[29]

The risk of bias, posed by the researcher as the research instrument and the intense involvement between by the researcher and the participants, has been a significant barrier to the acceptance of qualitative research by the biomedical academic community. Notwithstanding those concerns, by virtue of the focus on events in their natural context, qualitative research allows a depth of description that can be impossible to achieve in quantitative research and thus has clear value. A range of strategies have been developed to overcome the risks of bias, and to provide increased validity and reliability to qualitative research findings[30–32] (see Tables 20.5 and 20.6).

The majority of qualitative research studies in healthcare are based on either in-depth interview techniques or focus-group studies.[33] The advantage of both of these techniques over quantitative methods, such as questionnaires, is related to the conversational context in which the interview or focus-group takes place. In-depth interview questions can extend beyond the investigator's initial hypotheses, and there is less potential for a 'gap' in meaning between the question and the answer, the so-called 'Type III' error where the wrong question is answered (see[17], p. 29).

20.4 **Ethics, deception, and conflicts of interest**

There are important ethical issues to address in research involving human participants, particularly when the research offers no specific advantage to the participant.

20.4.1 **Risks and benefits**

In research that offers no specific advantage to the participants there must be minimal if any risk associated with participation. One of the assumptions underlying simulation is that it causes no harm, but that is unproven. In research involving the evaluation of

Table 20.5 Validation techniques in qualitative research

Technique	Description
Triangulation	The use of more than one measure (data source and type, method of investigation, researcher, or theory) to corroborate the investigator's interpretation, or to identify outliers that contradict the developing theory.
Theoretical/purposive sampling strategies	Participants who have particular characteristics are selected. A deliberate search is made for contradictory, outlying, or negative cases that may challenge the conclusions. Care is also taken to ensure that the sample is representative. Subjects are sampled until 'saturation' is reached (no new themes are evident).
Respondent validation	Research participants check the transcript of their interview and later give feedback regarding the analysis and conclusions.
Check for researcher effects	Personal and intellectual biases that have shaped the researcher's thinking are explicitly stated, including the relationship between researcher and subjects, and the context of the research.
Check the meaning of deviant cases (outliers, extreme cases, contradictory findings)	Theory that is developed, must be able to explain disconfirming evidence and rival explanations adequately explained.

Source: data from Miles MB, Huberman AM, Saldana J. Drawing and verifying conclusion, *Qualitative Data Analysis: A Methods Sourcebook*, 3rd edn. SAGE Publications, Inc.; 2014, pp. 275–322, and Pope C, Ziebland S, Mays N. Analysing qualitative data, *British Medical Journal* 2000;320(7227):114–116.

Table 20.6 Evaluation of reliability in qualitative research

Method	Description
Coder reliability	When data care classified (coded) into different phenomenological categories, inter-coder and intra-coder reliability should be checked.
Clear audit trail	A clear description of the process of data collection and analysis, including the relationship between these processes, so that the reader can decide if the process is valid, and could potentially replicate the study.
Replication	The theory developed should be confirmed with further data, and the existing work should be replicable by another investigator.

Source: data from Miles MB, Huberman AM, Saldana J. Drawing and verifying conclusion, *Qualitative Data Analysis: A Methods Sourcebook*, 3rd edn. SAGE Publications, Inc., 2014; pp. 275–322, and Pope C, Ziebland S, Mays N. Analysing qualitative data, *British Medical Journal* 2000;320(7227):114–116.

performance, there could be unforeseen potential risks attributable to the participant's emotional response to the experience, or even the potential for negative transfer of incorrect learning from the simulator to the clinical environment. The risks can be difficult to determine and this requires careful and unbiased peer review during the planning stages.

20.4.2 **Information and consent**

The provision of sufficient information for participants to make a free choice to participate in the absence of coercion is a fundamental ethical principle. However, research involving human behaviour is fraught with a dilemma caused by the potential for the provision of information to alter participants' subsequent performance. A controversial solution is to undertake some form of deceptive research. The spectrum of deception ranges from total misrepresentation of the purpose of the research, through to failure to mention all the details and to undertake covert or unobtrusive measures. The practice is controversial because it breaches participants' trust, and participants cannot give *bona fide* consent. For those unfamiliar with the concepts of deception, it is worth reading about the obedience experiments of Stanley Milgram. Three criteria have been suggested in the justification of deceptive studies (see [20], p. 503): the investigators need to convince external reviewers that there is no alternative, that the degree of deception is warranted, and that the magnitude of potential harm is low. To minimize potential harm, participants should be appropriately debriefed after the experience, although 'appropriate' debriefing is ill-defined. For example, by whom should it be done and when? From the perspective of the participant it should be done at the end of the experimental session, whereas from the perspective of the investigator, it should be after all participants have been studied. The extent of any harm and the effectiveness of the debriefing should probably be evaluated during a pilot study.

Even in the presence of full information, if there is an unequal relationship between the investigators and the participants, then there is a risk of consent being given with a degree of coercion. For example, numerous studies have been undertaken by specialist anaesthetists using anaesthesia registrars (trainees) as the experimental participants. In special relationships such as these it can be difficult to ensure that consent is freely given, and for participants to be confident that they can withdraw at any time without prejudice. One solution is to engage a third party in the recruitment process to ensure that those who decline to participate remain anonymous to the investigators.

Another problem with research in the simulation environment is the presence of conflicts of interest. A conflict of interest is defined as any situation in which an investigator may have an interest or obligation that can bias, or be perceived to bias, a research project (see [20], p. 536). There are numerous examples in the anaesthesia literature where investigators have undertaken research using equipment in which they have a financial interest. When the investigator stands to gain in a material way based on the research findings (such as an increase in sales if their product is shown to be effective), it is better for the research to be undertaken by third parties who do not have a financial interest in the tool being studied.

20.5 **Conclusion**

The purpose of this chapter is to provide an introduction to simulation-based research and to emphasize common concerns and flaws in experimental methods. Many of the problems that arise in simulation-based research relate to difficulties caused by the need to measure theoretical constructs rather than physical quantities, and the need to ensure that the measurement tools are valid and reliable. The need to ensure that there is appropriate experimental control, with the measurement of relevant covariates, requires a clear understanding of the related literature. It is important to calculate statistical power, first to determine sample size, and second to appropriately analyse negative finding (e.g. no difference between treatments). Qualitative research is playing an increasing role in research that is examining social phenomena, and as with quantitative research, there is a need for rigorous attention to validity and reliability. Ethical considerations are particularly critical in research where there is likely to be no direct benefit to the participants, and where there is often a power imbalance between the investigator and the participant. These are frequent considerations in simulation-based research, particularly where participant performance is under investigation, and so the ethical concerns should be addressed as part of the initial assessment of the feasibility of a research project.

References

1 **Rosenthal R, Rosnow RL**. Essentials of behavioral research: methods and data analysis. 3rd edn. Boston, MA: McGraw-Hill; 2008.

2 **Kazdin AE, editor**. Methodologic issues and strategies in clinical research. Washington, DC: American Psychological Association; 2003.

3 **Denzin NK, Lincoln YS, editors**. Handbook of qualitative research. 4th edn. Thousand Oaks, CA: Sage Publications; 2011.

4 **Miles MB, Huberman AM, Saldana J**. Qualitative data analysis: a methods sourcebook. 3rd edn. Thousand Oaks, CA: Sage; 2014.

5 **Denson JS, Abrahamson S**. A computer-controlled patient simulator. JAMA 1969;**208**:504–508.

6 **Abrahamson S, Denson JS, Wolf RM**. Effectiveness of a simulator in training anesthesiology residents. J. Med. Educ. 1969;**44**:515–519.

7 **Gaba DM, Howard SK, Flanagan B, Smith BE, Fish KJ, Botney R**. Assessment of clinical performance during simulated crises using both technical and behavioural ratings. Anesthesiology 1998;**89**:8–18.

8 **Garden AL, Robinson BJ, Kappus LJ, Macleod I, Gander PH**. Fifteen-hour day shifts have little effect on the performance of taskwork by anaesthesia trainees during uncomplicated clinical simulation. Anaesth Intensive Care 2012;**40**:1028–1034.

9 **Allan CK, Thiagarajan RR, Beke D, Imprescia A, Kappus L, Garden A, et al**. Simulation-based training delivered directly to the Pediatric Cardiac Intensive Care Unit engenders preparedness, comfort and decreased anxiety among multidisciplinary resuscitation teams. J. Thorac Cardiovasc Surg. 2010;**146**:646–652.

10 **Garden A, Robinson B, Weller J, Wilson L, Crone D**. Education to address medical error—a role for high-fidelity patient simulation. N Z Med J. 2002;**115**:132–134.

11 **Howard SK, Gaba DM, Fish KJ, Yang G, Sarnquist FH**. Anesthesia crisis resource management training: teaching anesthesiologists to handle critical incidents. Aviat Space Environ Med. 1992;**63**(9):763–770.

12 **Garden AL, Robinson BJ, Arancibia CU, Carron TJ, Monk S, Vollmer J, et al**. Unrecognised malfunction in computerized patient simulators [letter]. Br J Anaesth. 2004;**93**:873–875.

13 **Lejus C, Magne C, Brisard L, Blondel P, Asehnoune K, Pean D**. What is the accuracy of the high-fidelity METI Human Patient Simulator physiological models during oxygen administration and apnea maneuvers? Anesth Analg. 2013;**117**(2):392–397. Epub 2013/06/08.

14. Weller J, Henderson R, Webster CS, Shulruf B, Torrie J, Davies E, et al. Building the evidence on simulation validity: comparison of anesthesiologists' communication patterns in real and simulated cases. Anesthesiology 2014;**120**(1):142–148. Epub 2013/08/02.

15 Cheng A, Hunt EA, Donoghue A, Nelson K, Leflore J, Anderson J, et al. EXPRESS—Examining Pediatric Resuscitation Education Using Simulation and Scripting. The birth of an international pediatric simulation research collaborative—from concept to reality. Simul Healthc. 2011;**6**(1): 34–41. Epub 2011/02/19.

16 Cheng A, Hunt EA, Donoghue A, Nelson-McMillan K, Nishisaki A, Leflore J, et al. Examining pediatric resuscitation education using simulation and scripted debriefing: a multicenter randomized trial. JAMA Pediat. 2013:1–9. Epub 2013/04/24.

17 Kirk J, Miller ML. Reliability and validity in qualitative research. Newbury Park, CA: Sage Publications; 1986, 87.

18 Tashakkori A, Creswell JW. Editorial: the new era of mixed methods. J of Mixed Methods Res. 2007;**1**(1):3–7.

19 Higgins JPT, Altman DG, Sterne JAC, editors. Assessing risk of bias in included studies. In: Higgins JPT, Green S, editors. Cochrane handbook for systematic reviews of interventions version 510 [updated March 2011]. The Cochrane Collaboration; 2011.

20 Kazdin AE. Research design in clinical psychology. 4th edn. Boston, MA: Allyn and Bacon; 2003.

21 McGaghie WC, Issenberg SB, Petrusa ER, Scalese RJ. Effect of practice on standardised learning outcomes in simulation-based medical education. Med Educ 2006;**40**(8):792–797.

22 DeVellis RF. Scale development theory and application. 3rd edn. Applied Social Research Methods Series;26. Bickman L, Rog DJ, editors. Thousand Oaks, CA: Sage Publications; 2012.

23 Standards for educational and psychological testing. 6th edn. Washington, DC: American Educational Research Association; 2014.

24 Clark L, Watson D. Constructing validity: basic issues in scale development. In: Kazdin AE, editor. Methodological issues and strategies in clinical research. Washington, DC: American Psychological Association; 1995, 207–231.

25 Devitt JH, Kurrek MM, Cohen MM, Fish K, Fish P, Noel AG, et al. Testing internal consistency and construct validity during evaluation of performance in a patient simulator. Anesth Analg. 1998;**86**:1160–1164.

26 Cohen J. A power primer. Psychol Bull. 1992;**112**:155–159.

27 Cohen J. Statistical power analysis for the behavioural sciences. Hillside, NJ: Lawrence Erlbaum Associates; 1988.

28 Miles MB, Huberman AM, Saldana J. Chapter 1. Introduction. Qualitative data analysis: a methods sourcebook. 3rd edn. Thousand Oaks, CA: Sage; 2014, 3–16.

29 Corbin J, Strauss A. Basics of qualitative research: techniques and procedures for developing grounded theory. 3rd edn. Thousand Oaks, CA: Sage; 2008.

30 BMJ. Editor's checklists 2014 (1 November 2014): <http://www.bmj.com/about-bmj/resources-authors/article-types/research/editors-checklists>

31 Miles MB, Huberman AM, Saldana J. Chapter 11. Drawing and verifying conclusion. Qualitative data analysis: a methods sourcebook. 3rd edn. Thousand Oaks, CA: Sage; 2014, 275–322.

32 Tong A, Sainsbury P, Craig J. Consolidated criteria for reporting qualitative research (COREQ): a 32-item checklist for interviews and focus groups. Int J Qual Health Care 2007;**19**(6):349–357. Epub 2007/09/18.

33 Sofaer S. Qualitative research methods. Int J Qual Health Care 2002;**14**(4):329–336. Epub 2002/08/31.

Chapter 21

Airway training devices

Cindy Hein, Cyle Sprick, and Harry Owen

Overview

- There are many devices to assist education and training in airway management. Choice of aids needs to be based on learning objectives and the level of skill of students or trainees.

- Airway training using simulators can be structured to provide the most efficient training but this training must be integrated with clinical training for it to be most effective. Motivation is required to achieve superior performance.

- Airway training models do not always replicate normal anatomy or may not allow practice guidelines to be followed. This can interfere with learning by students and trainees and adversely impact on clinical care.

- Perceptual focusing is common during crises, so advanced airway training must stress when to abandon attempts and also emphasize rescue techniques for when ventilation cannot be achieved promptly.

- Expertise in airway management is very dependent on context and setting, so assessment of competence requires a range of scenarios in different settings. Simple additions or modifications can be made to patient simulators to increase the degree of challenge or complexity.

- Video feedback is routinely used during 'full mission' simulation. Video feedback of procedures and interventions attempted by novices on simple-skill trainers is also effective, and enhances learning and skill retention.

21.1 Introduction: changing the way airway management is taught

All medical, nursing, and paramedic training programmes require their graduates to be proficient in basic airway management. Postgraduate training programmes of acute-care disciplines require acquisition of more advanced airway interventions. Airway skills have been taught in a range of settings (see Box 21.1) including some unethical use of patients and animals in the past,[1] but thankfully good ethical guidelines are now almost universally in place.

> ## Box 21.1 Past and present settings and materials used for teaching and training airway interventions
>
> - Humans
> - Cadavers
> - Newly deceased (in the emergency room)
> - In coma (in intensive care units (ICUs))
> - Prisoners of war
> - Undergoing routine anaesthesia (in the operating room (OR))
> - Manufactured difficulties or simulated complications (in the OR)—this has given rise to adverse outcomes
> - Recovering from anaesthesia (in the post-anaesthesia care unit (PACU))
> - Simulated patents (for minimally invasion training such as head positioning, etc.)
> - Animals
> - Small and large live animals (e.g. dogs, kittens)
> - Dead animals (e.g. white deer)
> - Simulators
> - Skill trainers (bench models, desktop/small simulators, medical phantoms, etc.)
> - Whole-body manikins
> - Computer-controlled patient simulators
> - Virtual reality (VR) simulators

The sections of this chapter outline basic airway training devices useful for all health professionals and airway training devices that support learning advanced airway interventions. Regular review of training curricula is necessary because guidelines do change in both content and emphasis. For example, the recommendations on endotracheal intubation in resuscitation were changed when it became apparent that attempts to intubate the trachea could themselves contribute to mortality.[2] These guidelines and recommendations should be readily available for trainers and trainees to refer to.

21.2 Education in airway care

Teaching methods have been strongly influenced by theories of the way that motor skills are learned and how expertise is developed. The three-stage theory of motor skill acquisition proposed by Fitts and Posner[3] remains widely accepted as the basis for acquisition of psychomotor skills. The three stages provide a sound basis for designing airway skill teaching that accommodates the transition from novice to expert.

21.2.1 Cognitive stage (novice)

In this stage, the novice learns the sub-tasks (steps) needed to perform the skill or complete the task. Understanding and mastering individual steps or sub-tasks occurs at different rates, so performance will appear halting and erratic. This stage has been referred to as being 'consciously incompetent'. Skill trainers are ideal at this stage providing a low-cost platform for repetitive practice of particular steps and sequences.

Demonstration of steps by the trainer, videos, posters, and display models enhance learning. Systems and devices that facilitate observation and recording of elements of the learner's performance help the trainers provide specific feedback. 'Practice makes permanent', so skill trainers must provide an accurate representation of real life to ensure only correct behaviour patterns are laid down.

21.2.2 Integrative stage (advanced beginner/trainee)

Practice and feedback facilitates progress to this stage where the learner must still think about performance but can move between steps more 'fluidly' and can cope with minor variations. Practitioners in this stage can be thought of as being 'consciously competent'. Whole body manikins are good to use at this stage because they require clinically appropriate actions and positioning.

21.2.3 Autonomous stage (competent)

The practitioner no longer needs to think about the steps, readily adapts to different conditions, can accommodate interruptions, and can divide attention with other tasks. This is the stage of being 'unconsciously competent' but this can lead to lapses and other errors. High-fidelity simulators and a system to record performance and replay it for review are most appropriate at this stage; however, the optimal educational design is yet to be determined.[4]

21.3 Aids for teaching and learning airway management

A large variety of airway devices and skill trainers have been developed for airway management. Many are very good; some, less so. The key message is to understand the limitations of each device and tailor their use to the skill and needs of the learners.

Some airway devices function differently in simulators to the way they perform in patients. The maker of the McCoy laryngoscope, for example, has specifically warned against using it in simulators. Also, when the airway anatomy of a model departs from the normal range, performance of airway devices based on patient size can be a problem. The upper airway of the SimMan UPS has been reported to be unrealistically short,[5] so recurrent training only on this simulator could lead to unintended and unwanted clinical behaviours.

21.3.1 Basic life support

Key airway/ventilation skills in basic life support (BLS) are: identifying and removing airway obstruction, opening the airway using head tilt/chin lift or jaw thrust manoeuvres, identifying signs of life (i.e. normal breathing), insertion of an oropharyngeal airway, and artificial ventilation using expired air techniques or a self-inflating resuscitator.

21.3.1.1 Basic airway manoeuvres

A comparison of basic airway trainers revealed that many had shortcomings. Some design features that made it easy to make and clean the models or to open the airway impacted on realism and meant that only stylized psychomotor skills were used by learners.[6] This may limit transfer of skills and contribute to poor performance in an actual emergency. Also, most models appear young, fit looking, and have good teeth, whereas most people requiring resuscitation are old and overweight and many have poor dentition or dentures. The better models have soft features, articulation between head and neck, and a palpable mandibular angle (see Box 21.2).

21.3.1.2 Artificial ventilation

While ventilation by first responders at sudden cardiac arrest may be less important than once thought, there will always be a need for this, particularly in trauma care, resuscitation from drowning, and after return of spontaneous circulation. Basic training models must have a visible chest rise but models for healthcare professional training should be able to indicate volume and flow to provide feedback on performance as hypo/hyperventilation can be harmful, particularly during cardiopulmonary resuscitation.[7]

Using differently shaped face masks and adding a beard to models are good ways of increasing difficulty with mask ventilation. The models need to be disinfected when mouth-to-mouth or mouth-to-mask techniques are being taught. The risk of student-to-student

---

Box 21.2 Useful features for a model for teaching and assessing basic airway management

+ Realistic size and appearance
+ Head tilt and chin lift can open airway (needs a chin that lifts and a head that tilts)
+ Palpable mandible that can be felt to move with a 'jaw thrust'
+ Exhalation from the mouth (look/listen/feel)
+ Stomach insufflation or other indication of overzealous ventilation
+ Range of difficulties (obesity, facial hair)
+ Easily cleaned between students

spread of infection is very low[8] but students with a respiratory illness or open sores should be taught separately from the rest of the group.

Two inexpensive devices, both from O-Two Medical Technologies, can help improve training in artificial ventilation. The Mini Ventilation Training Analyzer (<http://otwo.com/training-aids/ accessed online 2014/05/16>) is a system that demonstrates the impact of too rapid lung inflation during artificial ventilation. The device has a stylized lung and stomach and, while appropriate ventilation causes only lung inflation, overzealous ventilation causes progressive filling of the stomach bag. The other device is also from O-Two—a self-inflating resuscitator which has a spring-loaded mechanism that operates to limit pressure and flow when the bag is squeezed too fast (<http://otwo.com/smart-bag-mo-manual-resuscitator/>). The auditory and tactile feedback it gives makes it an excellent training tool.

Prior to 2010, peak resuscitation organizations recommended cricoid pressure during bag and mask ventilation in resuscitation, as well as in emergency intubation, to reduce the incidence of gastric regurgitation. However, if the cricoid pressure is applied in the wrong place, wrong direction, wrong amount of force, or at the wrong time, the technique leads to distorted anatomy, reducing ventilation and potentially making airway insertion difficult.[8] A recent meta-analysis[9] demonstrated that commercial and/or investigator constructed trainers are equivalent in significantly improving cricoid pressure performance, particularly where feedback mechanisms are available, but retention of this skill is limited.

21.3.2 Advanced airway interventions

21.3.2.1 Supraglottic airway devices

The original Supraglottic Airway Device (SAD) Laryngeal Mask Airway (known as the LMA Classic (<http://www.lmaco.com/>)) has a related range of reusable and single-use devices, and several manufacturers have brought out their own versions.

Typically, it is not easy to insert a correctly sized LMA in airway training models and when the cuff of the LMA is inflated the device does not rise up as it does in patients. This may encourage trainees to use a smaller LMA than ideal. Difficulties in insertion are exacerbated by inadequate lubrication of both the device and the airway model. The CPaRlene model (<http://www.eNasco.com>) has a useful feature arising from the shape of the pharynx and larynx. If the LMA used is smaller than recommended, some air often passes into the stomach providing a good demonstration of why following the manufacturer's guidelines on sizing is important. The C-Trac (Teleflex Medical Australia) is a video-enabled intubating LMA that can also help demonstrate issues associated with using an LMA of the wrong size.

Recently, there has been an explosion in innovation and design of SADs (also referred to as Extraglottic Airway Devices (EADs)) which may not perform well in the current airway trainers—e.g. the SLIPA™ and i-Gel have this problem. SAD manufacturers should be encouraged to sponsor development of training models to support realistic device training.[10]

21.3.2.2 Endotracheal intubation

Endotracheal intubation (ETI) is widely considered to be the ultimate airway intervention and is sometimes referred to as the 'gold standard'. There are several elements to consider in education on ETI: basic skill training, ETI in the difficult airway, rescue from the failed intubation, and skill retention.[11] See Box 21.3 for a list of features to look for in simulators for teaching endotracheal intubation.

21.3.2.2.1 **Technique** Observation of the trainee's actions can assist the trainer to provide specific feedback on technique. Video feedback provides insight into technique that assists learning[8] and can also improve skill retention.[12] Some technique traits are easy to see and record—e.g. rotating the laryngoscope (and levering on the teeth) and poor posture during intubation, which can have a big influence on success.[13] Without special aids, the view the trainee or student has of the larynx can only be guessed by the teacher. Ambu make an intubation trainer (<http://www.ambu.com/>) with an open side for visualizing intubation and there is an inferior Chinese copy of this (see Figure 21.1).

21.3.2.2.2 **Visualization** Other ways for the instructor to view the larynx during intubation training include placing a fibre-optic scope in the nasopharynx to view intubation or installing a small camera in the nasopharynx of an airway trainer. Miniature cameras are inexpensive but the short distance between camera and glottic opening means that

---

Box 21.3 Features to look for in a simulator for teaching endotracheal intubation

- Dimensions similar to human anatomy—including distance from teeth to vocal cords and vocal cords to carina
- Epiglottis moves realistically during laryngoscopy
- Has realistic-looking vocal cords
- Has palpable upper airway cartilages (thyroid and cricoid)
- Shape of upper airway changes with external force applied to airway cartilages
- Allows practice of additional measures to confirm intra-tracheal placement such as the Oesophageal Detector Device (ODD) (see Box 21.4) and intra-tracheal ridges
- Can see chest rise with lung inflation
- Lung auscultation in axillae (not apices)
- Epigastric auscultation
- Allows capnography measurement of carbon dioxide (CO_2)
- Range of difficulties, e.g. limited mouth opening, limited neck movement, prominent upper incisors, etc.

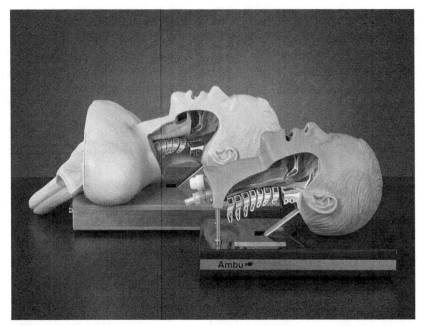

Fig. 21.1 A tale of two airway trainers. One device is from a Scandinavian medical equipment manufacturer and has been refined over several years. The other is made in China and appears to be a copy with some modifications and rough edges—*caveat emptor*!
Reproduced by permission of Ambu/AS (Ambu.com). Copyright © 2015 Ambu A/S (Ambu.com).

a 'close-up' lens is required for focus and this can cost more than the camera. A propriety training aid, the ET-View™, is an endotracheal tube with a miniature USB camera at its tip (<http://www.etview.com/>). It must be connected to a computer but it is easy to use the system and it does provide a large and clear image on the screen. Unfortunately, the ET-View trainer is both expensive and available only in an 8.0 mm ET-tube when a 7.0 mm endotracehal tube (ETT) is the largest size recommended for many airway models.

A number of systems designed to facilitate intubation of patients can be used to assist ETI training through demonstrating laryngeal anatomy. We have used the Glidescope (<http://verathon.com/products/glidescope-video-laryngoscope>), the Truphatek EVO2 (<http://www.truphatek.com>), the C-Trac (previously at <http://www.lmana.com>), the AirTraq (<http://www.airtraq.com>), the King Vision (<http://www.kingsystems.com>), the AP Advance (Venner Medical: <http://www.vennermedical.de>), and the Pentax AWS (Ambu) to demonstrate airway anatomy of patient simulators. Some video-laryngoscope systems are currently being introduced into anaesthesia—e.g. McGrath® laryngoscope (<http://www.aircraftmedical.com/index.htm>) and the Pentax AWS-S100 Airway Scope (<http://www.pentax.co.jp/english>)—and they may be useful training aids.

The AirwayCam is a unique system for demonstrating conventional laryngoscopy and intubation on a simulator and in clinical care but it has an appreciable learning curve of its own. In theory, the AirwayCam would give the trainer a trainee's eye view of the airway.

21.3.2.2.3 **Model variety** There is some evidence that learning intubation is more efficient if models that are easier to intubate are presented before more difficult airways.[14] Novices learn more from a successful intubation than an unsuccessful attempt. Once a particular airway has been mastered, little is gained from repeated successful intubations; so, as experience is gained, health professionals need to be presented with more challenging airway simulations. Some models incorporate features that can make intubation more difficult but this needs to reflect the area the trainee is training to work in. For example, trismus is a common cause of difficulty in the pre-hospital setting, so models that have this feature are useful for paramedic student training. In anaesthesia, anatomy and pathology are more likely to be a cause of airway difficulty.

21.3.2.2.4 **Confirmation of intubation** ETI is supposed to improve patient outcome; however, recent evidence suggests that there is an unacceptably high incidence of errors in airway management[8, 15] in pre-hospital settings and emergency departments, even after training. The results of such an error such as unrecognized oesophageal intubations is very serious but even a relatively minor error during intubation can cause problems, e.g. mild hypoxaemia from main stem bronchus intubation can give rise to major injury in a trauma patient with head injury.

There are many methods of confirming correct ETI and students should use those listed within resuscitation council and anaesthesia guidelines but be aware that no one method is 100% fail proof. Not all guidelines list the same methods but a comprehensive list from the Australian Resuscitation Council (ARC),[7] the American Heart Association (AHA) Inc.,[16] the European Resuscitation Council (ERC),[8] and the American Society of Anesthesiologists (ASA)[11] can be created (see below) and used during training of ETI (see Box 21.4 and Figure 21.2).

When training in ETI skills, confirmation methods must be practised and become second nature. However, there is no one skill trainer available today that allows all of the

---

Box 21.4 Methods of confirming correct intubation

- Visualize ETT passing through the vocal cords
- Feel the clicks of a bougie on tracheal cartilages (if used)
- Utilize an ODD
- Visualize continuous bilateral chest expansion
- Auscultate the epigastrium ('breath sounds' should not be heard)
- Auscultate over lung fields bilaterally in axillae to determine adequate and equal breath sounds
- Observe $ETCO_2$ by either continuous waveform or colorimetric device

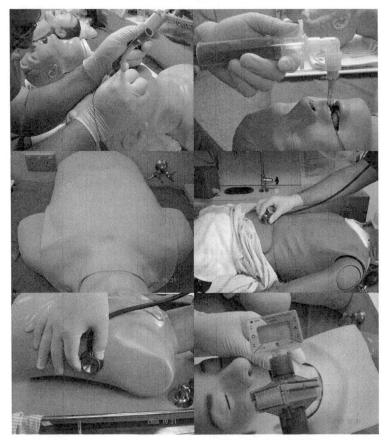

Fig. 21.2 This sequence of images shows the sequence of steps used to confirm endotracheal intubation. The ODD is typically used during resuscitation from cardiac arrest and must be used before artificial ventilation.

methods listed to be performed. High-fidelity simulators (e.g. METI's Human Patient Simulator® (HPS) (<http://www.meti.com/blog/>)) come close but are very expensive and certainly not widely available for basic training. Students and trainees can be informed of limitations of the simulators (e.g. the LMA doesn't rise up on inflation of the cuff) but this then reduces the value of the training.

Looking for chest rise is an important sign after intubation but for novices a model without a chest can have some value, seeing one lung lying limp while the other inflates provides a good lesson on the need to control how far the tube is advanced beyond the cords. Once this is understood, further practice requires a model with a thorax and epigastrium that makes the trainee go through confirmation of successful intubation in the correct manner. Beware of models that encourage poor practice like the Laerdal® Airway Management Trainer (<http://www.laerdal.com/au/>) that has auscultation points only over lung apices. Once this has been mastered, a model that allows the difficulty of intubation to be increased is very desirable—e.g. the AirSim Multi (Trucorp (<http://www.trucorp.com/>). In our unit we use at least five models in basic ETI training, including the simulators mentioned above. Recurrent practice in recognizing signs of correct intubation make it more likely that oesophageal intubation will be identified.[8] The sequence of ETI confirmation can be seen in Figure 21.2.

When a misplaced ETI occurs in training, it should be recognized quickly and the 'patient' extubated immediately and if a second attempt to intubate also fails, the 'patient' should be ventilated by other means (face mask, SAD, cricothyrotomy, etc.). This ensures that skill learning incorporates use of alternative skills that would be utilized in clinical practice. Students should also be aware that, in some circumstances, methods of confirming correct intubation can produce false-negative results such as in the case of pulseless or poorly perfused patients with little or no $ETCO_2$ being detected. This error (referred to as a Type II error) may lead to an ETT that is properly placed, being unnecessarily removed.

21.3.2.2.5 **How much intubation practice is needed?** The rate of learning ETI can be quite different between trainees and some may never become competent. Published studies vary of how many intubations are required,[17] but it would be better to track the acquisition of skills of individual practitioners than rely on a particular number of attempts.[18]

There are several questions about ETI that need to be asked: can practitioners become competent in ETI through practice on patient simulators alone? This is most important for non-anaesthesia healthcare professionals who do not have good access to patients undergoing ETI as part of their clinical care.[19] For practitioners who need to maintain a very high level of expertise in airway management techniques, is there an optimal mix of simulator training and clinical exposure? This is very relevant to anaesthesia providers who will be presented with some very difficult airways that must be managed quickly and correctly to avoid morbidity and mortality. Techniques learned during simulation need to reflect local policies because they will quickly be extinguished if they are not reinforced by clinical experience.[18]

21.3.2.3 Trans-tracheal ventilation

Occasionally, ventilation cannot be achieved without bypassing the upper airway and using a trans-tracheal technique to access the airway. In an emergency, this is best achieved by cricothyrotomy (cricothyroidotomy) and there are several training aids and models made specifically for this purpose. It is certainly possible to make a training aid from discarded items or inexpensive components from a hardware store and there is much to recommend this approach for familiarization with equipment for trans-tracheal ventilation and the steps of the procedure. Skill trainers and whole-body patient simulators are needed when the task is being practised in context and 'when' is being learned as well as 'how'. All the models have limitations but some have a more lifelike feel than others; an example of this is the Smiths Medical Tracheostomy Head (<http://www.smiths-medical.com/>) that has 'skin' that moves, wrinkles, and stretches.

21.4 **The challenge of airway competence**

There have recently been several publications indicating that specialists and trainees in acute-care disciplines do not have the skills needed for difficult airway management.[7, 8, 16, 20] Deaths due to airway mismanagement have prompted official recommendations for teaching and maintaining skills to avoid patient injury from hypoxia.[21] It is clear from these reports that repeated attempts at intubation are dangerous and training needs to reflect this. If trainees are allowed to make multiple attempts at intubation in a skills lab then they are being set up to transfer this undesirable behaviour to the OR or ED. Difficult airway management (DAM) guidelines have been developed by many organizations and every hospital with trainees should have a range of skill trainers that can be used to teach DAM. Teaching should be based on national guidelines and local variations should be avoided.

Video feedback can help identify errors and provide insight into improving performance,[12, 22] so should be a routine part of simulation training to gain the most from training time. To take advantage of the range of airway simulators available for use, training should be embedded in clinical curricula; however, cognitive bias must be considered.[23]

There are several courses that include airway care teaching (e.g. Advanced and Immediate Life Support (ALS/ILS) courses: <http://www.resus.org.au/als_ils/>). The airway training in these courses is quite short but useful in relation to the desired outcome.

21.5 **Airway training devices in the future**

Training using simulators have become essential in airway management training, falling into three distinct categories. One is teaching basic airway management to all health professionals. Automated systems that provide feedback have been developed for this in the same way that systems have been developed to guide external cardiac compression during CPR. Resusci Anne Simulator® (<http://www.laerdal.com/au/>) provides real-time feedback on ventilations and compressions.

Another category is providing a way of developing skills in advanced airway interventions for anaesthetists and other specialists. VR has been increasingly used for this. Sophisticated VR airway simulators that can effectively prepare trainees for clinical procedures on patients exist now[24] with recent advances in VR simulators for cricothyroidotomy training.[25]

The third category includes health professionals who need to provide effective airway care occasionally and often in difficult settings. Pre-hospital ETI has such a high failure rate[ARC 7, 8, 16] and thus the 'occasional intubator' will increasingly be expected to undertake simulation for skills maintenance. Laryngoscopic skills decay rapidly and it is possible that another device or intubating system that has less skill decay over time will become more widely used.[26]

An emerging category is Google Glass, an innovative device that has been trialled in various clinical situations. One medical centre in Boston, US, is using Google Glass to '. . . facilitate hands-free communications and to expedite workflow . . ', while at a Rhode Island hospital, doctors are connecting it with off-site specialists while they are still in the ED.[27] Google Cardboard is an inexpensive VR system for Android phones. Advances like this may evolve into more readily accessible airway training.

21.6 **Conclusion**

Airway-skills teaching has to be designed to cater for all adult learning styles and to adapt to the rate of learning by participants. Content has to be relevant to engage learners, so their background and achievements must be ascertained when the teaching is being planned. Most healthcare practitioners want to provide better care, so relevant links that can be made to actual clinical care can be helpful. Training that may lead to negative transfer must be avoided.

Teaching should be based on published guidelines rather than personal opinions and use the best available equipment rather than local 'fixes'. Outcome of patient care is dependent on the 'weakest link', so all steps need to be included in teaching.

Deliberate, repeated skills practice is important to develop 'unconscious competence' so that working memory is freed up for situational awareness and other tasks. There is no one device that provides everything needed for airway-skills teaching, so quality education and training will require airway-teaching facilities to have several different skill trainers and patient simulators.

There are many aids for teaching airway skills and choice should be determined by the learning objectives of the teaching or training. There is no one model or device that can be recommended over another and some that are useful for one group may not be as useful for another. Budgets for airway skills and simulation training facilities will need to reflect this now and in the future.

References

1 World Medical Association. World Medical Association Declaration of Helsinki: ethical principles for medical research involving human subjects. JAMA 2013;**310**(20):2191–2194.

2 **Cummins RO, Hazinski MF**. Guidelines based on the principle 'First, Do No Harm'. New guidelines on tracheal tube confirmation and prevention of dislodgement. Resuscitation 2000;**46**:443–447.

3 **Fitts PM, Posner MI**. Human performance. Brooks/Cole Publishing Company;1967.

4 **Kennedy CC, et al**. Advanced airway management simulation training in medical education: a systematic review and meta-analysis. Crit Care Med 2014;**42**(1):169–178.

5 **Hesselfeldt R, Kristensen MS, Rasmussen LS**. Evaluation of the airway of the SimMan™ full-scale patient simulator. Acta Anaesthesiol Scand 2005;**49**(9):1339–1345.

6 **Rosenthal E, Owen H**. An assessment of small simulators used to teach basic airway management. Anaesth Intensive Care 2004;**32**(1):87–92.

7 Australian Resuscitation Council. Equipment and techniques in adult advanced life support. Guideline 11.6 Dec 2010, 2010: <http://www.resus.org.au>

8 **Nolan JP, et al**. European Resuscitation Council guidelines for resuscitation 2010. Resuscitation 2010;**81**(10):1219–1276.

9 **Johnson RL, et al**. Cricoid pressure training using simulation: a systematic review and meta-analysis. BJA 2013.

10 Hein C, Owen H, Plummer J. A proposed framework for deciding suitable extraglottic airway devices (EAD) for paramedics to use. Resuscitation 2010;**81**:914.

11 Committee on Standards and Practice Parameters: the American Society of Anesthesiologists. Practice guidelines for management of the difficult airway: an updated report by the American Society of Anesthesiologists Task Force on management of the difficult airway. Anesthesiology 2013;**118**(2):251–270.

12 Hein C, Owen H, Plummer J. A training program for novice paramedics provides initial laryngeal mask airway insertion skill and improves skill retention at 6 months. Simul Healthc 2010;**5**(1):33–39.

13 Matthews AJ, Johnson CJH, Goodman NW. Body posture during simulated tracheal intubation. Anaesthesia 1998;**53**(4):331–334.

14 Plummer J, Owen H. Learning endotracheal intubation in a clinical skills learning centre: a quantitative study. Anesth Analg 2001;**93**(3):656–662.

15 Cook TM, Woodall N, Frerk C. Major complications of airway management in the UK: results of the Fourth National Audit Project of the Royal College of Anaesthetists and the Difficult Airway Society. Part 1: Anaesthesia. Br J Anaesth 2011;**106**(5):617–631.

16. Neumar R, et al. Part 8: adult advanced cardiovascular life support: 2010 American Heart Association guidelines for cardiopulmonary resuscitation and emergency cardiovascular care. Circulation 2010;**122**(18 suppl 3):S729–S767.

17 Owen H, Plummer JL. Improving learning of a clinical skill: the first year's experience of teaching endotracheal intubation in a clinical simulation facility. Med Educ 2002;**36**(7):635–642.

18 Graham CA. Advanced airway management in the emergency department: what are the training and skills maintenance needs for UK emergency physicians? EMJ 2004;**21**(1):14–19.

19 Johnston BD, Seitz SR, Wang HE. Limited opportunities for paramedic student endotracheal intubation training in the operating room. Acad Emerg Med 2006;**13**(10):1051–1055.

20 Cook TM, et al. Major complications of airway management in the UK: results of the Fourth National Audit Project of the Royal College of Anaesthetists and the Difficult Airway Society. Part 2: intensive care and emergency departments. Br J Anaesth 2011;**106**(5):632–642.

21 Department of Health Western Australia— Office of Safety and Quality in Healthcare.. From death we learn. Lessons from coronial findings: a very difficult airway (Dec 2008): <http://www.safetyandquality.health.wa.gov.au/>, accessed online 04/08/2014.

22 Farquharson AL, et al. Randomized trial of the effect of video feedback on the acquisition of surgical skills. Br J Surg 2013;**100**(11):1448–1453.

23 Park CSMD, et al. Training induces cognitive bias: the case of a simulation-based emergency airway curriculum. Simul Healthc 2014;**9**(2):85–93.

24 Goldmann K, Steinfeldt T. Acquisition of basic fiberoptic intubation skills with a virtual reality airway simulator. J Clin Anesth 2006;**18**(3):173–178.

25 Proctor MD, Campbell-Wynn L. Effectiveness, usability, and acceptability of haptic-enabled virtual reality and mannequin modality simulators for surgical cricothyroidotomy. Mil Med 2014;**179**(3):260–264.

26 Maharaj CH, et al. Retention of tracheal intubation skills by novice personnel: a comparison of the Airtraq and Macintosh laryngoscopes. Anaesthesia 2007;**62**(3):272–278.

27 No authors listed. Emergency providers see big potential for Google Glass. ED Manag 201;**26**(5):55–58.

Part 3

Applied simulation

Chapter 22

Cardiopulmonary resuscitation and training devices

Sheena M Ferguson and Anthony R Lewis

Overview

- The availability of passive and low-fidelity tools for a simulation lab is extensive and varied.
- Factors which influence your selection include course frequency, course size (number of manikins needed), durability, cost, portability, and level of functionality.
- Provide a variety of devices and stretch the learning and practice of effective interventions; consider having several different manikins.
- Rotate learners through several stations to practice different manikins; each can add something different to the learning experience.
- Select the right tool for the learning objective.
- There has been a rapid increase in the use of tablet-based devices for simulation.
- Safety, flexibility, and adaptability are key features of tablet-based devices.
- Simulation of cardiopulmonary bypass is challenging and 'Orpheus' is a dedicated simulation solution.

22.1 Introduction to cardiopulmonary resuscitation and training devices

There are numerous passive manikins and partial-task trainers available on the market (Ambu, Armstrong, Gaumard, Laerdal, Limbs & Things, Lifeform, Nasco, Simulaids, etc.) to augment the range of low- to high-fidelity full-body human simulators. The numbers of products available is extensive and recent website such as KeyIn (<www.keyin.to>) publish validated reviews of them. Customer service and post-purchase assistance varies tremendously. The end of this chapter includes a resource section; this information is provided as a service, not an endorsement of any particular product.

The routine training of the healthcare professions and the community training of the public have given rise to the widespread use of basic cardiopulmonary resuscitation (CPR) manikins over the last few decades. Manikins are now so affordable, portable, and low-tech (e.g. the Styrofoam versions) that community instructors are able to purchase their own personal sets for CPR training. As additional courses were developed in first aid, intermediate, and advanced life support, additional passive trainers have become more and more available. Over time, greater fidelity, more interventions, and increased features have been added allowing the products to become more realistic. However, by their very nature such trainers are passive and automation is negligible. The basic-level task trainers are specifically useful for the acquisition of psychomotor skills, rather than focusing on any comprehensive simulated physical response for the student to interpret. Decisions about the best tools for a particular simulation centre must be made with consideration of many factors.

22.2 Cardiopulmonary resuscitation

CPR manikins that allow ventilation and compressions cover a wide range of simulation options. High-fidelity, full-body simulators provide one of the highest degrees of realism for CPR situations, in that they demonstrate chest rise, return breath, generate pulses, are able to be defibrillated, and other features. These are suited for small learner numbers with a high instructor-to-student ratio. These simulators are also limited in their portability. For large groups of students or routine courses, the passive trainers or low-fidelity systems can be optimal. Early on at the inception of CPR training, the passive manikins which provided the greatest student and instructor feedback were the 'Annies' by Laerdal in the early 1960s. When CPR training became more stringent, the electronically recording 'Annies' that recorded the number and depth of compressions and the number and depth of ventilations became the manikin of choice. This same version also had an audible 'tick-tock' tone so that the novice could have a reference for how quickly to compress. These manikins did provide the student with a more lifelike physical work-out for simulating CPR, but as the philosophical approach to education has changed over the years, the rigidity of this type of exercise fell out of favour. A review of the recall and implementation of CPR by the public identified that laypersons often felt pulses when they were absent and didn't feel pulses when they were present. A reduction in the complexity of the sequence and the number of steps was needed. The 'perfect' recorded strips model was retired and performance standards were simplified. Since actual people requiring CPR did not have recorders, the emphasis was on chest compression as fast as the provider could provide and generating an adequate pulse became the new standard for performer feedback. These 'Annies' are still very common as they are robust and make excellent rescue victims when they are no longer needed for CPR, because of their weight which more closely simulates an actual victim and the sturdiness of the material from which they were made.

Simulation of compressions and ventilations during CPR, specifically in terms of difficulty and rigour, can be a complex and perplexing dilemma. Novices may lack real-world experience to be able to make a comparison with simulated CPR. Some experienced CPR providers feel that the more substantial manikins are more realistic but others disagree. The variety of manikins on the market and the inter-manikin differences can be viewed as reflecting patient variability. That is, there are variations that mimic the particulars of the clinical situation and the range of pathologies that can be encountered clinically.

At the lower end of the spectrum, although quite functional, are the Styrofoam, pillow, or inflatable models. These are lightweight and highly portable and affordable, though being somewhat featureless in terms of anatomical landmarks and providing any feedback to the student. This requires additional emphasis by the instructor to demonstrate or simulate anatomical features on students or use alternate methodologies.

In summary, there is a wide variety of manikins on the market. Looking at the range of vendor catalogues in the United States, there are at least 47 different types and models of devices for CPR training.

22.3 **Manikin selection**

There are many factors to consider when purchasing CPR manikins for a simulation lab. The director will need to determine the portion of the budget that will be directed towards such items. The determining factors in this assessment will include the focus of the simulation centre itself. If the centre will be supporting community activities such as public programmes for a training CPR, then a larger number of manikins will be needed. Recent guidelines from the national organizations that have developed CPR training programmes is for each student to have their own manikin; this is very different from previous recommendations that the student: manikin ratios were 6:1.

The selection of a manikin should also include a clear plan for managing infection control. While some centres may still provide each student with their own manikin face (to swap out between testing), this requires an area for decontamination on-site or a decontamination (sterile processing) programme for off-site location. Most centres avoid this time and expense by using a disposable airway or shield of some type. The complexity and time to replace a disposable airway, as well as the actual cost of these disposable airways, should be a factor in the selection process.

Additional considerations may extend to portability issues, manikin weights (select more weight for simulation exercises if rescue is involved, less weight if routine transport to external venues is planned). The size of the manikins, as well as the size and weight of the cases, are all important when mobility is a part of the centre's scope of activities.

The durability of the device should also be considered. Styrofoam or lightweight plastics will not endure high-utilization situations. Alternatively, the sturdier and heavier weight manikins can withstand many thousands of hours of use. Some of the manikins in the 'BATCAVE' (Albuquerque, University of New Mexico) are still very usable a decade later and were in the moderate price range when purchased. An equipment log with purchase date, service history, and descriptions of problems with each manikin is essential.

Another consideration is the ability to repair a manikin and the cost of the repair. In some manikins the cost of the repair approaches the cost of the manikin. When considering purchase, look at the number of movable parts and the materials of which the manikin is made. Inquire with the sales representative about the warranty, a list of replaceable parts, labour charges, and note where the manikin needs to be shipped for repairs. 3D-printing technology has become cheaper and more user-friendly over recent years and many organizations can now print replacement parts locally. If your manikins are going to be portable, assess the costs, weight, and functionality of storage cases. Finally, inquire about the composition of the manikins to identify latex-allergy risk. This emerging problem is so important that it should be a prime consideration. Manikin diversity on the market today allows the educator to tailor their purchases to the needs of their students. Manikins are available in a wide range of sizes and colours. The paediatric sizes include 'premie' (premature baby) (e.g. Gaumard), newborn, toddler, child, adolescent, as well as adult ranges. For in-hospital settings, many of the manikins can be altered to include tracheostomy tubes, gastric tubes, casts, and a variety of other devices. Manikins can also be ordered in a variety of skin tones, and may include ethnic skin features. Manikins are available that simulate a variety of patient conditions, such as the series that represent obese patients.

One other element manikin selection in CPR would be the basic life support scenarios, such as choking. Manikins with physical obstructions are available on the market. These manikins can also be obese or pregnant and are available in a variety of age ranges as well. An object is connected around the manikins' neck by a barely visible nylon thread to prevent them from getting lost or separated from the manikin. A properly delivered abdominal thrust relieves the obstruction and the student has a visual cue of the airway obstruction being relieved. See Box 22.1 for a list of features to consider before purchase

Box 22.1 Features to consider prior to CPR mannequin purchase

- Budget allowance and manikin cost
- Course frequency and size
- Types of learners (laypersons, healthcare professionals)
- Specialty situations or care
- Infection control components
- Ease and cost of disposable airway/shield use
- Durability of the manikin (latex-free)
- Portability (manikin cases)
- Repair ability and cost
- Diversity and ranges
- Additional BLS features (choking feature, obesity, skin tones)

of CPR mannequins. The relative importance of these factors will vary with the centre's mission, customer base, and budget.

22.4 **Defibrillators**

22.4.1 **Devices**

The cornerstone of CPR training is airway, breathing, and circulation (A,B,C). D has traditionally been defibrillation. The Gaumard virtual series includes a virtual defibrillator in their low-fidelity computer interface-based systems. Many centres have had substantial difficulty obtaining either enough defibrillators for training or having the current version. To begin, assess what your lab needs. Novices becoming familiar with defibrillation may not need the newest version, whereas rapid response or code teams may benefit from the same models they will encounter in a clinical situation. Assess your centre's affiliations: an academic medical centre may present different opportunities than a smaller school. Be aware of changes in healthcare organizations in your community that are downsizing or expanding as these often present opportunities for acquiring equipment. Often, the sheer size of the institution's purchases can (i) assist in negotiating a stripped-down version of a newer model, (ii) a trade-in of an older model for a newer one, and (iii) a shifting of resources within the organization to allow for an exchange for an older but still functional unit from a low-use area.

22.4.2 **Safety**

A major consideration is safety of staff and participants. Should a simulation centre defibrillator be fully functional? There are several schools of thought on this topic. Some centres use full energy at the recommended levels. Proponents argues are that the students know that 300 joules (higher settings) takes longer to reach than 2 joules (lower settings). The student has the benefit of audible (the energy whine) and visual cues (red lights) on the defibrillator. They learn to look for these when troubleshooting in a clinical situation. Opponents argue about the potential danger of an accidental discharge with student or faculty injury. The responsibility of the faculty is enormous and there must be little room for student misadventure. Given the numbers of times defibrillators are used in many centres, the wear and tear on each defibrillator is very high.

Other labs use live energy but at a vastly reduced energy, usually the lowest setting. Proponents argue for a safer environment, and the ability to have audible (though the time to a full charge is very short and this may result in learning incorrect procedures) and visual cues. On the other hand, the student (later the practitioner) not expecting charging to take so long may believe the machine to be dysfunctional. Note that newer defibrillators may have reduced charge times compared with earlier models.

A third solution is to disengage the discharge route from the defibrillator. The audible and visual cues are intact but there is no electrical discharge. Clinical engineering at the hospital will be able to assist with this modification. This preserves all of the positive arguments previously discussed, but with none of the disadvantages. The caution in this scenario is that a defibrillator thusly disabled must not find its way into a clinical situation. It should have appropriate labels affixed. There may be some centres where the defibrillators are never turned on or charged but the students lose many of the opportunities for learning.

22.4.3 Semi-automatic external defibrillators

The widespread implementation of semi-automatic external defibrillators (SAEDs) in public areas mandates their incorporation into CPR curricula. These devices that are widely known as automatic external devices are actually misnamed, because they are not automatic and require operator initiation of the electrical discharge based on a system prompt. Nonetheless, they are in widespread use, and can be found at most airports, large shopping centres, sports venues, and industrial facilities. In CPR training, most vendors that produce these devices for use in the community produce and market training versions of their SAED.

Organizations that are responsible for guidelines (e.g. the American Heart Association, the European Resuscitation Council) alter their recommendations on CPR, first aid, and emergency care based on the latest research findings assessed by the International Liaison Committee on Resuscitation (ILCOR). The early versions of SAEDs were often not easily altered. Their thrifty cost and limited alterability necessitated a repurchase of newer models to allow instructors to use them in training with the more recent guidelines. Hence, programmability and the ability to update via a chip or other method are important. If the parent organization is planning a large purchase of SAEDs, discussions with the vendor should include the trainers being included in the training package. The ability to change or select different scenarios assists the instructor with having to take out the 'verbal staging' and allows the student to respond to the situation. The durability of the casing is important for good value in length of service. The padded cases that come with some of the SAEDs does prevent damage as some of the plastic cases do not hold up well to repeated use. The ability to use both AC and DC power assists with the variability of having long sessions or the need for portability to areas without electrical outlets. Be warned that some devices may use an unusual or expensive battery. The SAED warranty, access to repairs, and again upgradeability, should also be considered. If the community has selected a standard public vendor, for familiarity and training effectiveness, this also plays a part in the product selection if community training is part of the centre's mission. Otherwise, the model that the organization is using internally is the obvious choice. Finally, the importance of assessing the cost, durability, and functionality of the SAED training pads cannot be overstated. Some training pads are very flimsy and not repairable. Others are much more robust. The costs can vary considerably. The stickiness or ability to clean the manikins after use is also a factor. Centres that use a large number of these training pads should consider using Velcro tabs to apply the pads to the manikin. Such skin tone Velcro packets are inexpensive and barely visible. Box 22.2 lists some factors that should guide purchase of a SAED device. The relative importance of these factors will vary with the centre's mission, customer base, and budget.

> **Box 22.2 Factors to consider when purchasing a SAED**
>
> ◆ Upgradeability with algorithm guidelines
>
> ◆ Cost per unit
>
> ◆ Programmability with different scenarios
>
> ◆ Carrying case type and cost
>
> ◆ Durability of the material
>
> ◆ Electrical and/or battery-powered
>
> ◆ Warranty and repair ability
>
> ◆ SAED brand used internally and/or in the community
>
> ◆ SAED training pad cost and durability

22.5 Cardiac auscultation simulation

Harvey® has been a presence in the medical simulation community for approximately 40 years.[1] At 96 pounds, Harvey is a moderately mobile half-body human simulator, capable of simulating a variety of human vital functions: breath sound auscultation in six areas (see also Chapter 25), cardiac auscultation in nine areas, 30 different signs of cardiac disease, digitally driven impulses for pulses, and various amplitude and intensity of findings that provide opportunities for the novice to the competent learner. There is also a built-in functionality that allows Harvey to 'speak' via an instructor through a speaker providing a history-taking feature. The system includes a stand-alone system for an independent learning opportunity in addition to the usual group-learning experiences that manikins provide, which can be used with learners from a variety of health professions' programmes.

22.6 Mobile simulation technology

The popularity and functionality of tablet computers has increased in recent years. Concurrently, there has been a rapid development of tablet-based applications that simulate patient monitors and defibrillators. Mobile technology also includes devices which use various connection options to link a control and a display unit.

22.6.1 Devices, applications, and connectivity

22.6.1.1 Devices

These can be divided into tablet and non-tablet devices.

Tablet devices can be categorized by their operating system. The three main operating systems are iOS (Apple), Android (Google), and Windows (Microsoft).

The iOS system runs exclusively on Apple devices such as the iPad, iPod Touch, and iPhone. Since its launch in 2010, there have been six versions of the iPad, all with a 9.7 inch screen size. The iPad Mini was released in 2012 and has a smaller screen size of 7.9 inches. The Android operating system (OS) is based on Linux and is an open-source licence developed by Google. The Windows 8 OS is developed by Microsoft. Many manufacturers utilize both the Android and Windows 8 OS on phones and tablet devices. Consequently, the screen sizes are more variable.

Non-tablet devices are usually bespoke hardware solutions. Many stethoscope simulators utilize this technology as well as SimCentral with the SimOxy, SimCap, and SimObs devices.

22.6.1.2 Applications

Applications, or 'apps', are the software programs which run on portable devices. Although tablet devices often have features such as location detection, cameras, and Internet connectivity, they are typically less powerful than personal computers and run on battery. The development of mobile apps can exploit novel features of the tablet but the developer is often constrained to the hardware specifications and configurations of the tablet. User interface design is a key component of mobile app development. Ease and simplicity of use is fundamental to successful app development.

22.6.1.3 Connectivity

Internet connectivity is a key feature of mobile devices. A tablet can connect directly to the Internet via a SIM card using a mobile network such as 3G or 4G. Alternatively, the tablet may connect via a wireless network. A wireless network is provided by a wireless router which, in turn, is connected to the Internet. **Bluetooth** is another connectivity option but this is mainly used to transmit and receive audio to other devices such as speakers and microphones. **Zigbee** is similar to Bluetooth and is more suited for control and monitoring.

Connectivity is important as it not only allows devices to connect to the Internet but it also allows devices to connect to each other. This feature is exploited by many tablet-based simulation applications such that one tablet becomes the controller and the other tablet becomes the monitor. The screen output of the tablet can also be streamed or mirrored to a larger screen using a wireless network and an additional device such as Apple TV or Google Chromecast.

22.6.2 Specific simulators

22.6.2.1 Tablet-based simulators

SimMon was one of the first tablet-based patient monitor simulator applications. The same application is installed on iOS devices and the simulator can be run as a stand-alone monitor or installed on two devices allowing remote control. The first version of SimMon displayed numeric values of heart rate, oxygen saturations, blood pressure, and respiratory rate. Subsequent versions have added waveforms for each of these parameters as well as end-tidal carbon dioxide. There is no defibrillator feature in SimMon.

Simulation Monitor is similar to SimMon in that it runs on all iOS devices. In addition to SimMon, Simulation Monitor also has patient sounds and an image bank of radiology images and ECGs. Blood results can also be displayed. There is a defibrillator feature but the controls do not mimic a defibrillator control panel.

Dart runs on iOS devices and on a laptop. As well as the features in the above applications, there is the ability to create scenarios which can be saved and run again.

ALSi (iSimulate Pty Ltd) runs on two iPads and uses one iPad as a controller (the facilitator) and the second iPad as the student display. Different modes can be selected allowing the display to mimic a patient monitor, defibrillator, or AED. All of these modes have been designed to mimic a real-life device as closely as possible allowing this application to be used extensively in Advanced Cardiac Life Support (ACLS) courses instead of a live defibrillator. This has inherent safety benefits as no live energy is used when the shock button is pressed. ALSi also has features which are usually seen on high-fidelity simulation solutions such as multi-parameter trending, the ability to create scenarios, a fully editable blood result function, display of any image or video file, and the ability to import and export scenarios to other ALSi users.

22.6.2.2 AED simulators

ALSi includes an AED simulator but there are many other applications which mimic AEDs.

22.6.3 **Non-tablet-based simulators**

SimCentral produces three mobile simulation devices, all utilizing a handheld control unit which communicates via ZigBee to a small display unit. The display unit can show oxygen saturations and pulse rate (**SimOxy**), end tidal carbon dioxide (**SimCap**), and vital signs (**SimObs**). Many manufacturers of stethoscope simulators also utilize bespoke hardware, which allows a control unit to communicate with a device connected to a stethoscope allowing the educator to manipulate the sounds heard by the student.

22.6.4 **Benefits of mobile devices**

The ease of use and portability of mobile devices makes them ideal for many aspects of training and teaching. Tablet devices also allow the display and storage of presentations, images, and videos. Hence, they are very useful for impromptu and 'Just-in-Time Teaching' (JiTT) if the educator has prepared material on the device for such occasions.

22.7 **Cardiopulmonary bypass simulation**

22.7.1 **Rationale for the use of simulators in cardiopulmonary bypass training**

Cardiopulmonary bypass (CPB) is characterized by a relatively low frequency of rapidly evolving but potentially serious critical incidents. In a recent American study, Stammers and Mejak[2] surveyed the results of more than 650,000 perfusions carried out at nearly 800 institutions and reported that serious injury resulting from perfusion-related incidents occurred in approximately one in 2,000 cases.

22.7.2 'Orpheus'—a high-fidelity perfusion simulation system

'Orpheus' is a high-fidelity patient simulator (manufactured by Terumo) specifically intended for use in the domain of CPB practice. It is a hybrid system comprising a computer-controlled hydraulic model of the human circulation and a suite of real-time computer models which continuously calculate various cardio-respiratory, thermal, and pharmacodynamic parameters within the patient. In addition, the system supervisor (trainer) can use the simulator control program to initiate a variety of systemic failures (power, gas, circuit, and oxygenator) or to deliver a series of audiovisual cues to the perfusionist (trainee). The system is designed to interface with any modern heart-lung machine (HLM), patient-monitoring system, and CPB circuit.

22.7.2.1 Description of the 'Orpheus' perfusion simulation system

The principal components of the 'Orpheus' perfusion simulation system are the:

- Hydraulic simulator
- Electronic control unit
- Simulator control software
- Failure devices
- Trainee screen
- Recording system

These components are shown in Figures 22.1 and 22.2.

The hydraulic simulator is a 'single' circulation comprising two chambers (atrium and ventricle) together with appropriate resistances and capacitances. In addition, the device includes a thermal mass which corresponds roughly to the size of a 70 kg patient, a myocardium which can be perfused with a cardioplegic solution, and a pleural cavity which can accumulate lost blood. The hydraulic simulator can be physically connected to any CPB circuit, HLM, and patient-monitoring system.

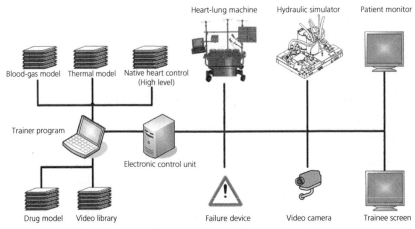

Fig. 22.1 The principal components of the 'Orpheus' perfusion simulator.

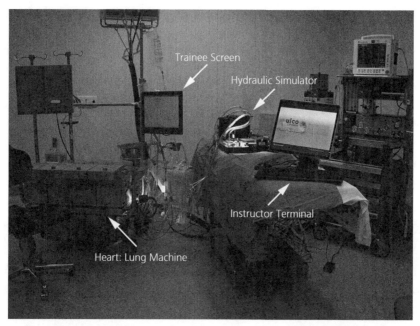

Fig. 22.2 The 'Orpheus' simulator. The electronic control unit is under the operating table and is not well seen.

The electronic control unit (ECU) is the interface between the trainer's computer and the hydraulic simulator. It translates commands from the trainer's computer into activity in the hydraulic simulator or the failure devices. In addition, it provides the basic behaviour of the simulator including the cardiac rhythm, myocardial contractility, and atrial activity.

The principal functions of the simulator control program include the:

♦ Running of the real-time drug, cardio-respiratory, and thermal models

♦ Control of the hydraulic simulator

♦ Streaming of audiovisual prompts

♦ Recording of the trainee's responses

♦ Recording of the physiological and hydraulic data

♦ Initiation (and termination) of system failures

The control program can either be run on the host computer or on a remote, networked device.

22.7.2.2 Other functions of the simulator control program

The simulator control program is also used for high-level control of the hydraulic model. It can be used to change parameters such as myocardial contractility, systemic vascular resistance, pulse rate, and cardiac rhythm.

A library of audiovisual clips can be streamed to the trainee's screen by the simulation controller. The clips show the surgeon undertaking manoeuvres such as cannulation, decannulation, and aortic cross-clamping. The simulator incorporates a video-recording system which records the trainee's responses and a physiological and hydraulic data-recording system which outputs to an 'Excel'™ spreadsheet.

A wide variety of system failures can be initiated (and terminated) by the simulation controller. These failures include:

♦ Oxygen supply failure

♦ Oxygenator failure

♦ Electrical supply failure to the HLM, heater/cooler, and patient monitor

♦ Air-locking of the venous line

♦ Kinking of the venous line

♦ Occlusion of the arterial line

The trainee screen is a touch-screen terminal which is attached to the HLM. The terminal provides:

♦ The results of blood-gas analysis

♦ The results of activated clotting time measurement

♦ A drug-administration interface

♦ A view of the surgical field

The 'Orpheus' perfusion simulator is distributed with a series of scenarios which have been developed for use with the system.

References

1 Karnath B, Thornton W, Frye AW. Teaching and testing physical examination skills without the use of patients. Academic Medicine: Journal of the Association of American Medical Colleges 2002;**77**(7):753.

2 Stammers AH, Mejak BL. An update on perfusion safety: does the type of perfusion practice affect the rate of incidents related to cardiopulmonary bypass? Perfusion 2001;**16**(3):189–198.

Chapter 23

Respiratory medicine and respiratory therapy

Brian Robinson

Overview

◆ Clinical simulation-based education and training is established in respiratory care for competency skills assessment and developing critical thinking.

◆ Training in the areas of respiratory care and assessment is achieved with a variety of breath sound simulators and computer-based arterial blood gas training programmes.

◆ There are many patient simulators, mannequins, part-task trainers, and lung/breathing simulators for teaching respiratory care skills.

◆ Respiratory care skills include oxygen administration, airway management, respiratory support, and ventilation that are not limited to health professionals.

◆ Mannequins and virtual reality technologies are available for chest drain insertion and care through to the use of flexible fibre-optic bronchoscopy.

◆ No single simulation device currently exists for the training and assessment in all aspects of respiratory medicine and associated therapies.

◆ Combinations of devices and clinical training and assessment techniques are required to provide comprehensive coverage.

23.1 Introduction to respiratory medicine and respiratory therapy

Simulation-based education and training has become established in respiratory care[1] and is recognized to enhance competency skills assessment.[2] Clinical simulation is considered an important strategy for developing critical thinking in respiratory care training and in the intensive-care setting.[3, 4]

The aim of this chapter is to provide examples for using simulation and skills-based teaching methods focusing on the respiratory care of patients. It is intended for all health specialties that provide respiratory care of patients and provides examples to facilitate undergraduate and postgraduate learning. These may extend to multidisciplinary or interprofessional learning and provide opportunities for certification or credentialing assessments.

When looking through catalogues and websites, there is a vast array of part-task clinical trainers, mannequins, and simulators applicable for clinical training and respiratory care. The issue that often confronts the trainer, the teacher, or instructor is selection of the most suitable device. The frequent problem is the gap that exists between the learning objectives and the capabilities of the device. Often, the role of a clinical training facilitator is to bridge those gaps. Although an array of respiratory care mannequins or training devices exists, effective learning will occur when use is appropriately matched to the intended learning outcomes.

The following sections describe the varieties of part-task trainers, mannequins, and simulators available for clinical respiratory teaching and training. These have been divided into three sections focusing on learning outcomes: respiratory assessment, clinical respiratory skills and therapies, and clinical decision-making regarding the care of a patient. Because there is a large and expanding range of training devices and software on the market it is likely that some devices may not be described here. The training devices, software, and methods described are provided as examples and by no means comprehensive.

23.2 Respiratory assessment

23.2.1 Respiratory rate and breathing patterns

Respiratory rate and breathing pattern have been historically key features of patient assessment. However, against this setting is the reported inability of health professionals to reliably and correctly recognize significant changes to respiratory rates and patterns in the spontaneously breathing patient.[5, 6] This has become notable in multiple studies and has a significant effect on patient risk and outcomes with numerous studies indicating the inability for nurses to detect and respond to the deteriorating patient, particularly in the ward setting, has a significant effect on patient safety.[7–9] Included among the key reasons is the displacement of clinical observation by automated measurement; the latter being a better fit to the complex high workload of the clinical environment where the pulse oximeter has become the respiratory monitor.[5, 7] As a result, the pathophysiological significance of altered respiration is commonly misinterpreted, unreported, or ignored. Education is required, especially for nursing graduates, to understand the significance of key physiological measurements and observations.[9]

This lack of appreciation of the respiratory assessment appears reflected in the physical presentation of respiration in commercially available patient simulators. In general, manufacturers use simple pneumatic mechanisms that generate bilateral or unilateral rise and fall of the sternum although several paediatric or neonatal simulators providing abdominal movements indicating airway obstruction. It is reasonable to say that these clues lack clinical fidelity or subtlety and frequently teaching using patient simulation relies on clues presented using monitoring or through instructors rather than direct observation. Given that patient morbidity and mortality can be detected and prevented through the skilled and appropriate assessment of respiration, it is surprising that manufacturers have not succeeded to simulate realistic accessory muscle, intercostal muscle, and diaphragm movement with paradoxical movement to replicate airway obstruction.

Despite these simulation limitations, courses have been developed, evaluated, and clinically validated in the recognition and management of the deteriorating patient, in which altered respiration is emphasized as a key principle of patient assessment. It is, therefore, noteworthy that these use either patient actors[10, 11] or mannequins.[12, 13]

23.2.2 **Breath sounds**

Teaching interpretation of breath sounds could be considered another core skill for respiratory assessment. Ward and Wattier[14] recently reviewed the available technology for teaching chest auscultation identifying the advantages and potential limitations of various devices and technologies. In considering training in the recognition and interpretation of breath sounds there are three major features, as follows.

23.2.2.1 Recognition of the breath sound

Students have a need to know how breath sounds are produced, how to use a stethoscope, and normal patterns and phases of sounds. This is most easily taught on the trainees themselves. For teaching recognition of abnormal breath sounds, several training devices are available. A variety of breath sound generators are available from manufacturers such as Laerdal (e.g. VitalSim with auscultation module) and Nasco (e.g. Heart and Lung Sounds Manikin, Auscultation Simulator) that have audio speakers and may also have listening points for auscultation with stethoscope. These sound generators can also be connected to mannequins for auscultation on the chest (e.g. Laerdal Nursing Anne). Compact discs, such as the 3M Learning Lung Sounds, Cardionics Learning Lung Sounds, or the Kyoto Kagaku Lung Sound Auscultation Trainer (LSAT), are interactive training programmes that are run on personal computers and also delivered via the Internet. These programmes display sonograms synchronized to each breath sound and they have the advantage of being useful for group learning and tuition but also provide self-directed learning packages. Cardionics also produce the PneumoSim Digital Breath Sound simulator that allows recorded and simulated breath sounds to be edited and altered for students to obtain better understanding of the inspiratory and expiratory components of the sound.

Wireless technology, combined with microelectronics, has allowed the development of electronic simulation stethoscope that allows a variety of breath sounds to be played to students or candidates participating in clinical assessments.[15] Cardionics has developed the SimScope WiFi, through which a library of breath sounds can be accessed from a computer and can be used with standardized patients or mannequins. Similar technologies are offered by other manufacturers (e.g. Lecat's Ventriloscope, Thinklabs Electronic

Stethoscope, and Sansa Shaker) with differences in the usability in clinical education and assessment of devices.[14]

There are also online open-source sound files that can be accessed via the Internet. Generally, the quality of inbuilt computer speakers is far from desirable for listening to breath sounds and may be improved using speakers with lower frequency response or headphones.

23.2.2.2 Where to listen to breath sounds

The major issue of teaching this skill is appropriate placement of the stethoscope to listen to breath sounds. The computer CD programs have instructional diagrams indicating where auscultation should be made. This may not equate to actually placing the stethoscope on a patient's chest and can be one potential advantage to using a mannequin. However, most training mannequins are recumbent and can usually be auscultated for breath sounds in four areas; generally, the left and right anterior chest and mid-axillary regions corresponding to the size and placement of speakers for manufacturing ease rather than clinically ideal regions. While these are suitable to emergency-management scenarios, they are deficient for advanced clinical assessment and diagnosis. Purpose-designed breath sound training mannequins are available (e.g. Nasco, Kyoto Kagaku, Cardionics) comprising paediatric and adult torsos that allow for the auscultation in up to 17 positions, including the posterior chest wall, and differentiate between listing locations. These trainers do not have respiratory movement to identify specific inspiratory and expiratory breath sounds. The Nasco Auscultation Trainer is a stand-alone unit that requires the use of the electronic SmartScope. Kyoto Kagaku and Cardionics use standard stethoscopes and the mannequins are connected to computers that combine screen-based and Internet-deliverable training packages. Harvey (Laerdal) is a simulator that enables breath sounds to be linked with cardio-respiratory sounds and pulses.

23.2.2.3 Interpretation of the breath sound

In the context of other clinical signs, this is perhaps the final step in this process. The interpretation of inspiratory and expiratory breaths sounds associated with chest movement should be an advantage of the high- and intermediate-fidelity patient simulators over the static part-task trainers. Currently, however, the breath sounds can only be auscultated on a limited number of anterior and mid-axillary positions in patient mannequin simulators and it is fair to say that the breath sounds available are of limited quality and quantity. The small speakers placed in mannequins are generally of the type that have higher frequency ranges than associated with breath sounds and this does not aid learning or interpretation. As described previously, the breathing movements and mechanisms of mannequin simulators are generally achieved by the hinged anterior rising and falling of the chest rather than in combination with lateral chest expansion. This causes noise artefact from the movement through the rubbing of dry plastics plus various click of solenoids, valves, etc., and the internal compressors of wireless simulators.[14] These sources of confusion and frustration for instructors and trainees are the opportunities for future patient simulator and respiratory mannequin refinement.

23.2.3 Percussion

Percussion of the chest wall is one other clinical skill used in respiratory assessment. Mannequins tend to have chest walls that do not lend itself to teaching these skills or allowing any form of interpretation. One simple but elegant method for teaching this skill is the use of 2-litre plastic paint tubs that are empty (to sound hyper-resonant), filled with large polystyrene beads (to sound normal) or filled with rolled oats (to sound dull). Percussing the lids allows students to learn to distinguish sounds.[16]

23.2.4 Interpretation of blood gas and acid-base balance

While education in the interpretation of blood gas and acid-base balance is generally run as case-based or problem-based learning scenarios, the interpretation and subsequent management of disordered blood gas physiology complements skill stations and scenarios in a setting of adult interactive learning. Simulated blood gas physiology is available in patient simulators and personal computer programmes.

The CAE Healthcare human patient simulator (CAE HPS) provides calculations of $PaCO_2$, PaO_2, pH, and SaO_2 but not HCO_3 or base excess. The blood gas values are indicative of the gases within the lungs of the simulator that are generated by a complex process involving the automatic detection of the gas composition and effectively the removal of O_2 that is replaced by a mixture of CO_2 and N_2 to simulate O_2 uptake due to metabolism. This gas composition is automatically adjusted for the measured minute ventilation and other variables including respiratory quotient, O_2 consumption, and an approximation of V/Q mismatch. Within the physical structure of the lungs of this simulator is dead space and functional residual volume, so alveolar gas composition and consequent changes can reflect ventilation. The gas concentration values are not adjusted for alveolar water vapour pressure. The effects of renal, haemoglobin, or plasma buffering mechanisms, metabolites (e.g. plasma lactate or 2,3-DPG), or body temperature on blood gas physiology do not appear to be modelled and, therefore, this feature of the CAE HPS should to be used cautiously when using the raw values for teaching or assessment. This complex system can also fail without recognition by users causing functional faults in the respiratory control of the simulator.[17] Several other CAE patient simulators similarly generate blood gas and acid-base balance physiology data but without the automatic detection of the O_2 and CO_2 concentrations or the measured volume of minute ventilation.

Computer software blood gas simulation programs based on physiological models are available. Blood Gases from Mad Scientist Software provides a tutorial program suited to self-directed learning. The Nottingham Physiological Simulator is a sophisticated and detailed program suited for research or teaching at the very advanced level.[18] These programs may be useful for generating realistic blood gas results that can be integrated into clinical simulation scenarios.

23.3 Clinical respiratory skills and therapies

23.3.1 Oxygen administration

Teaching oxygen administration allows an opportunity to distinguish between the different oxygen delivery modes and the effect of patient respiration. The high-fidelity patient simulators, such as the CAE HPS, have sophisticated pulmonary mechanisms that replicate O_2 uptake and CO_2 production. This can be controlled to create patient pathologies and ventilatory changes (e.g. patients with congestive heart failure or asthma) as well as an adjustable functional residual capacity (e.g. the effect of restrictive respiratory disorders such as pregnancy, morbid obesity, or kyphosis).

23.3.2 Airway management

For more information on airway management, see Chapter 22. The opportunities for airway management in the setting of respiratory care may involve, but is not restricted to, the following.

23.3.2.1 Nasopharyngeal airway (NPA)

This commonly used therapy requires training with appropriate mannequins. The cutaway head mannequins, such as the Ambu Airway Management Trainer, allow the nasopharyngeal vault to be visualized, which can be ideal when demonstrating positioning of the NPA, the importance of appropriate NPA size selection, and the correct and incorrect insertion techniques. Most airway-management mannequins can be used for training NPA placement, although mannequins with more accurate nasal anatomy, as in the Scopin II Broncho Boy Trainer, are desirable.

23.3.2.2 Endotracheal and tracheostomy tube management

Suctioning of secretions from the endotracheal and tracheostomy tube is a skill frequently taught and assessed. Appropriately intubated mannequins can be used in conjunction with suction, catheters (using both the simple catheter and closed suction systems), and gloves. Applying tracheal suction to the mannequins with exposed lungs, such as the Laerdal Airway Management Trainer, generates small reductions of the lung volumes and can demonstrate the concept of suction on the alveoli.

23.3.3 Respiratory support: bi-level positive airway pressure (BiPAP), continuous positive airway pressure (CPAP), and intermittent positive pressure breathing (IPPB)

Nursing and allied health professionals are increasingly more involved in providing non-invasive respiratory therapy. These therapies require a good seal between the patient and face mask, and one limitation frequently encountered is the difficulty in obtaining a quality seal between masks and the silicon or plastic face of mannequins. Despite this limitation, the high-fidelity patient simulators with pulmonary mechanics (e.g. CAE HPS) can be used to demonstrate non-invasive respiratory techniques. It is important that the instructor is practiced in the technique of placing the face mask on the mannequin to obtain a suitable seal and the students are aware that there will be subtle differences to using this technique on patients. Other manufacturers do not recommend using high-flow devices such as CPAP or BiPAP devices on their simulators (e.g. Laerdal SimMan). Mannequins can be utilized to demonstrate equipment static set-ups and those with a soft face and nose (e.g. Laerdal ALS Baby) can be useful for demonstrating paediatric nasal CPAP.

The RespiPatient (Ingmar Medical) comprises an adult head that can be ventilated via endotracheal tube or face mask; a lung that can be adjusted for airway pressure or compliance. This is by way of a computer-controlled low-resistance large-volume piston, sold as the ALS 5000 Breathing Simulator, which simulates the respiratory air flows of spontaneous breathing and can also be manually ventilated. It has sophisticated lung modelling that replicates pressure flow curves associated with changes in respiratory compliance (e.g. pneumothorax) and airway resistance (e.g. bronchospasm). Ingmar Medical also produces the QuickTrigger, which, when coupled to other test lungs (e.g. Ingmar RespiTrainer or QuickLung), can also be used to simulate spontaneous breathing.

23.3.4 Ventilation

The CAE HPS is a high-fidelity simulator originally developed for use in anaesthesia and, as a result, has sophisticated mechanisms capable of generating change to airway resistance and lung compliance appropriate for healthy patients and patients with respiratory dysfunction or pathology. Recently, simulators such as the Laerdal SimMan 3G and the Gaumard HAL S3201 have been developed with similar physical capability. This allows application of intermittent positive pressure ventilation (IPPV) on the simulator to be ventilated using modern electronic controlled ventilators. Other patient simulators have lungs that do not have these mechanisms; instead, they have simple lungs (i.e. passive filling bags) that, when inflated, result in chest rise. The compliance of these lungs is restricted by the weight of the mannequin chest wall and elastance of chest skin. This compliance is typically very low at around 25 ml/cm H_2O (or approximately one-third the compliance of the usual adult human at 70 ml/cm H_2O). Ventilating these intermediate fidelity simulators using a modern ventilator with typical patient settings results in activation of high peak pressure and low tidal volume alarms. These compliances are acceptable and not discernible when manually ventilated with a resuscitation bag.[19] The Ingmar Medical RespiTrainer, and the RespiPatient, as mentioned, are also alternatives.

23.3.5 Chest drain insertion and management

There are a variety of training devices for the treatment and management of pneumothorax. These range from stand-alone devices that can be used for training needle thoracotomy (e.g. Simulaids Pneumothorax Simulator, Laerdal Pneumothorax Trainer) through to devices for chest drain insertion, securing, and dressing (e.g. LifeForm Chest Tube Mannequin, SimCentral Super Annie II, Simulab TraumaMan, Pharmabotics Chest

Drain Simulator). The METI and Laerdal range of simulators also allow for needle thoracotomy and chest drain insertion procedures to be performed. Several of these mannequins (Nasco Chest Tube Mannequin, SimCentral Super Annie II) can also be used for training in the care and trouble shooting of the chest drain by connection to underwater seal drains and demonstration of swinging and bubbling associated with normal and abnormal chest drain function. This not only provides training opportunities but also creates opportunities to assess students' understanding of chest drain function, critical-patient management, and diagnostic skills. Several professional organizations also provide online training resources for self-directed learning in chest tube insertion and thoracic drain management.

23.3.6 **Bronchoscopy**

Flexible fibre-optic bronchoscopy (FOB) is generally associated with respiratory physicians, ear, nose, and throat (ENT) and cardiothoracic surgeons, anaesthetists, and intensive-care specialists. It is often used to assess patients in the intensive or critical setting and, in several health systems, FOB is also performed on patients with intubated tracheas by non-medical health professionals. Because FOB is a difficult clinical skill to acquire, it lends itself to simulation and part-task trainers, and there are a variety of methods for training in this technique with several anatomical and non-anatomical training devices available. The various product and resources for simulation-based bronchoscopy training have been described and published reports reviewed in depth by Kastelik and his colleagues.[20]

Examples of anatomical training devices are airway-management trainers to which a bronchial tree can be added (e.g. Laerdal Airway Management Trainer, SimMan and AirMan, Scopin II Broncho Boy Trainer, and TruCorp AirSim). Non-anatomical training devices (Pharmabotics Oxford Training Box, Replicant Dexter Endoscopy Training System) focus on the acquisition of learning the psychomotor skills required for FOB. Virtual reality systems consist of a PC with software modules, an interface device connected to a proxy bronchoscope, and providing training scenarios presenting computer-generated airways. Examples of these include the CAE EndoVR Simulator, ORSIM, and the Simbionix BRONCH Mentor and BRONCH Express. The virtual reality simulators include bronchial aspiration, lavage and ultrasound training module are provided with self-directed learning modules and can potentially provide assessment of endoscopy skills prior to patient contact.[20–22]

23.4 **Clinical education in respiratory care**

The design of scenarios has been covered elsewhere in this book (see Chapter 14) and two examples highlighting decision-making and teamwork issues are presented here (examples 1 and 2). Providing students and trainees with sufficient information to enable structured learning may require appropriate laboratory and clinical tests (e.g. blood gas and electrolytes results, ECG printouts, chest X-rays, etc.). Decision-making is considered an important proficiency in respiratory care and both case studies and clinical simulation are potentially important strategies towards making better decisions.[3] In the future, respiratory care will probably involve more procedures and health professionals will require more extensive training where competency assessments will become common.[23] Patient simulation can facilitate the acquisition of procedural skills required for the care of mechanically ventilated patients.[24] This is a preferred method of learning that is not associated with differences in knowledge learnt when compared with online education.[25] It should also be recognized that airway and ventilatory care is not limited to the high-acuity healthcare setting and many families provide respiratory care in home settings. Whiting and O'Loughlin[26] have described a programme of teaching clinical procedures, including tracheostomy suctioning, emergency change of tracheostomy tube, and invasive and non-invasive ventilation, to non-healthcare professionals caring for family members. The opportunities that exist for respiratory medicine and respiratory care are strongly weighted in favour of using simulation as it has the potential to be used in skills training as well as competency skills and decision-making assessments in a broad range of health professional and care-provider groups.

23.4.1 Example 1: introduction to CPAP training

Nursing-led triage can influence the early application of CPAP to reduce the need for tracheal intubation and assisted ventilation.[27] Demand for CPAP therapy can increase the requirement for structured training programmes. Patient simulators provide an opportunity for training and advanced acute-care nursing education that include discrete didactic lectures, clinical skills training, and problem-based learning. Suggested topics include:

1 respiratory assessment

2 oxygen therapy

3 blood gas interpretation

4 airway management

5 setting up CPAP equipment

6 patient scenarios

The patient scenarios could include respiratory distress or respiratory failure that consolidates learning processes featuring a patient with defined pathology (e.g. congestive heart failure) including:

1 Patient assessment: history, respiratory and cardiovascular functions, hydration status, consciousness, pain and/or other symptoms, and then repeating these assessments within a dynamic scenario.

2 Oxygen therapy: matching appropriate oxygen delivery with oxygen demand.

3 Blood gas interpretation: determining the respiratory and metabolic status of the patient and potential management plan(s).

4 Airway management: anticipating and planning appropriate airway management for loss of consciousness or preparation for elective rapid-sequence intubation and controlled ventilation.

5 Medication: planning for the administration of appropriate drug therapies.

6 Applying CPAP therapy: ensuring the equipment set-up is understood, used appropriately, and effective communication with the patient regarding the course of the treatment.

7 Team management: allocation of a team leader, verbalization of patient care plan and management, allocation of team members to specified areas of responsibility, clear direct communication within the team, and anticipation and planning.

23.4.2 Example 2: positive pressure ventilation in ICU setting

A skills competency programme for respiratory physiotherapists introduced to provide out-of-hours cover for the intensive-care unit, consisting of:

1 Airway management: open and closed suction of the endotracheal tube.

2 Intermittent positive pressure ventilation to clear secretions.

The IPPV skills training that focuses on:

1 Manual IPPV technique.

2 Equipment used for IPPV.

3 Potential complications and considerations for the causes of increased airway pressure during IPPV: failure of equipment, migration of tube to endobronchial intubation, mucus plug in lung or tube, or pneumothorax.

4 Airway management: anticipating, recognizing concomitant physiological changes (e.g. oxygen saturation, heart rate, blood pressure), and planning appropriate management in response to increased airway pressure.

23.5 Conclusions, future directions, and developments

It is important to recognize that applying simulation to respiratory-care training and assessment is not a new concept. The first commercially available resuscitation training mannequin, the Laerdal Resusci Anne, was manufactured around 60 years ago for the purpose of training and assessing airway management and ventilation skills in addition to cardiac compression. Sim One, the first computer-controlled patient simulator, was developed in the mid-1960s and initially focused on training and assessment of skills acquisition in anaesthesiology residents.[28, 29] Sim One was reported to be useful in the training of ventilator use and patient ventilation in medical, nursing, and allied health professionals and students.[30]

Today, simulation manufacturers continue to be developing new products with wide ranges of capabilities and applications, including those for respiratory care.[31] Models of patient care will also change; patients' length of stay in hospital will reduce while the intensity of in-hospital treatment will increase, and patient care will move from the hospital to the home requiring an ever-increasing range of training capability and accessibility. Clinical educators and trainers should consider who will be providing patient care and the setting of that care, while matching the training and simulation technology to the clinical skills alongside the development of appropriate assessment methods. Simulation also has the potential to inform the choice of respiratory therapy to be used.[32]

There will be developments in the range of products for training in respiratory assessment and care. Some of the advances may include the colour changes to skin and mucosa, lung and airway secretions, or improving chest movement to indicate respiratory difficulties that were the planned additional features for Sim One.[28] There may be the integration of existing technologies and the development of new technologies. We may see further development of self-directed learning, virtual reality, and automated training assessment similar to those available for resuscitation training.[33] It will be intriguing to observe future advances in the technical advances of simulation and the development of health-professional and non-health professional skills training.

References

1 **Weinstock PH, et al**. Towards a new paradigm in hospital-based pediatric education: the development of an onsite simulator program. Pediatr Crit Care Med 2005;**6**:712–713.

2 **Tuttle RP, et al**. Utilizing simulation technology for competency skills assessment and a comparison of traditional methods of training in simulation-based training. Resp Care 2007;**52**:263–270.

3 **Hill TV**. The relationship between critical thinking and decision-making in respiratory care students. Resp Care 2002;**47**:571–577.

4 **Sinz EH**. Partial-task-trainers and simulation in critical care medicine. In: Dunn WF, ed. Simulators in critical care and beyond. Des Plaines, IL: Society of Critical Care Medicine; 2004, 33–41.

5 **Hogan J**. Why don't nurses monitor the respiratory rate of patients? Br J Nurs 2006;**15**:489–492.

6 **CliftonSmith T, et al**. Breathing pattern disorders and physiotherapy: inspiration for our profession. Phys Ther Rev 2011;**16**:75–86.

7 **Odell MT, et al**. Nurses' role in detecting deterioration in ward patients: systematic literature review. J Adv Nurs 2009;**65**:1992–2006.

8 **Liaw SY, et al**. A review of educational strategies to improve nurses' roles in recognizing and responding to deteriorating patients. In Nurse Rev 2011;**58**:296–303.

9 **Purling A, et al**. A literature review: graduate nurses' preparedness for recognising and responding to the deteriorating patient. J Clin Nurs 2012;**21**:3451–3465.

10 **Smith GB, et al**. Impact of attending a 1-day multi-professional course (ALERT™) on the knowledge of acute care trainee doctors. Resuscitation 2004;**61**:117–122.

11 **Featherstone P, et al**. Impact of a 1-day inter-professional course (ALERT™) on attitudes and confidence in managing critically ill adult patients. Resuscitation 2005;**65**:329–336.

12 **Fuhrmann L, et al**. A multi-professional full-scale simulation course in the recognition and management of deteriorating hospital patients. Resuscitation 2009a;**80**:669–673.

13 **Fuhrmann L, et al**. The effect of multi-professional education on the recognition and outcomes of patients at risk on general wards. Resuscitation 2009b;**80**:1357–1360.

14 **Ward JJ, et al**. Technology for enhancing chest auscultation in clinical simulation. Resp Care 2011;**56**:834–845.

15 **Sherman JJ, et al**. Physical assessment experience in a problem-based learning course. Am J Pharm 2011;**75**:Article 156.

16 **Wearn A**. Teaching, learning and assessing clinical skills: does one size fit all? Second International Clinical Skills Conference, Monash Centre. Prato: Italy; 2007.

17 Garden AL, et al. Unrecognised malfunction in computerised patient simulators. Br J Anaesth 2004;**93**:873–875.

18 Hardman JG et al. A physiology simulator: validation of its respiratory components and its ability to predict the patient's response to changes in mechanical ventilation. Br J Anaesth 1998;**81**:327–332.

19 Gough JE, et al. Tactile assessments of lung compliance are not reliable. Acad Emerg Med 1999;**6**:761–764.

20 Kastelik JA, et al. Developments in simulation bronchoscopy training. Open J Resp Dis 2013;**3**:154–163.

21 Ost D, et al. Assessment of a bronchoscopy simulator. Crit Care Med 2001;**164**:2248–2255.

22 Martin KM, et al. Effective non-anatomical endoscopy training produces clinical airway endoscopy proficiency. Anesth Analg 2004;**99**:938–944.

23 Hess D. Training and education challenges for the twenty-first century: respiratory care competency and practice. Respir Care Clin N Am 2005;**11**:531–542.

24 Jansson MM, et al. Human patient simulation education in the nursing management of patients requiring mechanical ventilation: a randomized, controlled trial. Am J Infect Control 2014;**42**:271–276.

25 Corbridge SJ, et al. Online learning versus simulation for teaching principles of mechanical ventilation to nurse practitioner students. Int J Nurs Educ Sch 2010;**7**:Article 12.

26 Whiting M, et al. Training high: a clinical skills initiative for families and staff. Nurs Educ & Young People 2012;**24**:30–33.

27 MacGeorge JM, et al. The experience of the nurse at triage influences the timing of CPAP intervention. Accid Emerg Nurs 2003;**11**:234–238.

28 Denson JS, et al. A computer-controlled patient simulator. JAMA 1969;**6**:712–713.

29 Abrahamson S, et al. Effectiveness of a simulator in training anesthesiology residents. J Med Educ 1969;**44**:515–519.

30 Hoffman KI, et al. The 'cost-effectiveness' of Sim One. J Med Educ 1975;**50**:1127–1128.

31 Spooner N, et al. Medical simulation technology: educational overview, industry leaders, and what's missing. Hosp Top 2012;**90**:57–64.

32 Marjanovic N, et al. Evaluation of manual and automatic manually triggered ventilation performance and ergonomics using a simulation model. Resp Care 2014;**59**:735–742.

33 Dong Hoon L, et al. The usefulness of a 3-dimensional virtual simulation using haptics in training orotracheal intubation. Biomed Res Int 2013;Article ID 534097 doi:10.1. 1155/2013/534097

Websites of products referred to

3M PPE Safety Solutions:
<http://solutions.3m.com>
Adam,Rouilly Limited:
<http://www.adam-rouilly.co.uk>
Ambu USA:
<http://www.ambuusa.com>
CAE Healthcare:
<http://www.caehealthcare.com/eng/>
Cardionics:
<http://www.cardionics.com>
Dexter Endoscopy:
<http://www.dexterendoscopy.com>

Enasco:
<http://www.enasco.com>
IngMar Medical:
<http://www.ingmarmed.com>
Kyoto Kagaku:
<http://www.kyotokagaku.com>
Laerdal Medical:
<http://www.laerdal.com>
Madscientist Software:
<http://www.madsci.com>
ORSIM:
<http://www.orsim.co.nz>
Pharmabotics:
<http://www.pharmabotics.com>
Simbionix:
<http://www.simbionix.com>
SimCentral:
<http://www.simcentral.com.au>
Simulab:
<http://www.simulab.com>
Simulaids:
<http://www.simulaids.com>
Trucorp:
<http://www.trucorp.co.uk>
Lecat's Ventriloscope:
<http://www.ventriloscope.com>

Chapter 24

Simulation in critical care

Joshua S Botdorf, Julie A Schmidt, William F Dunn,
and Kianoush Kashani

Overview

- Curriculum design should start with consideration of institutional and departmental needs.
- Simulation exercises can be added to existing curriculum or created *de novo*.
- Procedural training should incorporate 'Mastery Learning' concepts in requiring demonstrated proficiency of learners.
- Recognized certification courses and local curricula can be a source of development of simulation scenarios.
- Simulation development should have the consumer in mind.
- Critical care simulation exercise learning goal fall within one of three classic domains: communication/attitudinal skills, finite technical skills, and cognitive skills.

24.1 Introduction to simulation in critical care

Dr William Mayo stated 90 years ago, 'There is no excuse today for the surgeon to learn on the patient.' These words hold true to all facets of medicine. The promise of simulation within healthcare is to provide such a learner-centric, psychologically safe environment for training without jeopardizing patient safety. Caring for those in duress is a situation when teaching and risk of learner error does not afford optimized educational opportunities. Simulation in the field of critical care allows safe learning experiences and development of proficiency. This chapter covers the role of simulation training within the disciplines of critical care. It has been written for the educator, either associated with a simulation centre or training programme. The intention is to provide a framework in which critical care simulation can be adapted to existing curricula or *de novo* curricula might be developed. As described, simulation-based scenarios and workshops in critical care can provide powerful experiences which (cognitively) imprint long term. Such experiences (pending appropriate modifications) are broadly applicable across learner levels and disciplines. Considerations are discussed regarding the planning of curriculum and scenarios within the cognitive, procedural, and communication skill domains.

24.2 **Where to start**

Developing a simulation programme with a focus on critical care requires reflection and planning prior to development and implementation. As a starting point, vision and mission statements, both institutional and departmental, should be considered, as follows:

- developing vision and mission statements
- identifying the important learning goals and objectives
- detecting and determining scenarios and workshops that need to be provided

Goals and objectives should be clearly developed and concisely stated. This applies to both course curriculum and workshop series, in addition to the individual educational offerings. For instance, the Mayo Clinic 'Critical Care Boot Camp' course is an introductory curriculum for critical care fellows as opposed to medical students, residents, or nurses. In the majority of time, the intent of design is for advanced fellows and seasoned practitioners. However, a major strength of simulation as an educational endeavour includes its interdisciplinary potential. As such, much of the curriculum described herein (i.e. the Mayo Clinic Critical Care Boot Camp) can be modified by a competent simulation educator toward applications across a broad spectrum of learners. Sources to guide development of workshops include institutional practices and standards, ongoing quality improvement and quality-assessment demands, recognition of knowledge deficits at varying levels of training, and standardization of skills. When resources are available, education professionals can be of great assistance in incorporating educational theory and refining learning objectives.

24.3 **Planning process**

Critical care, like all specialty specific simulation, has its own particularities to consider in the planning phase. The course purpose should be considered first in the design. Common directives include teaching procedural techniques, assessing for competency, and creating learning environments to stimulate further learning and discussion. Areas to consider in planning involve sites of instruction, materials and resources available, staffing, assessment/demonstrated proficiency tools, and the consumers. Incorporating concepts of 'process engineering' will aid in the design of achievable goals. Standardized (and 'best') practices, such as those emanating from specialty societies serve as a rich opportunity for learning, whether as pre-briefing, scenario content, debriefing, or take-home reflective exercises.

24.3.1 **Site and materials**

Sites of instruction for critical care are unbounded. Dedicated simulation labs offer standardized environments. Advantages may include accessibility to low- and high-fidelity mannequins and trainers, audiovisual resources, simulation staff, and standardized equipment and environments. Starting the planning process involves knowing what resources and items are available to the educator and understanding what items are necessary for the simulation activity to be successful. *In situ* environments have certain advantages, including environmental realism and reinforcement of prior concepts within an experience unanticipated by the learner. When items such as medications or other expensive consumables are needed, substitutes can be used as alternatives. While seemingly cumbersome, mannequins and audiovisual equipment can be made portable, allowing the simulation lab to be brought to the clinical environment.

24.3.2 **Resources and staff**

Consideration of resources includes staff availability for attending physicians/consultants, house staff, medical students, nurses, respiratory therapists, non-nursing care providers, standardized patients, educators, and simulation centre personnel. The use of different hospital employees (or emeritus staff) is valuable in creating the simulation experience. Involving various participants, not only as trainees but also during set-up and implementation of simulation exercises, adds significant value to the curriculum. There is great benefit in involving allied health staff as standardized patients within the exercise. Having healthcare-literate staff allows for greater improvisation and replication of medical presentations. Utilizing any group has associated costs, whether it is the cost of recruiting clinical staff in a non-clinical environment or the cost of maintaining a standardized patient pool or supporting the salary of dedicated educators. Seeking and encouraging volunteerism among interested individuals with regards to simulation can be crucial in lowering associated costs. Allied health personnel and clinicians can also prove to be excellent resources in scenario development and management.

24.3.3 **Consumers and learners**

A wide variety of consumers may be attracted to simulation with a critical care focus. While traditional learners are considered house staff and medical students, the multidisciplinary management and team approach to critical care supports an array of learners. Nurses, respiratory therapists, nurse practitioners, physician assistants, and pharmacists all potentially benefit from simulation exercises. Minor alterations in maturely developed patient scenarios can allow for transferability between trainees with different backgrounds and disciplines. Scenarios are rarely a one-size-fits-all product; however, a scenario stem can possess several core elements that aid in set-up and implementation. Keeping this frame of reference of the intended consumer/learner and their level of experience and background can aid to the educational success. Considerations should include:

1 educational background:

   a physician, physician extender, nursing, respiratory therapy, pharmacy, paramedical

   b educational background: critical care versus other specialties, i.e. cardiology

2 specialty: internal medicine, anesthesiology, surgery, family medicine, etc.

3 experience: novice to expert

4 location of practice: tertiary-care centres, private-practice settings, rural settings, outpatient

5 participants: number of participants in the designed exercise and instructor-to-learner ratio

6 non-clinical consumer: researchers and those engaged in quality or cost assessments

7 patients: non-standardized or standardized patients

24.3.4 **Research and quality improvement**

Non-educational simulation, namely research and quality improvement, is an important portion of critical care simulation curriculum development. Simulated intensive care unit (ICU) environments can provide a standardized, reproducible environment to test: research protocols, proposed clinical aids (checklists), electronic medical records, order entries, and educational-based research. Advancement of quality-improvement initiatives via certification and credentialing of skills and procedures can be incorporated, as well as the evaluation of system responses, time sinks, and inefficiencies to high-quality care.

24.3.5 **Patient safety**

Patients are often the indirect consumers of simulation. An important model is patient-safety initiatives that are supported by simulation exercises. Implementation of best practices and standards of care can be reinforced through simulation and credentialing of common activities to mitigate their associated risks. The instruction of central venous catheters placement and the utilization of best practices are examples of such resources.[1] The standardization of the performance of central venous catheterization credentialing can be accomplished through mandatory ('mastery') standards of demonstrated proficiency which incorporate not only venepuncture skills but also institutional requirements pertaining to safety-based behaviours. Such mastery learning opportunities are relevant for trainees, established practitioners, and others. Similar types of high-value, high-expectation activities can be applied to many procedures at the onset of training, and regular simulation activities provide maintenance of skills. An additional method by which patient safety can be supported is through sentinel event reviews. Turning a sentinel or near-miss event into a scenario permits the learner the opportunity to learn from the event and to gain knowledge to avoid a future event from occurring.

24.3.6 **Mastery learning**

Concepts of mastery learning are being increasingly incorporated in simulation-based education.[2] Concepts of mastery learning include an emphasis on learning, rather than teaching. As such, the demonstration of acquired proficiency is always implied within a mastery learning curriculum construct. Such adult-learning principles were originally described within non-medical domains, as common to humanity.[3, 4] Mastery learning as applied to individual simulation-based instruction includes the following key principles[5]:

1 Baseline, or diagnostic testing.

2 Clear learning objectives, sequenced as units in increasing difficulty.

3 Engagement in educational activities (e.g. skills practice, data interpretation, reading, focused on reaching the objectives).

4 A set minimum passing standard (e.g. test score) for each educational unit.

5 Formative testing to gauge unit completion at a pre-set minimum passing standard for mastery.

6 Advancement to the next educational unit given measured achievement at or above the mastery standard.

7 Continued practice or study on an educational unit until the mastery standard is reached.

Mastery learning principles may be also applied at an organizational level. For instance, an organization may require that mastery learning-defined demonstrated proficiency is required as prerequisite training for all care providers performing central venous catheterization, or other procedures. When applied at an organizational level, simulation-based mastery learning key principles include the following[6]:

1 Define the baseline system state or problem, using valid metrics.

2 Establish clear targets of system (or individual) performance to measurable, defined organizational standards.

3 Create an actionable plan including simulation-based techniques within the available leadership toolbox, focusing on demonstrated proficiency standards of performance.

4 Formalize and standardize curricular components of simulation-based training.

5 Certify via demonstrated proficiency (e.g. within a simulation laboratory) the key variables identified, to mastery standards of performance.

6 Remediate via learner-centric non-punitive methods those not capable of first-time demonstrated proficiency in achieving the organizational standard(s).

7 Maintain organizational mechanisms to enhance and optimize simulation-based (and other) components of system improvement toward the established goal(s).

24.4 **Planning a curriculum**

Recognized courses and certifications may also drive course development. The American Heart Association's (AHA's) Adult Cardiac Life Support (ACLS) and Pediatric Advanced Life Support (PALS) certifications are two such offerings in which simulation outside the confines of the course can provide important opportunities to clarify concepts and engrain standardize approaches of care. Additional structured curricula to gain ideas for scenario development include the American College of Surgeons' Advanced Trauma Life Support (ATLS) course and the Neurocritical Care Society's (NCS) Emergency Neurological Life Support (ENLS) course. While we often consider simulation as a tool for education per se, the real impact of simulation within critical care specialty training is targeted at improving the patient experience and/or clinical outcome. As such, simulation is a potent safety-quality (i.e. practice) tool. Such 'non-educational' areas of significance include patient safety, quality improvement, and research. Educational subject matter generally includes cognitive skill development, finite technical skills, and communication skills.

24.4.1 Scenario construction

Simulation-based course construction will vary depending on many factors, including learner level, resources, formative versus summative learning goals, etc. A comprehensive simulation critical care curriculum will cover areas across disciplines. Areas for potential consideration that are core to the specialty of critical care should include the previously mentioned domains of communication, cognitive skills, and finite technical skills. Sample curriculum topics for house and nursing staff as utilized at Mayo Clinic are featured in Table 24.1.

Finite technical skills incorporate partial-task trainers to a large extent. Models, either professionally manufactured or locally fabricated, can be used for repetitive practice and technique instruction. Common objectives include acquisition of procedural consent, patient positioning, device/kit set-up, recognition of contraindications, indications, and complications.

Clinical synthesis (i.e. high-level decision-making requiring efficient integration of multiple key inputs) revolves around accurate syndrome recognition and timely application of interventions. Use of previously prearranged models or facilitator improvisational instructed simulators are of maximum value in these settings along with supporting staff to create lifelike, interactive experiences. Regardless of the intricacy of the scenario-based simulation, the debriefing process reinforces key concepts, which can be (by design) strengthened by post-simulation reflective experiences.

24.4.2 Simulation in critical care nurse training

Simulation is an important component of critical care nurse training at Mayo Clinic. Structured curriculum scenarios that focus on the care of haemodynamically unstable patients or those requiring critical intervention, such as respiratory failure, provide opportunities for novice nurses to practice in innocuous learning environments. Objectives of scenarios can also centre on completing daily tasks such as equipment safety checks (i.e. is the suction functioning, is there a bag valve mask in the patient's room), patient advocacy, and effective communication with providers. Specific cognitive skills can also be taught or evaluated during training, such as the administration of sedation, interpretation of haemodynamic measurements, anticipation of interventions, or execution of protocols.

Table 24.1 Curriculum for critical care trainees and allied health staff

	Critical care trainees	**Allied health staff**
Communication-based simulation	Emergency response training Adverse outcomes End-of-life discussions Patient hand-offs	Communicating with patients and family members Communication during sentinel events and dealing with bad news Communication during the grieving process Communication for administrative roles Communication for the preceptor Understanding the patient experience through simulated device use
Finite technical skills	Airway workshop Bronchoscopy workshop Thoracentesis & thoracostomy workshop Critical care ultrasound Critical care cardiac ultrasonography Interosseus access workshop Central venous catheter placement Paracentesis workshop Haemodynamic workshop	Set-up, management, and troubleshooting of devices Ventricular assist devices Chest tubes and drainage devices Using defibrillators and accessing code carts Haemodynamic monitoring lines Rapid infusers and infusion pumps Wall suction set-up Mechanical ventilator alarms Monitor use Intracranial pressure monitoring
Cognitive skills	Cardiac emergencies Mechanical ventilation workshop Neurologic emergencies workshop Recognition of shock and resuscitation Mechanical ventilation: troubleshooting and waveform analysis Procedural sedation	Caring for Haemodynamically unstable patients Conscious sedation Assisting providers with bedside procedures Early recognition of the deteriorating patient Prioritization of critical care patient needs Triaging sass casualty events Prioritization of patient care needs Patient assessment

24.5 Communication

Communication skills and development of team dynamics play a central role in critical care patient management. Communicating facts regarding critical illnesses is very stressful for providers, patient, and family. Simulation provides the opportunity for a safe environment, in order to work through difficult experiences with immediate mentored feedback. Experienced standardized patients are of value in this type of simulation experience to create genuine depictions of (preferably) real or hypothetical patient interactions. Patient empathy can be taught through simulation, as well, by allowing interdisciplinary learners to 'experience' common treatments that patients endure in the critical care setting.

In this section we review the main goals and objectives of a critical care simulation curriculum regarding communication skills, as practised at Mayo Clinic.

24.5.1 **Patient transitions of care**

The Joint Commission and National Institutes of Medicine have targeted patient hand-offs (handovers) and transitions of care as a quality of care index. With increased acuity of patients in the critical care unit, simulation of patient hand-off tools can stream-line care and create safer care environments. Potential scenarios to develop include: (i) physician-to-physician and nurse-to-nurse hand-offs, and (ii) communication in the context of in-house and outside hospital transfers. Real-life communications, such as those that happen at the change of shift, via phone, and from the operating room, can add to realism and applicability. Use of standardized tools such as checklists and Situation-Background-Assessment-Recommendation (**SBAR**) tools can also provide a framework for reflection and debriefing.[7]

24.5.2 **Breaking bad news and end-of-life discussions**

The responsibility of breaking bad news and end-of-life decision-making often falls to the intensivist. Understandably, these areas of communication can be difficult for trainees and early career nurses alike. Simulating these environments and creating discussion can be powerful learning opportunities. Having a defined 'mental model' framework from which to build is advantageous: the Setting up-Perception-Invitation-Knowledge-Emotions-Strategy/Summary (**SPIKES**) or the Background-Rapport-Explore-Announce-Kindling-Summarize (**BREAKS**) protocol are two such examples.[8, 9] Simulating the delivery of a terminal illness, the death of a patient to family members, and disclosure of adverse out-comes can easily be simulated with the aid of standardized patients. Beyond one-on-one communications, mock family conferences or scenarios requiring techniques utilized in conflict mediation and resolution could be included in the curriculum. At the cen-tre of these topics are concepts of relationship building; a useful basis for this approach is with utilization of the Partnership-Empathy-Apology-Respect-Legitimation-Support (**PEARLS**).[10]

24.5.3 **Interdisciplinary team training and team communications**

Interdisciplinary team training is essential for critical care providers. In a simulated environment, members of varying disciplines are able to practise and learn together. Inter-disciplinary team training courses often focus on low-volume, high-risk situations where rapidly formed teams must come together in a crisis situation to resuscitate or rescue a patient. Participants can be recruited from physicians, advanced practice providers, re-spiratory therapists, nurses, pharmacists, and other key team members to enhance learn-ing of those involved. Effective team communication leads to high-functioning teams and successful resuscitation events. An example of a resource to be utilized by instructors and course developers is the **TEAMSTEPPS** curriculum developed by the Agency for Health-care and Research and Quality (AHRQ).[11]

The primary objectives of team training courses should focus on enhancing the com-munication and teamwork skills of interdisciplinary members, all while trying to promote a sense of cohesiveness. Unannounced simulations can be an effective way to do this, whether *in situ* or during an organized class in a simulation centre. Calling learners to a mock code event, either at the start of the course or unexpectedly during a lecture, can create spontaneity and a sense of urgency. This helps simulate the unpredictable elements that happen during true medical emergencies, where chaos and poor communication can quickly predominate orchestrated teamwork. Secondary objectives should focus on team member roles, positions, equipment, algorithms, and site-specific resources. One of the challenges for emergency response teams is the improbability of responding to actual events with the team that trained together. All team members should leave a course knowing the responsibilities of their own roles. Creating tension during a simulation scenario through misplaced or malfunctioning tools can reinforce the need to know the location of emergency equipment and troubleshooting skills. While trainers need to teach the learners, the importance of being familiar with emergency equipment and resources, creating debriefing opportunities about situational awareness, fixation errors, and communication among team members carries a very high value.

24.6 **Finite technical skills**

24.6.1 **Airway**

Consistent with mastery learning theory, airway simulation (and related experiential learning) training can be formed from a composite of non-invasive and invasive approaches. The resulting mosaic of training experiences constitutes the building blocks of partial tasks that build into clinical competence. The learning of airway skills can be initiated with training of proper airway assessment. A subsequent session includes oxygen delivery systems such has nasal cannulas, tents, and masks. Providing opportunities to engage in the trial of devices provides the learners not only the opportunity to demonstrate safe use and set-up, but also allows first-hand experience of the devices and understanding of the patients' experience. Expanding into invasive options, the use of airway task trainers (nasopharyngeal and oropharyngeal) are excellent tools in the application of advanced airways; a range of endotracheal tubes and supraglottic devices can be simulated. Many high-fidelity mannequins have the capability to create difficult airway situations. Animal and human tissue specimens can offer even greater levels of anatomical reality and its variations. Simulation is generally a positive experience in the training of airway devices and is associated with improved outcomes, compared with non-simulation intervention. In addition, learners have greater satisfaction with animal and cadaver models compared with synthetic mannequin models.[12] Optimally, learners should be exposed to a variety of invasive approaches including direct laryngoscopy, videolaryngoscopy, and fibre-optic laryngoscopy. Simulations can be expanded from mastery of technique to full-fledged simulations that include airway management from start to finish with demonstration of rapid sequence intubation, management of the difficult airway, and simulation of complications (dental injury, oesophageal intubation, pharmacologic effects).

24.6.2 **Bronchoscopy**

Simulation can provide an effective means of education in training of bronchoscopy. Simulation models are many, and require vigorous forethought in leveraging advantages while understanding limitations of each simulator tool. Simulators range from virtual-reality bronchoscopy simulators, partial-task trainers made of varied materials, mannequins, and animal or human cadaveric tissue. Virtual-reality bronchoscopy simulators have the advantage of simulating pathology and patient response (e.g. cough). Additionally, they can provide feedback in the case of airway touches and trauma, topical sedation usage, and appropriateness of interventions. Despite the common penchant for high technology, a recent systematic review and meta-analysis found that cadaveric tissue models and partial-task trainers tend to be more satisfying than virtual simulators.[13] Simulation exercises should focus on proper techniques with repetition and the development of 'muscle memory' (i.e. consolidating a specific motor task into memory through repetition) to attain bronchial segments. The validated Bronchoscopy Skills and Tasks Assessment Tool can serve as a guide for competency-based testing and curriculum development.[14]

24.6.3 **Thoracentesis and tube thoracostomy simulation**

Simulation can also improve the skills of the trainee with regards to thoracentesis.[15] Proper use of equipment, procedural technique, patient positioning, anatomical landmarks, and use of ultrasound should be emphasized. Tube thoracostomy and pleural drainage catheter placement can be simulated with commercially designed partial-task trainers and animal or human cadaveric models. By utilizing the human cadaveric torso, in addition to thoracentesis, multiple simulations can be achieved including advanced airways, bronchoscopy, and tube thoracostomy. Alternatively, a large rack of ribs from the local butchery can provide an inexpensive option to mannequins and partial-task trainers.[16]

24.6.4 **Critical care ultrasound**

The importance of critical care bedside ultrasonography has been increasingly recognized in the last few years, and has evolved into a critical skill for newly trained Intensivists. While published studies have not substantiated the role of simulation-based education in ultrasound practice, structured curriculum in training has become a necessity to expediently train novice learners.[17–19] Simulation-based exercises can be employed utilizing standardized patients, animal models, ultrasound models, or with the use of ultrasound simulators. Basic skills can be broken into three domains: thoracic, abdominal, and vascular. Curriculum can be started with image acquisition with advancement to goal-directed applications and protocols. The availability of dedicated, experienced faculty is crucial, as guided instruction with real-time coaching provides a model for education.

Critical care cardiac ultrasonography continues to be incorporated into the practice of critical care. Simulation-based training in transthoracic and transoesophageal cardiac ultrasonography has the potential to expedite the learning process. Basic skills can be broken into image acquisition from standard views, with a focus on 2D cardiac ultrasonography followed with an introduction to M-Mode, Doppler, and colour Doppler waveform technologies. Image interpretation and pathological finding discussions with focus on critical illness issues is another important aspect of such workshops. Advanced topics may then focus on the critical care cardiac ultrasonography incorporation into clinical decision-making. Training standards have been developed by several societies with the development of a consensus statement that can be of guidance.

24.6.5 Interosseous access workshop

Rapid access to the interosseous space for the infusion of fluid and medications can be simulated with relative ease. A variety of task trainers exist from basic, modified bone models to advanced partial-task trainers and mannequins for humerus, tibia, and sternum sites. Adaptable devices can be added to instructor- and model-driven simulators. Beyond indications and contraindications, proper use of equipment and patient positioning can be emphasized. Validated evaluation tools have been developed for assessment.[20]

24.6.6 Central venous catheter placement

Central venous catheter placement should be an early component of all critical care specialty training curricula due to the frequency of use. Training via simulation enhances patient outcomes in a cost-effective manner.[21–23] Simulation exercises and evaluation can be constructed around established guidelines.[1] Several partial-task trainers and instructor- and model-driven simulators are available. Techniques gained in ultrasound simulation can readily be adapted with regards to ultrasound physics, vascular anatomy, and ultrasound device use. Important criteria to consider with the development of a central venous catheter placement scenario include antiseptic technique and infection prevention, vascular ultrasound use, and education and technique training of device placement.[24] Additionally, catheter maintenance and its care can be reviewed. Ideally, an objective assessment tool is applied to the learners and certification of proficiency is granted.

24.6.7 Paracentesis simulation

Paracentesis can be taught with the use of simulators, with learners reaching demonstrated competence.[25] Several partial-task trainers exist. In-house-designed models can be more difficult to design and build as opposed to home-made thoracic models. The use of ultrasound for detection of a fluid packet and roll-out of vessels underneath the needle insertion site should be emphasized. Beyond the basic technique of a diagnostic or therapeutic paracentesis, diagnostic peritoneal lavage can be demonstrated.

24.6.8 Haemodynamic monitoring

Haemodynamic simulation can be presented to cover intra-arterial pressure, central venous pressure, cardiac output, and pulmonary artery pressure monitoring. Simulation course components can be divided into two areas. The first component focuses on the technical aspects of setting up the system. The subsequent focus is data interpretation and management. Invasive arterial device monitoring use should include demonstrating monitor set-up, zeroing transducers, square wave testing, identifying over- or under-dampened waveforms, introduction to cardiac output and stroke volume variation, and troubleshooting devices. Pulmonary artery catheter use should include patient positioning, insertion distances, interpretation of waveforms, and placement technique. A combination of high-fidelity mannequins, monitor simulators, and screen-based simulators could be used for this purpose. Data interpretation can be incorporated into demonstrative simulation or be expounded upon through scenario development in the context of identification and management of shock states.

24.7 Additional cognitive integration skills

24.7.1 Cardiac emergencies

Cardiac emergencies can be all-encompassing of cardiac pathology. The AHA's ACLS is the prototypical resource. Longitudinal and course refreshers can be of benefit in the retention of skills.[26] Instructor-driven simulators with linked monitors are of great value and can allow for varied and impromptu scenarios that can be modified based on the trainees' analyses, responses, and interventions. Beyond the application of classic algorithms, scenarios can be expanded to include a variety of problems leading to cardiac emergencies, such as respiratory failure, pericardial effusion, pneumothorax, and shock. Assessment objectives can include rhythm assessment, proper protocol use, ACLS pharmacology, team communication, leadership skills, proper use of equipment, and post-arrest management. In addition to the use of mannequins and the design of simulated emergencies, screen- and game-based computer software programs have the flexibility and depth to operate as simulation supplements as well and platforms have been extended to even include mobile devices.

24.7.2 Mechanical ventilation simulation

Basic and advanced mechanical ventilation workshops can readily be incorporated into a simulation curriculum. Objectives of such workshops are to demonstrate and experience (as feasible) invasive and non-invasive mechanical ventilator circuits, set-up of basic and advanced modes, waveform analysis, and troubleshooting. It is of benefit to have learners try various modes via mouthpieces and nose clips and with non-invasive masks. Demonstration of modes can be done with a test lung or high-fidelity mannequins. Several screen- and game-based products have been developed that allow feedback with ventilator-setting modifications. Important aspects of demonstrative exercises include a review of available alarms and interpretation of waveforms. Scenarios can readily be developed using mannequins or ventilator simulators to challenge the learner with deteriorating patients. This is particularly beneficial in more advanced trainees. Simulated events can include equipment malfunction, airway and endotracheal tube obstruction, refractory hypoxemia, air trapping, and pneumothorax. Scenarios could be conducted individually or several simultaneously to simulate the real situation for high-intensity ICUs.

24.7.3 **Neurologic emergencies**

Simulation-based educational courses in neuro-critical care are of value across disciplines. Areas for consideration for simulation include acute stroke, management of elevated intracranial hypertension, status epilepticus management, coma assessment, and brain-death examination. Standardized patients and simulators can be used in hybrid scenarios to create the appropriate fidelity regarding neurological diseases. The recently developed ENLS course produced by the NCS can serve as a guide for curriculum development.[27]

24.7.4 **Recognition of shock and resuscitation**

Simulation of resuscitation can align across disciplines to include shock and sepsis states, cardiac life support, trauma resuscitations, and paediatric-based cases. Learner objectives should emphasize the recognize deterioration in physiologic states through assimilation of multiple lines of data from haemodynamic, respiratory, radiologic and laboratory sources, and simulated physical information. Focus should be placed on interpretation, analysis, and incorporation of the data into an implementable plan with appropriate timing of interventions. Model-driven simulators have a niche for these scenarios, but instructor-driven simulators have the advantage of adaptability and freedom to change the direction of the simulation midcourse. In a review of simulation-based resuscitation studies, areas that seemed to enhance the value of the scenarios included the use of booster sessions, team dynamics, leadership skills, debriefing, and feedback.[28] Simulating care of the deteriorating patient can also enhance interdisciplinary communication and teamwork. Scenarios, by design, can focus on early recognition of deterioration while simultaneously providing an opportunity to engage in effective team communication through both active practice and debriefing. Standardized approaches endorsed by professional societies (e.g. the Surviving Sepsis Campaign) can be readily integrated and reinforced.[29]

24.7.5 **Procedural sedation**

Procedural sedation can be simulated with the use of an instructor-driven simulators. The American Society of Anesthesiologists practice guidelines for sedation and analgesia by non-anesthesiologists can serve as a framework for scenario development.[30] Important facets of instruction will be pre-procedural assessment, the development of a sedation plan, anticipation, and management of complications. Complications can be simulated and assessments can be graded. A focus on communication can also be highlighted by creating stressful conditions with an antagonistic or hurried proceduralist. Having attending staff to serve as the proceduralists and allied healthcare staff to act as nurses heightens the authenticity of the workshop. Due to the potential risks involved to the patient, assessment for credentialing and maintenance of privileges can be incorporated into the simulation.

24.8 **Conclusion**

Simulation should be an integral component of critical care education across disciplines and backgrounds, including physicians, nurses, and the allied health fields. During the planning process, considerations unique to critical care should be made for sites, materials, educational resources, staff, and consumers. Curriculum development should draw from standardized courses, international and society directives, and local needs. The role of simulation lies in the education of cognitive-, manual-, and communication-based skill sets. A cohesively designed course should aim to enhance communications of providers and proficiency with infrequently performed services and procedures.

Acknowledgements

This chapter is dedicated first to the hundreds of critical care trainees and nurses at Mayo Clinic that have incorporated simulation-based training within a mentored learning experience recognizing the 'virtual' sanctity of the patient as human being, central to our professional goals in optimizing outcome. Second, this chapter is dedicated to those that strive for educational excellence beyond the norm, recognizing that the truest value of our work is (paradoxically) measured often in unmeasurable, but incredibly important, ways. Regardless of the conflicting forces impacting healthcare education and delivery globally, it is the desire of the co-authors that the reader strives to be first an individual of immense value, rather than personal success.

References

1 **Rupp SM, Apfelbaum JL, Blitt C, et al**. Practice guidelines for central venous access: a report by the American Society of Anesthesiologists Task Force on Central Venous Access. Anesthesiology 2012;**116**(3):539–573.

2 **Issenberg SB, McGaghie WC, Hart IR, et al**. Simulation technology for health care professional skills training and assessment. JAMA 1999;**282**(9):861–866.

3 **Skinner BF**. The evolution of behavior. J Exp Anal Behav 1984;**41**(2):217–221.

4 **Airasian P, Bloom B, Carroll J, et al**. Mastery learning: theory and practice: Holt Rinehart & Winston; 1971.

5 **McGaghie WC, Siddall VJ, Mazmanian PE, et al**. Lessons for continuing medical education from simulation research in undergraduate and graduate medical education: effectiveness of continuing medical education: American College of Chest Physicians Evidence-Based Educational Guidelines. Chest 2009;**135**(3 Suppl):62S–68S.

6 **Cook DAMDM, Brydges RP, Zendejas BMDM, et al**. Mastery learning for health professionals using technology-enhanced simulation: a systematic review and meta-analysis. Acad Med 2013;**88**(8):1178–1186.

7 Improvement IfH. SBAR Toolkit: <http://wwwihiorg/resources/Pages/Tools/SBARToolkitaspx>

8 **Baile WF, Buckman R, Lenzi R, et al**. SPIKES–a six-step protocol for delivering bad news: application to the patient with cancer. Oncologist. 2000;**5**(4):302–311.

9 **Narayanan V, Bista B, Koshy C**. 'BREAKS' protocol for breaking bad news. Ind J Palliat Care 2010;**16**(2):61–65.

10 **Barnett PB**. Rapport and the hospitalist. Am J Med 2001;**111**(9B):31S–35S.

11 Quality AfHaRa. TeamSTEPPS: National Implementation: <http://teamsteppsahrqgov/>

12 **Kennedy CC, Cannon EK, Warner DO, et al**. Advanced airway management simulation training in medical education: a systematic review and meta-analysis. Crit Care Med 2014;**42**(1):169–178.

13 **Kennedy CC, Maldonado F, Cook DA**. Simulation-based bronchoscopy training: systematic review and meta-analysis. Chest 2013;**144**(1):183–192.

14 Davoudi M, Osann K, Colt HG. Validation of two instruments to assess technical bronchoscopic skill using virtual reality simulation. Respiration 2008;**76**(1):92–101.

15 Wayne DB, Barsuk JH, O'Leary KJ, et al. Mastery learning of thoracentesis skills by internal medicine residents using simulation technology and deliberate practice. J Hosp Med 2008;**3**(1):48–54.

16 Ching JA, Wachtel TL. A simple device to teach tube thoracostomy. J Trauma 2011;**70**(6):1564–1567.

17 Sekiguchi H, Bhagra A, Gajic O, et al. A general critical care ultrasonography workshop: results of a novel web-based learning program combined with simulation-based hands-on training. J Crit Care 2013 Apr;**28**(2):217.

18 Sekiguchi H, Suzuki J, Gharacholou SM, et al. A novel multimedia workshop on portable cardiac critical care ultrasonography: a practical option for the busy intensivist. Anaesth Intensive Care 2012;**40**(5):838–843.

19. Sidhu HS, Olubaniyi BO, Bhatnagar G, et al. Role of simulation-based education in ultrasound practice training. J Ultrasound Med 2012;**31**(5):785–791.

20. Oriot D, Darrieux E, Boureau-Voultoury A, et al. Validation of a performance assessment scale for simulated intraosseous access. Simul Healthc 2012;**7**(3):171–175.

21 Barsuk JH, McGaghie WC, Cohen ER, et al. Simulation-based mastery learning reduces complications during central venous catheter insertion in a medical intensive care unit. Crit Care Med 2009;**37**(10):2697–2701.

22 Barsuk JH, Cohen ER, Feinglass J, et al. Use of simulation-based education to reduce catheter-related bloodstream infections. Arch Intern Med 2009;**169**(15):1420–1423.

23 Cohen ER, Feinglass J, Barsuk JH, et al. Cost savings from reduced catheter-related bloodstream infection after simulation-based education for residents in a medical intensive care unit. Simul Healthc 2010;**5**(2):98–102.

24 Moureau N, Lamperti M, Kelly LJ, et al. Evidence-based consensus on the insertion of central venous access devices: definition of minimal requirements for training. Br J Anaesth 2013;**110**(3):347–356.

25 Barsuk JH, Cohen ER, Vozenilek JA, et al. Simulation-based education with mastery learning improves paracentesis skills. J Grad Med Educ 2012;**4**(1):23–27.

26 Ko PY, Scott JM, Mihai A, et al. Comparison of a modified longitudinal simulation-based advanced cardiovascular life support to a traditional advanced cardiovascular life support curriculum in third-year medical students. Teach Learn Med 2011;**23**(4):324–330.

27 Smith WS, Weingart S. Emergency Neurological Life Support (ENLS): what to do in the first hour of a neurological emergency. Neurocrit Care 2012;**17**(Suppl 1):S1–3.

28 Mundell WC, Kennedy CC, Szostek JH, et al. Simulation technology for resuscitation training: a systematic review and meta-analysis. Resuscitation 2013;**84**(9):1174–1183.

29 Dellinger RP, Carlet JM, Masur H, et al. Surviving Sepsis Campaign guidelines for management of severe sepsis and septic shock. Intensive Care Med 2004;**30**(4):536–555.

30 American Society of Anesthesiologists Task Force on Sedation and Analgesia by Non-Anesthesiologists. Practice guidelines for sedation and analgesia by non-anesthesiologists. Anesthesiology 2002;**96**(4):1004–1017.

Chapter 25

Simulation for teamwork training

Geoffrey K Lighthall, Nicolette C Mininni,
and Michael DeVita

Overview

- A crisis is an unplanned life-threatening event is which there is a mismatch between the level of resources available, and those that a patient needs to regain stability. These events occur every day in the healthcare setting.

- In today's healthcare settings, managing a patient in crisis requires a team of multi-disciplinary professionals performing both technical and non-technical skills that can be learned and perfected through simulation training.

- Different models of teamwork have been formulated and developed via simulation training.

- Crisis resource management (CRM) is based on human cognitive science, and provides a framework for understanding and improving upon performance in medical crisis. Situational awareness, proper communication, and effective leadership are foremost among CRM skills.

- Crisis team training directly addresses the roles and responsibilities of crisis team members and places a priority on choreography and efficiency of team processes.

- Some form of team training accompanies all interprofessional simulation programmes.

- A key component of effective simulation training is thoughtful feedback and debriefing.

25.1 Introduction to simulation for teamwork training

The early years of simulation highlighted the fact that some aspects of medical training, such as practice of event management, communication, and teamwork, may be best accomplished in settings outside the actual workplace, or at least in the absence of real patients. The need for specific teamwork training is highlighted by the improved outcome following the introduction of new forms of patient-care teams. A prominent and timely example is the medical emergency team (MET), a physician-led rapid response team that was first described in Australia by Lee, and then in the United States by DeVita.[1, 2] METs and rapid response teams (RRTs) are pre-organized groups of professionals and equipment that are dispatched to a patient's bedside anywhere within a hospital. Teams are implemented with the intent of swiftly identifying critically ill patients outside the intensive care unit, and then to immediately provide critical care resources to correct the 'needs-resources' mismatch. The goal of rapid response systems (RRSs) are to make sure that patients are: (i) identified as early as possible; and that (ii) experts in critical care evaluate these patients as quickly as possible in order to optimize patient outcomes.[3] Clear communication with ward staff, rapid gathering and sharing of information, formation of diagnostic impressions, and implementation of therapeutic plans are aspects of teamwork that characterize high-performance teams.

Crisis resource management (CRM) has come to define the cognitive and teamwork skills that facilitate management of medical events bearing a high risk to patient well-being. There are various definitions for crisis, but for purposes of this discussion, a crisis is defined as an unplanned life-threatening event in which there is a mismatch between the ambient level of resources and those that a patient needs to regain stability.

Resources should be thought of in the broadest sense to include a wide range of personal, psychological, and material components that can be mobilized to improve a patient's course. The requisite skills for managing crises include understanding the situation, its evolution and various solutions, and how to engage and coordinate with others in order to arrive at a solution. These, as well as the acquisition of additional information and help, communicating with co-workers, and making back-up plans are examples of CRM skills that can influence the overall outcome of the situation. The key points of CRM are listed in Table 25.1. Behavioural skills such as these have been labelled 'non-technical', in contrast to medical knowledge and procedural proficiency, which represent 'technical' skills.

Training in CRM or behavioural skills is most applicable to fields of medicine that commonly encounter crises or high risk unplanned events, high stress, diagnostic or therapeutic ambiguity, or time pressures. CRM training is based on the premise that both technical and non-technical skills are essential to critical-event management and should be developed in parallel. However, this realization has come only recently, lagging a century and a half behind the traditional paradigm of care that emphasizes knowledge and skill of the individual as the basic target of training and evaluation. Implicit to the traditional model is that those that excel will have the best outcomes. However, under stress, there is no guarantee that even the best plan will be implemented without some additional abilities in managing a diverse set of personnel, understanding one's own limitations under stress, and without deliberate attention to communication, contingency planning, and effective leadership.[4] Interest in such behavioural skills has come not from prospective evaluation of these components, but from the realization that a significant number of medical mishaps are traceable to the absence of these skills.

25.2 Origins of crisis resource management in aviation and medicine

The role of non-technical skills and their relationship to patient outcomes, which was explored in the late 1980s and 90s, had a striking resemblance to findings from research into aviation disasters of the prior decade. Inquiry into accidents revealed that in the majority of crashes implicating pilot error, it was not manual skills that were lacking, but deficiencies in leadership, teamwork, communication, and planning.[5, 6] Consideration of the evolution of cockpit resource management in commercial aviation and its entry into medicine provides an informative perspective on the use of patient simulation systems, and to what may turn out to be their 'higher calling'.

The transfer of cockpit resource management concepts to medicine occurred in contrast, largely in the absence of the public's awareness of errors and mishaps and their contribution to mortality, with little scrutiny of regulatory agencies calling for solutions, and with no organized front of patients, hospitals, or insurers clamouring for ways to minimize patient risks. David Gaba and colleagues at Stanford University realized the power and applicability of aviation-based cockpit resource management programmes to their work in medical anaesthesiology, and ended up creating a realistic patient simulator, curricula and research programmes aimed at understanding and improving decision-making of anaesthesiologists during operating crises.[7]

While interactive software-based simulators were available,[8] the hands-on simulator was able to 'recreate the anaesthesiologists physical, as well as mental, task environment'.[9] This was considered an important adjunct to the computer trainers that assessed only **knowing what to do**. With the entire environment at hand, participants had to balance manual as well as cognitive tasks, and manage such at the same time as maintaining communication with surgeons and managing distractions. The curriculum resulting from these efforts eventually became known as anesthesia crisis resource management (ACRM).[7, 10, 11]

The early years of simulation highlighted the fact that some aspects of medical training may be best accomplished in settings outside the actual workplace, or at least in the absence of real patients. It further highlighted the value of simulation as an entry point into understanding the non-technical or behavioural aspects of patient care.

25.3 Crisis resource management: core concepts

CRM offers a framework for understanding and improving on human performance in medical crises; as such, it is intended to complement pre-learned 'technical' skills of diagnosis and disease management and related procedures. Despite the intangible nature of an **approach** rather than a **set method**, a set of recurring concepts can be identified in the published reports from programmes that have implemented CRM-based curricula (Table 25.1).

There is no dogmatic list of CRM principles in either aviation or medicine. Rather, individual training programmes, hospitals, and disciplines may choose to emphasize certain

Table 25.1 Skill sets applicable to critical-event management

Technical skills	*Non-technical skills*	
Medical knowledge and its application	**Decision-making and cognition**	**Team and resource management**
Physical examination	Knowledge of the team and environment	Taking a leadership role
Data evaluation	Anticipation and planning	Calling for help early
Differential diagnosis	Wise allocation of attention	Communicating effectively
Knowledge of therapeutic plans and pathways	Use of all available information and confirmation of key data streams	Distributing the workload
Hands-on skills	Use of cognitive aids (e.g. checklists, reference materials)	Mobilization and utilization of all available resources

concepts over others and develop their own set of 'rules' or 'principles' applicable to that practice environment. Understanding the antecedents and contributing factors to critical events and 'near misses' within an institution is an important starting point for understanding the workplace, its inhabitants, and the training content that is likely to carry the greatest impact.

25.4 Using simulation systems to provide crisis resource management training

Critical event simulations can accommodate a diversity of training goals; however, the impact of each course is likely to be greater if one does not attempt to 'do it all at once'. The applicability of simulation systems to clinical education can be described by a spectrum of activities listed according to increased complexity:

+ Simple skill acquisition (central line placement).
+ Dynamic skill acquisition (airway management—dynamic because it involves decisions integrating pharmacology, anatomy, patient state and monitor data).
+ Pattern recognition and diagnosis.
+ Management of a disease process—as single discipline trainees or as a team.
+ Team management of a disease process—forming a team and initial stabilization.
+ Team management of an evolving or complex disease process.

CRM skills are certainly most applicable to the last three items on the list, although one might argue that at every juncture of training, one should be reminded that the practice of medicine is always a team endeavour. The true value of a simulated environment is that it raises the level of the event to one where team coordination can actually make a difference in actual patient outcome.

CRM training is typically coupled to scenarios where the medical management can be challenging (usually because of the need for very rapid assessment and intervention), but is not mysterious. If the diagnosis is too puzzling, valuable course time will be spent debating what really was going on, rather than concentrating on how a group can organize itself to deal with such a situation. Scenario design and length should be consistent with the goals of the exercise. Short scenarios are ideal for emphasizing the need to diagnose and intervene rapidly, something that is impossible if there is not good teamwork. That is, time constraints can force teamwork errors that need to be 'trained out'. Longer scenarios are also valuable, but require sustaining group attention on key problems and prevention of fixation on secondary problems.

Specific scenarios can be designed to address specific CRM points. By keeping the scenario simple, and focusing the training on a particular goal (teamwork), the participant should leave with a vivid experience that can serve as a model for managing similar situations in real life. Some specific suggestions are made in Table 25.2.

Table 25.2 Use of patient crisis simulation to address CRM concepts

CRM point	Scenario or condition	Rationale
Situational awareness	◆ Sepsis, obstetric disaster, bleeder, MI. Have arriving participant ask what's going on ◆ Diseases with secondary findings (i.e. Tachycardia in haemorrhage)	◆ Assesses ability to understand and verbalize nature of situation ◆ Assesses whether team maintains focus on primary abnormality
Leadership	◆ High-complexity cases with shifting needs (mechanical ventilation, procedures, CPR, etc.) ◆ Send in senior physician when junior physician (current leader) is doing an adequate job	◆ Assesses ability to focus on priorities while maintaining view of larger problems ◆ Set-up for power struggle—does leader support or take over? What is best for patient?
Use of cognitive aids	◆ Malignant hyperthermia ◆ Pulseless electrical activity	◆ Forces use of MHAUS* direction sheet ◆ Forces one to find list of 'five Ts and five Hs'**
Anticipation/acquiring help	◆ Haemorrhage, myocardial infarction, increased intracranial pressure ◆ Any rapidly deteriorating patient	◆ Requires engagement of others for definitive control—time sensitive disease processes ◆ Is patient receiving more attention or monitoring? ◆ Are junior-level trainees over their heads?
Check all data streams	◆ Pulseless arrest; equipment disruptions ◆ Pneumothorax, hypopnea, bronchospasm, heart murmur	◆ Requires examination of all sources confirming pulsatile blood flow ◆ Is a team member actually examining the patient?
Distribute the workload	◆ Sepsis or haemorrhage with several tasks to attend to—send in someone asking if they can help. ◆ Send in ECG tech or X-ray tech (= radiographer) who asks trainees to move away; Pt has PVCs (ventricular ectopic beats).	◆ Assesses leader's monitoring of workload and task pairing ◆ Assesses if anyone is watching patient

continued

Table 25.2 (continued) Use of patient crisis simulation to address CRM concepts

CRM point	Scenario or condition	Rationale
Prevent fixation errors	• Equipment malfunctions, pulseless patient • Novel, rare, or other problems with poor outcomes (malignant hyperthermia, machine malfunction, tamponade)	• Whether finding is related to overall situation, whether new information changes plans or are there overriding beliefs that all is fine • Can the team accept compelling information establishing a diagnosis?
Communication	• Data probes (information passed on to a single group member) • Send in extra people, create noise	• Assesses presence of healthy two-way communication, willingness of junior members to contribute information • Forces use of techniques such as readback that assure requests are properly received
Allocate attention wisely	• Pneumothorax, shock, tamponade, haemorrhage	• Cases requiring high-level of technical skill that may force senior leader to perform procedure (assesses whether leader gets other to do the procedure, watch patient, lead team)

* Malignant Hyperthermia Association of the United States

** American Heart Association Advanced Life Support algorithm

25.5 **Models for team training: strengths and weaknesses**

Highly functional teams exhibit coordinated behaviour directed towards a single goal, or a coordinated set of goals. Two models for coordination are hierarchical and non-hierarchical. In the former, a 'team leader' assigns responsibilities, coordinates activities, collects clinical data, analyses it, makes decisions, and gives directions for intervention. It is based largely on the cockpit resource management model where the 'captain' delegates responsibilities and makes decisions. In the latter, each member of the team has pre-assigned (sometimes self-assigned) roles and duties, and reports along predetermined lines in a non-hierarchical manner. In the latter model, when applied to medicine, there is no 'team leader' per se because the team members have pre-assigned duties, but there would be a 'treatment leader'—a person focused on what diagnostics and treatments are required. The distinction is that the 'team' leader has duties to both lead team **process** as well as **data analysis and treatment** decision-making. Critics believe that this can lead to a cognitive overload, and so prefer a 'treatment' leader who would only have responsibility for prioritizing data acquisition, performing data analysis, and decision-making regarding therapeutics. In the non-hierarchical model, the team members must know their roles and perfect their individual duties before the event for success to be achieved routinely. To improve specific skills that are embedded in a crisis response, multiple single-discipline simulation programmes have been implemented to perfect specific components of cardiac arrest management such as leadership, CPR, and defibrillator/pacer operation.[12–14] When designed well, these duties are coordinated, or choreographed, with others' duties to address prioritization and efficiency. Once designed, they can be taught and then practised to perfection. Benefits of this model include more rapid task completion, especially early in the response; planned coordination of activities; ease of teaching and assessing team performance because of objective; prioritized task load; and an equitable distribution of duties (planned avoidance of duty overload).

The more common hierarchical approach is somewhat more typical of cockpit resource management, and espoused by a number of authors, most notably Gaba and colleagues.[4, 9, 15] The non-hierarchical is based more on advanced trauma life support (ATLS), with its pre-assigned roles and responsibilities. In the setting of RRTs responding to a medical crisis, DeVita et al. has used the term crisis team training (CTT) to distinguish it from traditional CRM methodology.[16] Professionals trained using the CTT method have delineated roles and responsibilities, and a 'choreographed' response. In this model, responders self-assign to predetermined roles based on their skills, and then perform the duties ascribed to those roles. This pattern 'unloads' the treatment leader of the responsibility for team management and allows the leader to focus on patient needs instead.

Both models improve team performance. The common denominator of both models is that teams function better if the roles and responsibilities are clear and have been practised repeatedly. Simulation training to manage medical crisis has been documented to streamline the design of the response, master role clarity, and to optimize communication in order to create a unit that functions synergistically so that the team is more than the sum of its parts.

In both models, each scenario begins by one participant being given some patient information after which s/he needs to assess the patient. The initial participant is expected to identify whether there is a crisis, activate the team, and communicate the relevant information essential to proper treatment of the patient. Best practice involves video-recording the response enabling playback, analysis, and debriefing by the facilitator and participants. Comprehensive debriefing tools have been created to score participants on behaviours that fall into three categories: communication, organizational tasks, or therapeutic tasks.[17] The programmes typically do not focus on diagnosis and treatment of the crisis as much as maintaining focus on the impact of and how to organize quickly and communicate effectively. Trainees learn that teamwork leads to more rapid and accurate diagnosis and treatment.

25.6 **Debriefing and feedback**

The educational goals of the simulation experience are consolidated by an appropriate post-event debriefing. Different models exist for debriefing and include either a structured task-focused checklist[16] or a more reflective and open-ended style of debriefing; the type is highly dependent on the overall objectives of the simulation course. Straightforward events for which there are accepted protocols and principles (such as ACLS, sepsis, and malignant hyperthermia) may be more amenable to review by comparing team performance to known management principles and checklists. Complex events and crises for which the 'solution' is based on perception and judgement may be best explored by group discussions where the instructor provides some guidance, but often plays the role of the facilitator. CRM has taken the latter approach from its inception over 25 years ago; methods for facilitating post-event reflection have been described in a recent review and include[18]:

1   Guided consideration of **pros, cons**, and **alternatives** to witnessed actions.

2   **Technical-only debriefings**: involving checklists and a focus on task completion, as described above.

3   **The three-column technique**: in which discussion considers medical/technical, CRM/behavioural, and system-based aspects of the case.

4   **Plus-delta**: in which participants reflect on what went well, and which aspects of care may benefit from a different approach in the future.

5   **Debriefing with good judgement**: in which debriefing acknowledges that actions arise from different perceptions of a problem and frames of reference. **Inquiry** attempts to consider the participant's actions in terms of his/her frame of reference, and is compared with what actions would be **advocated** by the instructor, based on his/her point of view.[19]

Regardless of approach, experienced instructors are rarely satisfied with their debriefing style and are in constant search of techniques for improvement. Experimenting with different approaches is quite common, and is encouraged, as it is important for instructors to remain energized and challenged by the process. It is also important to recognize that participants often emerge from the simulation with questions in their mind, and these topics may not necessarily overlap with the debriefing 'agenda'. To maintain interest and to gain acceptance of the **planned educational agenda**, one may need to meet participants halfway and **accommodate their agenda**.

Video capture of the simulated event has been a valuable addition to most practices. Clark et al. report that participants recognize that reviewing the video-playback is the single most powerful teaching tool during the simulation exercise.[20] However, the presence of video and its technical requirements can be distracting and should probably be minimized or avoided in situations where it fails to stimulate discussion, or advance course objectives. Paul and Lane report that participants of one simulation training programme have advocated that debriefing time be increased to allow for more discussion.[21]

25.7 *In situ* training and assessment

Even with an established centre, the ability to conduct simulations in the actual workplace provides a valuable source of information and experience that can improve team and system function. Teams interacting with a native environment, including ward personnel, equipment, and electronic systems, can reveal deficiencies within the system as well as present unique novel challenges to group communication and problem-solving abilities. With cardiac and arrest and rapid response teams, success inevitably involves successful meshing between multiple hospital systems, such as patient detection and notification systems (the afferent arm), response team assembly and organization (efferent arm), and underlying policies and procedures.

In situ simulation can also be used as a probe to provoke errors (latent error detection), and to analyse or remediate prior errors through a simulated repeat of the event.[22, 23] The Johns Hopkins Children's Center uses simulation training as part of its quality-improvement effort for both the efferent and afferent arms of the RRS.[24]

Teamwork drills can also help correct behavioural sets or interpersonal behaviours. For example, some response team members may question being summoned, especially if the patient was not in cardiac arrest. They may make remarks such as 'this wasn't a real code' or 'I left the unit for this?' These types of remarks may cause the ward team to feel guilty or ashamed, and may create a barrier to future calls that may result in patient harm. The impact of the comments is usually unrecognized by the speaker. Simulation gives an opportunity to 'play it out' and refine or even script responses. For example, the phrase 'Thank you for calling, how can we help' is a mandated introduction for responders arriving on scene in some courses. This replaces 'Why did you call', which can be unintentionally threatening.

To identify attitudinal or cultural barriers to success, simulations have included scenarios where the patient has recovered by the time the team has arrived. A number of centres and disciplines have use *in situ* simulation to identify and mitigate sources of latent errors prior to their leading to patient harm, and as means of testing out new procedures, equipment systems, operating rooms, and other clinical environments.[25-29]

Operationally, to do an *in situ* simulation, a high-fidelity mannequin is taken to the room and is connected to any relevant equipment, after which the nurse is introduced to the patient and her clinical course, and told to respond to any problems as she would in real life. Pre-event cooperation from area managers is essential in determining a suitable location, time, and caregiver. Following introduction, an abnormality is introduced either by a 'family member' portrayed by simulation staff, or an electronic alert. Depending on the training goal, most scenarios involve a patient who is either medically unstable, or one in full cardiopulmonary arrest. If emergency teams are summoned, it helps to have a simulating staff member tell arriving personnel that 'this is a drill, treat it as if it were real'. The duration and extent of the simulation is dictated by the overall goal of the exercise for example, managing an arrest, calling for help managing an unstable patient, and transportation to OR or ICU, and is terminated according to the predetermined goal. Once the event is stopped, participants are thanked for their participation and asked to stay for a brief discussion. Debriefing then centres on the specific goals of the simulation, and must be focused because all the responders have been pulled away from other clinical duties.

Whether relevant to the goals of the simulation or not, participants are usually filled with questions on topics that interest them, so one should also recognize and accommodate these needs if it is possible to do it briefly. A great deal has been written on debriefing techniques, and the reader is referred to the discussion in Chapter 13. As with centre-based simulation, videotape is an effective adjunct to debriefing, and can often be accomplished with a small tripod-mounted video recorder, and a small video screen (or cables to the patient's TV) for playback. Some have suggested that the quality and fidelity of the *in situ* simulation experience obviates the need for a formal training centre.[26]

25.8 **Synthesis and conclusions**

Simulation systems and team-level training programmes owe their origin to data demonstrating a connection between medical errors, and failings in cognition and teamwork. CRM represents an analytic approach based on cognitive and social psychology that has been used in aviation and medical simulation training to understand and improve on human performance. Careful design of patient-crisis scenarios can facilitate the understanding and application of CRM concepts to the healthcare environment. Unlike retrospective studies that assess medical management error well after the fact, crisis simulations with debriefings can identify and correct errors in close to real time.

References

1 **Lee A, Bishop G, Hillman KM, Daffurn K**. The medical emergency team. Anaesthesia and Intensive Care 1995;**23**:183–186.

2 **DeVita MA, Braithwaite RS, Mahidhara R, Stuart S, Foraida M, Simmons RL**. Use of medical emergency team responses to reduce hospital cardiopulmonary arrests. Quality & Safety in Health Care 2004;**13**:251–254.

3 **Devita MA, Bellomo R, Hillman K, et al**. Findings of the first consensus conference on medical emergency teams. Critical Care Medicine 2006;**34**:2463–2478.

4 **Gaba DM, Fish KJ, Howard SK**. Crisis management in anesthesiology. New York, NY: Churchill Livingstone;1994.

5 **Helmreich RL**. Managing human error in aviation. Sci Am 1997;**276**:62–67.

6 **Cooper G, White M, Lauber J**. Resource management on the flightdeck: proceedings of a NASA/Industry workshop (NASA CP-2120). Moffet Field, CA: NASA Ames Research Center; 1980.

7 **Gaba DM**. Improving anesthesiologists' performance by simulating reality. Anesthesiology 1992;**76**:491–494.

8 **Schwid HA**. A flight simulator for general anesthesia training. Comput Biomed Res 1987;**20**:64–75.

9 **Gaba DM, DeAnda A**. A comprehensive anesthesia simulation environment: re-creating the operating room for research and training. Anesthesiology 1988;**69**:387–394.

10 **Cooper JB, Taqueti VR**. A brief history of the development of mannequin simulators for clinical education and training. Quality & Safety in Health Care 2004;**13**(Suppl 1):i11–18.

11 **Holzman RS, Cooper JB, Gaba DM, Philip JH, Small SD, Feinstein D**. Anesthesia crisis resource management: real-life simulation training in operating room crises. J Clin Anesth 1995;**7**:675–687.

12 **Lighthall GK, Mayette M, Harrison TK**. An institutionwide approach to redesigning management of cardiopulmonary resuscitation. Jt Comm J Qual Patient Saf 2013;**39**:157–166.

13 **DeVita MA, Schaefer J, Lutz J, Dongilli T, Wang H**. Improving medical crisis team performance. Critical Care Medicine 2004;**32**:S61–65.

14 **Fiedor ML, DeVita MA**. Human simulation and crisis team training. In: Dunn WF, ed. Simulators in critical care and beyond. Des Plaines, IL: SCCM Press; 2004, 91–94.

15 **Gaba DM, Howard SK, Fish KJ, Smith BE, Sowb YA**. Simulation-based training in anesthesia crisis resource management (ACRM): a decade of experience. Simulation and Gaming 2001;**32**:175–193.

16 DeVita MA, Schaefer J, Lutz J, Wang H, Dongilli T. Improving medical emergency team (MET) performance using a novel curriculum and a computerized human patient simulator. Quality & Safety in Health Care 2005;**14**:326–331.

17 DeVita MA, Lutz J, Mininni N, Grbach W. A novel debriefing tool: online facilitator guidance package for debriefing team training using simulation. Simulation in Healthcare 2006;1.

18 Fanning R, Gaba DM. Debriefing (Chapter 4). In: Gaba DM, Fish KJ, Howard SK, Burden AR, eds. Crisis management in anesthesiology. Second edition. New York, NY: Elsevier, Inc.; 2015, 65–78.

19 Rudolph J, Simon R, Dufrense R, Raemer D. There's no such thing as 'nonjudgmental' debriefing: a theory and method for debriefing with good judgment. Simulation in Healthcare 2006;**1**:49–55.

20 Clark EA, Fisher J, Arafeh J, Druzin M. Team training/simulation. Clinical Obstetrics and Gynecology 2010;**53**:265–277.

21 Paul G, Lane E. Inside the debriefing room: multidisciplinary rapid response team training findings revealed. Clinical Simulation in Nursing 2014;**10**:e227–233.

22 Hunt EA, Shilkofski NA, Stavroudis TA, Nelson KL. Simulation: translation to improved team performance. Anesthesiology Clinics 2007;**25**:301–319.

23 Hunt EA, Vera K, Diener-West M, et al. Delays and errors in cardiopulmonary resuscitation and defibrillation by pediatric residents during simulated cardiopulmonary arrests. Resuscitation 2009;**80**:819–825.

24 Hunt EA, Walker AR, Shaffner DH, Miller MR, Pronovost PJ. Simulation of in-hospital pediatric medical emergencies and cardiopulmonary arrests: highlighting the importance of the first 5 minutes. Pediatrics 2008;**121**:e34–43.

25 Kobayashi L, Parchuri R, Gardiner FG, et al. Use of *in situ* simulation and human factors engineering to assess and improve emergency department clinical systems for timely telemetry-based detection of life-threatening arrhythmias. BMJ Qual Saf 2013;**22**:72–83.

26 Weinstock PH, Kappus LJ, Garden A, Burns JP. Simulation at the point of care: reduced-cost, *in situ* training via a mobile cart. Pediatr Crit Care Med 2009;**10**:176–181.

27 Wheeler DS, Geis G, Mack EH, LeMaster T, Patterson MD. High-reliability emergency response teams in the hospital: improving quality and safety using *in situ* simulation training. BMJ Qual Saf 2013;**22**:507–514.

28 Lighthall GK, Poon T, Harrison TK. Using *in situ* simulation to improve in-hospital cardiopulmonary resuscitation. Jt Comm J Qual Patient Saf 2010;**36**:209–216.

29 Preston P, Lopez C, Corbett N. How to integrate findings from simulation exercises to improve obstetrics care in the institution. Semin Perinatol 2011;**35**:84–88.

Chapter 26

Surgical simulation

Roger Kneebone and Fernando Bello

Overview

- Surgical practice demands a complex mixture of knowledge, judgement, technical skill, and effective teamworking. But surgical practice is changing dramatically, with greatly curtailed training time.

- Simulation offers the opportunity to practise within a learner-centred environment that meets criteria for educational effectiveness yet avoids risk to patients.

- Simulation-based training should allow regular context-based practice, providing feedback within a supportive, learner-centred milieu. A theory-grounded curriculum should underpin surgical training and ensure a connection between clinical and simulation-based experience.

- Surgical simulators include physical models, virtual reality computer systems, and hybrids that combine the two.

- Increased computational power and advanced 3D modelling techniques make possible the combination of an individual patient's anatomy and pathology to generate personalized simulations.

- The context of learning is inseparable from the skills that are learned. Each surgical learning experience is unique and must be related to the specific needs of the learner.

- The relationship between fidelity of a simulation and its effectiveness is not a simple one. Levels of realism should be tailored to meet educational goals within practical constraints of cost and technical feasibility.

- Any new technology needs to be validated. The acid test for simulation is whether it maps onto clinical performance and leads to improved outcomes.

- Future developments include patient-specific simulation (uploading individual clinical data into simulations) and patient-focused simulation (using actors to play the part of patients within simulations and provide feedback from the patients' perspective).

- Multiscale integrative simulation from the nano to the macro scale, requiring trainees to deal with all currently available information about a patient and her state of health, represents the next big challenge in medical simulation.

26.1 **Introduction to surgical simulation**

Since the first edition, simulation in surgery has reached a tipping point. Earlier debates about **whether** simulation is effective have given way to discussions about **how** it can be made widely available. Yet, the term 'surgical simulation' continues to admit many interpretations, and widespread consensus remains elusive.

We start this chapter by painting a broad picture of what surgical simulation can offer and why it is widely used, outlining philosophical questions about its role within surgical education. As in the previous edition of this book, we distinguish between simulators and simulation. After summarizing key contributions from educational theory, we give an overview of current approaches. Finally, we highlight areas of likely growth and speculate about where these might lead in the future.

Technical expertise is so obviously essential to surgery that it tends to steal the limelight. For example, high-fidelity virtual reality (VR) simulation has focused on surgical techniques. However, technical skill is only one component of safe surgical practice. An overly technical emphasis can overshadow other elements of clinical care, where knowledge, decision-making, communication, and an awareness of clinical risk are equally important. Crucially, perhaps, a preoccupation with component skills and competencies can distract attention from the broader humanistic values of skilled, compassionate care and the education which underpins it.

One of our aims in this chapter is to highlight this wider landscape of clinical context. In it, we frame surgical simulation as an educational approach, rather than an activity confined to specialist centres. Our own innovations of hybrid, distributed, and sequential simulation raise new opportunities and challenges in response to a clinical, educational, and social landscape in continual flux. We frame simulation as a means of engaging clinicians, managers, patients, and those who care for them in collective encounters aimed at improving the quality and safety of care for all concerned.

26.2 **Background**

Major changes have taken place since the first edition of this chapter. Surgical simulation has moved from being a means of practising specific technical skills (often restricted to specialized centres and requiring complex and costly equipment), to becoming a mainstream component of every surgeon's training. In the United Kingdom, for example, a series of influential reports and policy documents have set out a mandate for simulation-based training.[1,2] The widespread move towards restriction of working hours on both sides of the Atlantic has given further impetus to finding alternatives to traditional 'learning through doing', whether in the operating theatre, the clinic, or at the bedside. The worldwide shift towards patient safety has provided further momentum. At the same time, exciting developments in the field of simulation itself have opened new avenues for simulation-based learning.

Surgery is an area where the arguments for simulation are very compelling. It seems obvious that novices should learn the basics of their craft on inanimate models before being let loose on patients. It is also evident that surgeons in training should continue to refine their techniques by practising within a safe environment. Perhaps the most powerful argument for simulation is the absence of an acceptable alternative.

Political and public pressure is mounting to make surgical training transparent, and patients are no longer willing to be practised on. Simulation offers the opportunity for safe, focused learning to complement and reinforce clinical experience. Yet, these apparently obvious truths conceal a more complex reality. Of course, technical skill is an essential component of any surgeon's work, but technical procedures are only a part of the story, and too much emphasis on technique can divert attention from other important aspects. Recent high-profile cases (such as the UK's Mid Staffordshire NHS Trust scandal) highlight the crucial importance of core values of care, compassion, kindness, and respect, and the catastrophic effects when they are absent.[3]

This unfolding phase of simulation-based practice and research marks a more subtle, nuanced, and critical approach to surgical simulation—one which takes into account the multiple perspectives of patients, clinicians, managers, and educationalists. Alongside technological advances in **simulators** (physical and computer-based apparatus), advances in our understanding of **simulation** (as a domain of educational practice and scholarship) are opening new horizons for the field.

26.3 **Simulation components**

Recent developments are challenging the assumption that effective surgical simulation requires a dedicated simulation centre. Although such centres can be highly effective (replicating complex clinical environments in minute detail), they are both scarce and costly. This limits the accessibility of simulation. Moreover, the organizational and economic imperatives of simulation centres are often different from those of clinical practice. Much can be achieved in other ways.

Alternative approaches include *in situ* simulation (locating simulations in authentic clinical settings such as hospital wards, intensive care units, and operating theatres)[4] and distributed simulation (DS).[5] The latter uses low-cost, portable alternatives to static centres to create a **sense** of a clinical setting without attempting to replicate every detail.[6] This provides a context where the social, technical, and educational elements of surgery can be interwoven. Although conceptually simple, this approach has proved highly effective in removing barriers of cost and access (see Figure 26.1).

26.3.1 **The procedure or operation**

This area has been dominated by simulators. Much development and investment focuses on apparatus for practising selected surgical techniques across a range of complexity. Latest advances include simulators supporting robotic surgery and new techniques of interventional radiology. Until recently, however, simulators focused on specific procedures and offered a relatively limited range of variants within a given intervention. Minimal access procedures, for example, relied on repeated performance of the same set of tasks.

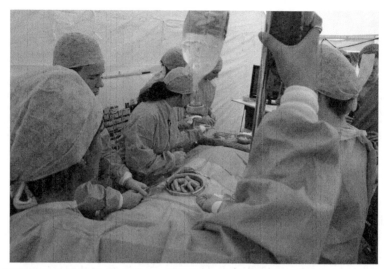

Fig. 26.1 Distributed simulation using customized prosthetic models.

This raised concerns that learners would 'play the simulator' without necessarily gaining skills that would improve their performance with patients. Many VR simulators now offer different levels of challenge, with a range of anatomical variants that may include both normal and pathological anatomy. Although not yet widespread, some simulators also include the possibility of practising patient-specific simulation. Nevertheless, simulation practice often takes place out of clinical context, and a 'formulaic' design can interfere with the suspension of disbelief.

26.3.2 **The professional setting**

Surgeons do not operate in isolation, but as members of a complex team with multiple viewpoints, priorities, and 'circles of focus'.[7] Effective functioning within the team is as important to a satisfactory outcome as technical expertise. Communication with anaesthetic, nursing, and other team members is essential to decision-making and high-quality care.[8, 9] Many of the stresses of operative surgery relate to the professional environment rather than purely technical problems.[10] A growing awareness of the complexity of 'normal' surgery emphasizes the need for simulation to address multiple perspectives simultaneously.[11]

Although an obvious focus of attention, an operation is only one component of the complex journey which all surgical patients undergo. From a patient's point of view, preoperative clinic assessment and investigation, the operation itself, postoperative care on ward or intensive care unit, discharge, and follow-up are part of a single experience, though they are often considered in isolation.

Building on DS, the concept of sequential simulation (SqS) frames clinical care as a **sequence** of interconnected elements rather than a single episode. Concatenating

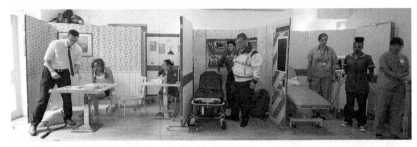

Fig. 26.2 Sequential simulation of a care pathway.

representative 'slices' of care (of which the operation is one) invites participants to identify which components of a care pathway are critical. SqS allows care pathways to be viewed, challenged, and remodelled as a collaborative endeavour, using DS to enact 'snapshots' of care (see Figure 26.2). Conceptually, this differs profoundly from the learning of procedures that are established and unproblematic.

26.3.3 **The patient experience**

For all its technical complexities, surgery is built on the same foundations as any other clinical field. Its crux is the relationship of care between two people—a clinician and a patient. Clinician–patient communication is crucial to all healthcare practice and demands sensitivity and awareness on the part of the clinician.

Our group's pioneering work with **hybrid simulation** (the combination of inanimate models and VR simulators with simulated patients) has expanded to include customized prosthetics, which create a powerful illusion of illness or injury in healthy human actors.[12] This allows the skills of clinical examination, communication, decision-making, and operative surgery to be fused. The effectiveness of simple hybrid simulation, in turn, has contributed to a growing international awareness that imaginative (and often inexpensive) approaches to simulation can create high levels of perceived realism without the need for elaborate technology.[13, 14]

26.4 **Educational theory**

In order to understand what simulation can achieve, and what its limitations are, some educational theory will be helpful.[15] If theory is ignored, there is a risk of providing simulators in a vacuum, without educational support. Although some learning will take place in such cases, there is a danger that it may not be effective. In each of the following categories, a brief overview of key theories is followed by a discussion relating to surgical simulation.

In a nutshell, surgical simulation needs to be actively managed and to have specific aims. Simulator technology is only part of a wider picture, with simulators being necessary, but not sufficient for effective simulation. It is important to pay attention to the conditions required for acquiring expertise, to provide tutor support when needed, to ensure that simulation-based experience integrates with the curriculum and maps on to actual clinical practice, and to create a supportive, learner-centred environment.

26.4.1 **Expertise**

The acquisition of technical skill is a most obvious use for simulation. The key to gaining expertise is sustained deliberate practice over a prolonged period. In the case of elite performers in other domains, a minimum of ten years is required.[16] Yet, simple repetition of a task is not sufficient. Practice has to be driven by a motivation to improve. Each learner needs a clear vision of what they are aiming for, together with the opportunity to practise repeatedly and gauge the effect of their practice. Knowledge of results and expert feedback is crucial here, if learners are not to develop bad habits.

26.4.2 **Tutor support**

Of course, much surgical learning takes place by observation, by experience, and by doing. Yet, a skilled tutor can help this process enormously. Lev Vygotsky (a Russian psychologist in the first half of the twentieth century) developed the concept of the 'zone of proximal development' (ZPD).[17] In the ZPD, a learner can solve problems 'in collaboration with more capable peers' even if unable to do so unassisted. This process is clearly seen in the operating theatre, with one-to-one teaching. But it can also take place within simulation. Tutor support may be personal, or it may involve educational technology. Simulation must form part of a curriculum which combines equipment with expert tuition. Most important of all, simulation needs to connect with the clinical reality it is designed to mirror.

26.4.3 **The context of learning**

Surgical simulation has a very practical aim—to improve patient care. So we must consider how the simulated universe maps onto the clinical one. Unless there is a clear connection between the two, simulation-based practice risks being out of touch with reality, with technical skills being learned but never applied.

Apprenticeship has been at the heart of surgical learning for generations, though restrictions in length of training are now challenging traditional models. A more contemporary view, based on the concept of communities of practice, frames learning as an integral part of social practice.[18, 19] In such communities, newcomers learn by joining a group of professionals who share a common aim and relations between peers are as important as relations between apprentice and master. According to this view, apprenticeship is as much about conferring legitimacy and establishing a professional identity, as about the transmission of knowledge and skill.

It follows from this that the context of surgical learning is crucial. If skills are practised out of context and there is no opportunity to apply them clinically, they will not feed into the communities of practice where clinical learning takes place. Therefore, simulation must set out to be relevant to the clinical activity in which learners engage after leaving the skills centre. Ideally, it should offer opportunities for 'just in time' learning, triggered by day-to-day clinical experience. This has implications for where simulation facilities are sited and how they are designed.

26.4.4 **The climate of learning**

Unlike the clinical environment, simulation is designed for the benefit of the learner. Rather than fitting learning opportunities around clinical care, the learning itself takes the spotlight. We know that the affective component of learning (whether positive or negative) has a powerful impact on participants. Effective simulation-based learning requires a supportive, learner-centred setting where all participants behave with respect and professionalism.

26.5 **Simulator technology**

Although only part of the wider picture outlined previously, simulator technology plays a vital role in the provision of simulation-based training. Such technology may be grouped in three main different types. Writing from a UK perspective, where the use of live animals for training has been prohibited for more than a century, we do not cover live animal simulations in our discussion. The final selection of which simulator(s) to use will depend on individual requirements and the proposed curriculum.

26.5.1 **Physical models**

Benchtop models are widely used within surgical training, especially at undergraduate and early postgraduate levels where they fulfil a useful function by allowing novices to practise tasks repeatedly. These models are made from a variety of plastic and latex materials. They address a range of clinical procedures (e.g. venepuncture, cannulation, urinary catheterization, basic suturing), as well as bowel and vascular anastomosis, hernia repair, and other commonly performed surgical tasks. They have the advantage of being able to interact directly with instruments and to show a range of tissue-handling characteristics.

Box trainers allow minimal access surgery procedures to be practised using endoscopic instruments. A covering of artificial skin allows port insertion and basic camera management, and a variety of tasks can be presented within the box. They are especially helpful during the early stages of training, since basic techniques such as camera handling, tissue dissection, and endoscopic suturing can be rehearsed repeatedly. Dead animal tissue can be used for practising more advanced procedures. Recent years have seen a surge in different types of box trainers based around the Fundamentals of Laparoscopic Surgery (FLS) programme, some of which are portable and compatible with smartphones, encouraging 'take-home' training of basic laparoscopic skills.

Advances in materials technology have drastically improved the level of realism that can be attained by bespoke models (see Figure 26.1), though these tend to be significantly more expensive than their less realistic, off-the-shelf counterparts. In comparison with VR computer simulators, physical models are relatively cheap. A major drawback is that the majority of these models are divorced from their clinical context and can lead to a reductionist approach to learning. They also do not incorporate facilities for objective performance assessment.

26.5.2 **Virtual reality (VR) computing**

The range of computer-generated simulations of surgical procedures has continued to expand, albeit at a slower pace while VR simulation companies have experienced a consolidation phase. The degree of available realism has also improved as a result of advances in computational power, visualization, and haptic interfaces, thus allowing learners to interact with a more convincing computer-based environment. Minimal-access procedures lend themselves especially to such simulations, as manipulating objects with surgical instruments, while watching a 2D screen, reflects the reality of minimal-access surgery.

A VR simulator consists of a manipulation station (using instruments which resemble those used in surgical procedures), a screen, and a computer. Learners choose procedures from a menu of varying levels of difficulty and performance metrics (e.g. time taken, bleeding encountered, errors made), and the procedure itself can be recorded automatically. Feedback based on these metrics is normally provided after the procedure, with or without a tutor's input.

The first generation of VR simulators focused on training basic skills by performing isolated tasks (e.g. pick and place, navigation) using abstract scenes and 2D representations of geometric solids. Systems like the original MIST-VR established a record of efficacy and were extensively validated.

The second generation focused also on basic skills, but attempted to achieve this by using more realistic procedural tasks, such as clipping blood vessels or intracorporeal knotting. In these programs, the background to the simulation or virtual environment looks much more like that of a real operation, with deformable tissues and realistic organ responses. The LapSim from Surgical Science was one of the first systems using this approach.

The third generation allowed entire procedures (e.g. laparoscopic cholecystectomy) to be simulated, providing anatomical variants to create different levels of difficulty. This was a significant advance in creating an environment that moved beyond psychomotor skill and began to include decision-making in a complex world. The LapMentor from Simbionix was a pioneer system offering force feedback-enabled laparoscopic training.

The current generation of VR simulators exhibits mostly incremental advances reflecting progress in computer graphics, design, interfacing, and visualization, as well as enhanced ergonomics, improved content and curriculum management, and better integration with simulated clinical settings. While minimal-access interventions continue to dominate, the range of specialities covered has expanded significantly and now includes otorhinolaryngology, orthopaedics, dentistry, and ophthalmology, among others.

While the trade-off between high visual fidelity and the simulator's ability to respond in real time to the manipulations of the operator still holds, a move towards highly parallelized computer architectures based around advanced GPU-processing has increased performance by orders of magnitude.

The cost of VR simulators and their need for specialized support continues to be a significant drawback to their wider adoption.

26.5.3 Hybrid simulators

These simulators combine a physical model (replicating the instruments as well as the anatomy interface) with a computer program (which creates interactive settings within which learning can take place). A key advantage of such technology is its potential for team training and for moving beyond the practice of isolated technical skills. The boundary between hybrid simulators and VR simulators is gradually becoming less well defined, with several VR simulators now providing further integration and able to also support team training.

26.5.3.1 Sophisticated patient manikins

Sophisticated patient manikins (Laerdal SimMan, CAE METIman/iStan) are computer-driven, full-scale model humans which present a range of pathophysiological variables and can respond to the administration of drugs, as well as give immediate feedback to a range of interventions. They are well established within anaesthetic training, for example, and increasingly being used in other domains including advanced life support training, operating room training, and paediatrics. Such simulators may be used within a dedicated educational facility (e.g. a training centre or simulated operating theatre) but also in the field. Portable manikins allow realistic disaster scenarios to be mounted in a range of authentic settings, enabling clinical assessment and casualty evacuation.

26.5.3.2 Hybrid endoscopy simulators

Hybrid endoscopy simulators (Surgical Science EndoSim, Simbionix GI Mentor) combine an authentic interface (the endoscope) with realistic VR displays of the endoluminal view seen by the operator. They simulate a range of diagnostic and therapeutic endoscopic procedures, including upper and lower gastrointestinal flexible endoscopy. A collection of virtual patient cases offers different levels of difficulty, allowing novice and intermediate learners to gain the basics of manipulative skill through repeated practice. Performance metrics are captured by the software and presented to the learner after each procedure.

26.5.3.3 Hybrid interventional endovascular simulators

Hybrid interventional endovascular simulators (CAE EndoVR, Mentice's VIST, Simbionix Angio Mentor) use sophisticated computer graphics and modelling techniques to produce synthetic live fluoroscopy images and simulate the interaction between vascular walls, catheters, and guidewires. Custom-made hardware interfaces using real catheters reproduce the crucial force feedback involved in such procedures. Current simulators offer a variety of cases covering a range of vascular procedures including coronary, neurovascular, renal, SFA and iliac artery interventions, carotid stenting, as well as more advanced interventions such as TEVAR and EVAR. The decision-making process is enhanced during the simulation by the display of vital signs, haemodynamic wave tracings, and patient responses that appropriately reflect the physiology.

As the range of simulators continues to expand, both in terms of functionality and procedures covered, specialized programmes making use of simulator technology are becoming established in some surgical specialties (e.g. laparoscopic surgery, orthopaedics). Given that the life cycle of individual simulators is relatively short (only a few years), it is crucial to have a clear educational strategy in place before selecting expensive simulator equipment.

26.6 **Simulation evaluation and validation**

It now seems clear that simulation has a central role to play within surgical education. Earlier arguments about whether simulation-based learning could transfer to clinical settings have now been largely settled. Yet, simulation remains a growth area (with major commercial potential) and new simulators and approaches to simulation are continually being released. Making sense of this diversity is a major challenge. Moreover, not all simulation is equally effective. Success demands a symbiotic relationship between users and developers. For surgical trainers and trainees, simulation must meet educational needs and improve clinical practice. For simulator developers, however, technical development and profitability are key drivers. This tension can lead to unhelpful confusion about who is leading and who is following. This may divert attention from the key tasks of identifying training needs and working collaboratively towards reliable and valid systems which satisfy them.

26.7 **Future developments**

The rapid pace of development in the fields related to simulator technology makes predicting the future impossible. Nevertheless, we believe that some currents are clear. There will be further symbiosis between users of simulators and their developers. Together with the acceptance and insistence by the public that all surgical professionals reach a required level of competence using simulation-based training before treating a patient, this symbiosis will serve as a catalyst for the more widespread use of surgical simulators. To support this use, simulator technology will continue to become more portable and cheaper, perhaps even following a 'Simulation App Store' model where simulation users can download simulator apps that can then be tailored and executed on a common **Smart Simulation Platform**.

Counterbalancing the experimental and exploratory nature of much simulation is a growing body of evidence relating to its impact. The need for consolidation, evaluation, and synthesis of evidence is obvious, and a rigorous scholarship of simulation is emerging.

Artificial and unhelpful separations between training, rehearsal, and clinical practice will be effaced, and a convergence between clinicians, industry, and the creative sector will develop new approaches to learning. At the same time, access to simulation will continue to expand. Until recently, the operating theatre was seen as the exclusive province of healthcare professionals. For obvious reasons of confidentiality and infection control, access to actual surgery must be strictly controlled, but simulation can offer a window into otherwise closed clinical worlds, opening new possibilities and inviting outsiders to witness (and participate in) the processes of surgery without jeopardizing patient safety.

Developments in simulator technology (especially the concept of low-cost lightweight DS) make it possible to present the world of surgery in non-traditional settings such as science fairs, arts venues, and music festivals. Boundaries between professional and public involvement with simulation will become erased, leading to more effective dialogue between those who need care and those who provide it.[20]

By reconfiguring notions of expertise, simulation can open the kinds of communication which break through disciplinary boundaries and challenge power gradients. Acknowledging that patients, carers, and clinicians have equally (though differently) valid perspectives, such events can bring about 'reciprocal illumination'.

26.8 Conclusion

Surgical simulation is here to stay. Yet, 'simulation' is a polyvalent term. In recent years, the focus has moved from procedural simulators to a broader perspective, acknowledging the complexities and ambiguities of surgery. Viewed as a mirror for surgical practice, simulation changes from being a vehicle for the transmission of knowledge and skills (where experts teach non-experts) into a forum for collaborative learning (where clinicians, patients, and those who care for them can learn from one another to bring about a change for all concerned).

This process seems certain to be a mainstay of surgical training in the future. These are exciting times, and the pace of change is breathless. Advances in computing and materials technology will increase the realism of skills-based simulators. A growing awareness of context will highlight the importance of teamworking and professionalism within the surgical environment. Developments such as *in situ* simulation and DS are pointing towards a democratization of simulation—a widening of its reach. Simulation will act as a nexus, where perspectives of patients, clinicians, and others come together to explore new approaches to surgery in its many forms.

Yet, a major challenge for any simulation is to ensure that learners' needs come first. Without a curriculum, there is a danger that technology will dominate learning and that educational goals will be eclipsed. Clear vision is essential to make wise use of simulation's enormous potential, and to ensure an equal partnership between pedagogy and technology.

Acknowledgements

We acknowledge the work of our many colleagues within and beyond Imperial College London; in particular, our collaborations with Debra Nestel, Gunther Kress, Ian Curran, and the invaluable contribution of our graduate students and researchers. We are grateful for the support of the London Deanery STeLI initiative, Health Education North West London, Wellcome Trust, Engineering and Physical Sciences Research Council (EPSRC), and Economics and Social Sciences Research Council (ESRC) in developing our work around simulation and engagement.

References

1 **Donaldson L.** 150 years of the Chief Medical Officer's annual report. Department of Health; 2008.

2 **Temple J.** Time for training. Medical Education England (MEE); 2010.

3 **Francis R.** Report of the Mid Staffordshire NHS Foundation Trust Public Inquiry. The Stationery Office; 2013.

4 **Patterson MD, Blike GT, Nadkarni VM.** *In situ* simulation: challenges and results. In: Henriksen K, Battles JB, Keyes MA, Grady ML, eds. New directions and alternative approaches. Vol. 3. Performance and tools. AHRQ publication no. 08–0034–3. Rockville, MD; 2008, 1–18.

5 **Kassab E, Tun JK, Arora S, et al.** 'Blowing up the barriers' in surgical training: exploring and validating the concept of distributed simulation. Ann Surg 2011;**254**(6):1059–1065.

6 **Kneebone R, Arora S, King D, et al.** Distributed simulation—accessible immersive training. Med Teach 2010;(32):65–70.

7 **Kneebone R.** Simulation, safety and surgery. Qual Saf Health Care 2010; **19**(S3):47–52.

8 **Lingard L, Reznick R, Espin S, et al.** Team communications in the operating room: talk patterns, sites of tension, and implications for novices. Acad Med 2002; **77**(3):232–237.

9 **Lingard L, Espin S, Whyte S, et al.** Communication failures in the operating room: an observational classification of recurrent types and effects. Qual Saf Health Care 2004;**13**(5):330–334.

10 **Wetzel CM, Kneebone RL, Woloshynowych M, et al.** The effects of stress on surgical performance. Am J Surg 2006;**191**(1):5–10.

11 **Kneebone R, Nestel D, Vincent C, et al.** Complexity, risk and simulation in learning procedural skills. Med Educ 2007;**41**(8):808–814.

12 **Tun JK, Granados A, Mavroveli S, et al.** Simulating various levels of clinical challenge in the assessment of clinical procedure competence. Ann Emerg Med 2012; **60**:112–120.

13 **Kneebone R, Nestel D, Wetzel C, et al.** The human face of simulation: patient-focused simulation training. Acad Med 2006;**81**(10):919–924.

14 **Kneebone R, Bello F, Nestel D, et al.** Learner-centred feedback using remote assessment of clinical procedures. Med Teach 2008;(30):795–801.

15 **Kneebone RL.** Clinical simulation for learning procedural skills: a theory-based approach. Acad Med 2005;**80**(6):549–553.

16 **Ericsson KA.** Deliberate practice and the acquisition and maintenance of expert performance in medicine and related domains. Acad Med 2004;**79**(10):S70–S81.

17 **Vygotsky LS.** Mind in society. Harvard University Press: Cambridge, MA; 1978.

18 **Lave J, Wenger E.** Situated learning. Legitimate peripheral participation. Cambridge University Press: Cambridge; 1991.

19 **Wenger E.** Communities of practice. Learning, meaning, and identity. Cambridge University Press: Cambridge; 1998.

20 **Tang J, Maroothynaden J, Bello F, et al.** Public engagement through shared immersion: participating in the processes of research. Sci Commun 2012;**35**:654–666.

Chapter 27

Simulation-based emergency medicine and disaster training

Mary D Patterson, John A Vozenilek, and Mark W Bowyer

Overview

- Simulation training is now a standard in emergency medicine as well as in disaster preparedness. The vast majority of emergency training programmes now utilize simulation in some way.

- These simulations may include multiple 'patients' and reflect the importance of surge and prioritization in emergency practice

- In addition to technical or procedural skill training, non-technical, interdisciplinary and *in situ* simulations have become increasingly important.

- Simulation provides a method of ensuring exposure to a standard set of critical and seasonal conditions as opposed to relying on chance or random patient presentations to the emergency department.

- The evaluation of competencies for emergency medicine trainees and the development of simulation-based certification processes for emergency medicine practitioners is a relatively new use for emergency medicine-based simulation.

- More sophisticated simulators present opportunities to develop and practise complicated decision-making and management skills as well as the management of multiple simultaneous patients.

- Restrictions in resident duty hours have resulted in simulation-based training replacing clinical experience in some circumstances.

- Simulation is becoming recognized as a valid tool for the evaluation of new facilities, systems, team, and processes before their actual use in the clinical environment and for disaster preparedness.

- The field is maturing but there is a need for additional evidence that directly links simulation training to improved patient outcomes

27.1 **Introduction to simulation-based emergency medicine and disaster training**

Simulation has found wide application as an educational and safety tool in emergency medicine (EM). By 2008, 91% of US emergency medicine training programmes utilized simulation and 85% utilized mannequin-based simulation.[1] In the last decade, published work in simulation has incorporated not only technical skills but significant work in non-technical skills and human factors work related to the evaluation of new facilities, new processes, and reconfigured teams.[2–6] The use of simulation has extended to disaster and mass casualty exercises as well.[7–9] There are a remarkable variety of cases and training events which fall within the purview of the emergency specialist. Since improved patient care and patient safety are generally the goals of EM simulations, the recognition of internal and external factors which can optimize or degrade patient care are key. Simulations often will focus on required skills in multiple simultaneous patient management (including mass casualty exercises). Paralleling simulation use in general, simulation is used increasingly to train and assess individual, team, and system competencies as well as to develop and evaluate new processes and new facilities.

Critical teamwork and communication skills (non-technical skills) are regularly incorporated in time-pressured critical emergency scenarios, and often these are now conducted in an interdisciplinary fashion. These simulations may include nurses, respiratory therapists, technicians, as well as medical specialties such as emergency medicine and surgery.[3, 10, 11] A further development in simulation-based emergency training is the setting for simulation-based training. Interdisciplinary simulation is now as likely to occur *in situ* (in the actual clinical setting) as in a simulation centre.[5, 12–16]

Simulations designed to meet the needs of the emergency-care provider may range from the patient with a minor illness or injury to the critical patient suffering a myocardial infarction. These and many other patients must be triaged, evaluated, and managed simultaneously. This is especially true of simulations constructed for disaster or mass casualty incidents. The 'open' format of the typical emergency department often leads to situations in which healthcare providers must simultaneously manage patient care and interact with the patient's family members. Using standardized '*moulaged*' patients concurrently with computerized mannequin simulators, therefore, provides obvious educational and experiential advantages. Another important aspect of emergency care is the concept of prioritization and 'flow' in times of crisis. Traditional modes for simulating these events include exercises on paper, computer-based exercises, and mannequin-type patient simulators, or any or all modes used in combination. These efforts can be effective not only for emergency practitioners, but also for the hospitals and systems in which they operate. The simulation of 'surge' (the influx of more patients than the system is equipped to handle) and the development of 'surge capacity', the solutions to an overwhelming influx of patients, are critically important in light of the concerns for pandemic disease and viral threats.[8, 9]

27.2 **Formal educational programmes**

As a relatively young specialty, much of the guidance related to curriculum and practice of EM in general originates in the United States, Europe, Australia, and New Zealand. In 2000, the American College of Emergency Physicians (ACEP) approved the first Model of the Clinical Practice of Emergency Medicine. The 2013 Model of the Clinical Practice of Emergency Medicine is jointly approved by the American Board of Emergency Medicine, ACEP, Council of Residency Directors, Emergency Medicine Residents Association (EMRA), Residency Review Committee for Emergency Medicine (RRC-EM), and the Society for Academic Emergency Medicine (SAEM).[17] Its original purpose, as defined in the document, is 'a listing of common conditions, symptoms, and diseases seen and evaluated in emergency departments'. As such, this document provides a framework for the types of cases or training that would be suitable for trainees in EM.

On a broader scale, a number of curricula have been developed that target not only physicians but the entire emergency team. This includes TeamSTEPPS (developed by the US Department of Defense and the US federal government) whose various versions may utilize simulation and may be used with a variety of acute-care teams.[18, 19] Additionally, a number of organizations have developed simulation-based curricula that focus on emergency teams, as well as relevant collaborations.[3, 20–22] These include simulation-based training focused on trauma patients in the emergency department or the emergency patient with a difficult airway.[6, 11]

27.3 **Technical skill training**

It has become generally accepted that providers should not perform their 'first' procedure of any type on an actual patient. There is a significant ethical drive to provide educational experiences for learners in a safe and controlled simulation environment. In addition, there is a growing body of information in the medical literature regarding the use of simulation for resident education. Reznek has written, 'Superior patient care and optimal physician training are often mutually exclusive in the clinical setting, and consequently live-patient training has several significant shortcomings'.[23] These limitations include the increased risk of complications for the patient, the inability to guarantee procedural opportunities (the presentation of a particular type of case or procedure is random or seasonal), the inability to provide repeated or graduated opportunities for practice of a particular procedure, and the ethical obligation to intervene if one sees an error in progress. There are no opportunities for a resident to learn from a mistake under controlled conditions without harm to a patient.[23] In EM, the development of competence is complicated by the sheer number of procedures and varied types of diagnostic and management challenges in which mastery must be attained prior to completion of training. One study on patient attitudes towards medical student procedures indicates that if the skill has been mastered on a simulator, patients are generally more accepting of medical students performing procedures on them.[24] Typically, the learner is 'prepped' with a variety of videos or screen-based simulations that reinforce the relevant basics of human physiology and anatomy.

Preparation of learners (providing detailed didactic information and expectations) prior to the immersive learning experience helps them extract and retain the greatest amount of educational value from simulation.

Particularly with respect to technical and procedural skills, a static model or task trainer is entirely sufficient during initial exposure and practice of various procedures. A learner who has never held a laryngoscope and does not know which hand to use, does not require a computerized manikin whose tongue swells or that simulates laryngospasm. A static task trainer is adequate for the initial introduction and practice of endotracheal intubation. Likewise, chicken legs suffice for the practice of intraosseous line insertion and other static task trainers provide an initial introduction to urinary catheter insertion or lumbar puncture. The progression from simple procedural skill practice on static models to the incorporation of critical thinking and teamwork skill practice with an interactive and more sophisticated dynamic simulator is entirely consistent with the principles of graduated challenges in simulation education. One novel approach to increasing the challenge of procedural task trainers is the creation of 'hybrid' simulations that place static or wearable task trainers (i.e. a complex laceration *moulage*) on standardized patients. The addition of standardized patients with whom the trainee must interact increases the clinical challenge associated with the educational experience.[25]

There is now published evidence that deliberate practice of certain skills, to a mastery learning (criterion-based) level utilizing simulation, results in improved patient outcomes. Barsuk's work on mastery learning of residents placing central lines demonstrated decreased central line associated blood stream infections, decreased number of attempts, and fewer complications when residents completed simulation-based mastery learning curriculum prior to performing the procedure on actual patients.[2, 26] Similar results have been demonstrated with mastery learning of other procedures.[27, 28]

The simulation environment allows for planning the cases to which a learner will be exposed providing an even distribution of the presentations irrespective of season or the influence of chance presentation. In a four-hour training sequence, a learner could manage four presentations of shock, ranging from septic, haemorrhagic, neurological, to cardiovascular, and receive a debriefing based on the specific learning objectives on each topic.

In the last 15 years, restrictions of resident duty hours in the United States have been implemented with the goal of improving patient safety and decreasing medical errors related to fatigue. These requirements have become more restrictive in the last several years and were not accompanied by a lengthening of postgraduate specialty training. Paradoxically, the decrease in clinical exposure increases the likelihood that an individual resident will finish training having cared for fewer patients, having less experience in managing critical conditions, and having performed fewer procedures for which technical competencies are mandated. One example of a response to this challenge is the development of an EM procedural simulation-based curriculum that allows EM residents to learn and master required common and uncommon procedural skills. An additional feature of this curriculum is the opportunity to apply successfully completed procedures in a simulated environment to the residency requirement of a minimum number of successful proced-ures.[29] This is especially useful for rarely performed procedures such as cricothyroidotomy. This regulatory requirement, though well intentioned, has diluted the practical clinical ex-perience and slowed the development of the critical thinking and decision-making skills of graduate physicians. The critical question is whether the widespread utilization of simula-tion training can in effect 'concentrate' the learning experience and promote an equivalent degree of competence with an overall decrease in clinical exposure.

27.3.1 Ultrasound simulation

EM has relied upon diagnostic bedside ultrasound for decades and has taken an increas-ingly active role in the preparation of residents and attending physician staff for the proper use of this powerful tool. Bedside ultrasonography in the emergency setting has been con-troversial, in part due to the misalignment of the goals of the emergency physician to rapidly obtain information in a specific area and the goal of a 'formal' ultrasound examin-ation where all available information via ultrasound is 'in scope'. A classic example is the focused bedside examination of the gallbladder, performed by the emergency physician to evaluate abdominal pain believed to be a result of cholelithiasis. The emergency physician explores the abdomen with a focus on the gall bladder. The diagnostic radiologist explores the abdomen for all potential causes and may, therefore, identify other pathology (e.g. liver findings) not within the focus of the bedside clinician.

The use of bedside ultrasonography has been increasing in range as new diagnostic tech-niques are formally described. Evaluations of the musculoskeletal system, eye, and the rapid evaluation of the heart and vena cava for fluid overload have become the routine subject matter of residency training within the last decade. In addition, the development of low-cost and highly portable technologies in ultrasound have created additional sub-stantial pressure to perform these investigations in the field and in the emergency depart-ment. This creates a need for refreshment of skills and development of new skills within the population of practitioners in professional status. That need is being filled, in part, through simulation.

The professional societies within the field have supported the creation of formal guide-lines for the acquisition of ultrasound skills and a rigorous curriculum for physicians in professional status, for fellowship trainees, and for residency programmes.[30] In 2011, the Academy of Emergency Ultrasound (AEUS) was founded as an international community of clinicians who are advocating for use of bedside ultrasound within emergency practice and who are creating new avenues for training and certification.[31]

Typical training includes didactic training coupled with direct observations of examin-ations by experts and/or recordings of ultrasound exams. Ultrasound simulator devices are currently in use for EM training and may become more frequently found in EM train-ing programmes. In several ways this movement toward a firm standard for new skills acquisition incorporating didactic practice in simulation and documented supervision of examinations with real patients is a model for developing knowledge, skills, attitudes, and judgements for other novel diagnostic and therapeutic workflows.

The currently available ultrasound simulator devices were initially intended to train registered ultrasound technicians. These devices create a facsimile of the ultrasonographic findings on a display as the trainee passes the 'ultrasound probe' across a mannequin instrumented with sensors. The simulator typically is housed within a unit which simulates the controls presented to the user on a real ultrasound device. In this way trainees may operate controls and fine-tune their skills interfacing with the device as well as practise the manoeuvres and hand-to-eye coordination required for successful ultrasonography.

The major advantages of these devices are that trainees may swiftly engage a number of normal variants, and abnormal findings, depending on the 'case' presented. Some simulators have an instructor mode, which allows the trainee to track and emulate the proper location of the ultrasound probe on the mannequin for a given exam. These devices may be used independently or in conjunction with other training and allow flexibility for scheduling. Patient models are not required and serious pathologies may be repeatedly simulated in a controlled training environment.

In 2001, ACEP created a policy statement entitled 'Emergency Ultrasound Guidelines'. This document (updated in 2011[30]), in combination with the previously published ultrasound curriculum by Mateer et al., may serve as a guideline for simulation-based ultrasound curricula.[32] To date, these devices produce fair to good fidelity, but still require augmentation with live patients or patient models to produce more realistic assessments of competency. The ACEP document predates the increased use of ultrasound simulators in EM training, and mentions that 'computer simulations of sonography can be useful additions in teaching and assessing the psychomotor component'. More explicitly, the document advocates the use of patient models, such as those who are on peritoneal dialysis, to simulate abnormal findings. Advances in computer-based training in ultrasound and the combination of motion and orientation sensors have created a new industry of highly portable training devices. Some of these are capable of producing lifelike ultrasound images in motion on laptops though a USB 'ultrasound probe'. This technology and others is likely to further expand the availability of simulation-based training in the field. Clearly, the computer-based ultrasound simulator will eventually find its way more formally into training.

27.4 **Non-technical training**

Non-technical skills can by categorized as individual critical judgement skills and team skills related to roles, responsibilities, leadership, communication, and cross-monitoring behaviours.

27.4.1 **Individual skills**

In addition to the need to develop knowledge and procedural skill expertise in EM, there is also a critical need to develop decision-making skills. Satish states that:

> treating patients often requires more than factual knowledge . . . The physician or medical team is thus often challenged by VUCAD (volatility, uncertainty, complexity, ambiguity and delayed

feedback). . . the medical decision maker may not possess the information processing skills that provide the needed mental model to perceive understand and respond optimally to such highly complex challenges.[33]

Satish has suggested that strategic management simulations may provide a way to assess strengths and weaknesses as well as train for these kinds of situations. Strategic management simulations are complicated simulations designed to assess the individual's response to stress and ability to process information and make decisions appropriately. These do not typically involve medical crises but complicated disasters like a dam break, which residents have described as 'just like dealing with multiple serious problems in the emergency department'.[34] While these types of simulations have been used widely in non-healthcare industries, their use in healthcare is limited.

For EM there is particular emphasis on the resident's achievement of the skills necessary to prioritize and manage the emergency care of multiple patients.[17] As such, immersive simulation centres which are used for emergency specialist training should present opportunities to engage the trainee with multiple patients sequentially or simultaneously.

Another concept that is particularly important in EM is the idea of cognitive bias and debiasing. Croskerry has written that the emergency physician is subject to approximately 30 cognitive biases.[35–39] Though simulation is not often recognized as a training tool to address bias, it has the potential to be a valuable in this domain. 'Garden path scenarios' are ones that are designed to present a case in which the elements of the simulation point to a typical diagnosis (perhaps a common or seasonal phenomenon, like a patient with influenza symptoms in the winter) but the scenario actually represents an alternative type of case; often one that is infrequent or more serious. This domain has not been well studied in simulation but would appear to have significant potential.

27.4.2 Teamwork and communication training in emergency medicine

The US Institute of Medicine report 'To Err Is Human' identified the emergency department as the area of the hospital that puts patients at the highest risk for adverse events.[40] The volume of patients, time pressure, and acuity of emergency department patients creates multiple opportunities for medical error. The emergency department shares many of the attributes of other high-risk domains:

- Problems are ill-structured.
- Information may be incomplete or conflicting.
- Situation is rapidly changing or evolving.
- There may be multiple conflicting goals.
- Time pressure may be intense.
- Consequences of error are grave.[41–43]

The Institute of Medicine suggested that simulation training and emphasis on teamwork and standardized communication skills are part of an effective strategy to improve patient safety in this high-risk environment. Crew resource management (CRM) training is often used interchangeably with teamwork training. In reality, CRM represents one area of teamwork training. Teamwork training also includes concepts of standardized communication, situation awareness, target fixation, etc. The adoption of CRM principles and teamwork training is gaining acceptance in a number of high-risk medical specialties. In EM, teamwork training of provider teams has been shown to decrease errors and improve team satisfaction.[44] The essential question is whether the incorporation of simulation training in teamwork training for high-risk endeavours improves performance, increases resilience, and decreases error as compared with teamwork training that does not involve simulation.[45–48] Given the expense, required resources, and intensive nature of simulation training, the answer is critical. The experience in other high-risk industries that employ simulation (aviation, nuclear power plants) suggests that the investment of time and assets in this type of training is worthwhile. However, the evidence is not entirely clear in many areas of medicine. Demonstration and proof of concept courses of simulation-based multidisciplinary teamwork training have been developed and implemented in EM.[19, 20] The participants believed that these courses were useful and would aid them in clinical care, but no clinical outcomes were measured. However a more recent study of simulation-based teamwork training in a paediatric emergency department was associated with a decrease in the number of preventable adverse events.[3]

A subset of the emergency-care team—the trauma team—has also participated in simulation-based training with positive results. This was a deliberate training of scenarios requiring the emergency team and trauma team (including surgeons and surgical trainees) to collaboratively care for patients. This recurring combined training resulted in improved care for trauma patients including reduced time for the patient to reach the CT scanner.[11]

In the simulation works referenced above, deliberate efforts were made to include concepts such as a shared mental model and back-up behaviours. While videos or didactic presentations may present or demonstrate these concepts, these methods do not create the emotional context of these concepts in a clinical situation. However, in a simulation one can recreate the situation, the crisis, and the emotions associated with an assertive statement. We have used the following simulation scenario on multiple occasions to embed this concept.

> A multidisciplinary team is caring for a 5-year-old boy with a severe head injury that requires rapid sequence intubation, and the team leader is scripted to insist upon using succinylcholine (suxamethonium) 'no matter what'. One of the nurses learns from the patient's mother that this child has a contraindication for using succinylcholine and needs to share this with the team and suggest an alternative medication. If the nurse is not able to convince the physician team leader to use an alternative medication, the patient suffers a ventricular arrhythmia secondary to hyperkalaemia.

Eighty per cent of the time the nurses do not succeed in successfully asserting their concern on their first experience with this scenario. In debriefing this scenario, we find that the nurses inevitably describe great emotional difficulty in 'speaking up' to a physician. This is disquieting to the nurses and the physicians. It allows for sharing of potential solutions around this type of issue as well as the opportunity to practise the behaviour in a safe setting. It is doubtful that traditional didactic presentations about the authority gradient and assertive statements would engender the same degree of realism or urgency and, more importantly, allow for the practice of this important behaviour.

Simulation also provides a way to examine the adaptive capacity of the emergency department (ED) team and the ED system. Though patient-safety initiatives have tended to emphasize the reduction and even the elimination of errors, a sole emphasis on this aspect of safety ignores the reality that as human beings we will make mistakes. High-reliability organizations, such as air-traffic control and nuclear power plant crews, emphasize a pre-occupation with failure and concepts such as 'cross-checking' to capture and mitigate errors as well as recover from errors.[49] As specialists studying human factors begin to look at healthcare, opportunities to develop and practise these skills are beginning to emerge from the study of actual events, including near misses.[50] Simulation scenarios provide an opportunity to 'plant' or script mistakes and errors and allow emergency teams to develop the skills of cross-checking and discovery of and mitigation of errors. Emergency simulation scenarios can include such features as broken equipment (bag valve masks, blood pressure monitors, cables, etc.) or incorrectly labelled medications or blood products. While these defects may appear obvious to the observer, the team in the midst of a crisis may take some time to identify and rectify these issues. These types of simulations reflect a high-reliability culture of sensitivity to operations and preoccupation with failure.[51] With respect to simulation and safety training, Salas et al. have written:

> The use of content-valid scenarios is critical in environments (such as health care) where errors if not corrected in a timely manner can have catastrophic consequences . . . Scenarios may also be crafted so that trainees can experience these errors and observe the consequences so that those behaviours can be recognized in the future.[48]

This also promotes team problem-solving and coordination when faced with a medical error as opposed to team paralysis when faced with unexpected difficulties.

27.5 Human factors and the emergency department

Time work studies have been used in other industries to assess the efficiency of personnel and the optimal placement of equipment. Simulation is now routinely used to assess new clinical environments, new processes, and new equipment. In one paper evaluating the use of simulation for this purpose, 18 latent threats were identified related to equipment placement or absence, communication systems, and procedural space. Fourteen of these issues were corrected before opening the unit for patient care.[15] In a similar fashion, simulation can be used to evaluate new clinical processes and new team configurations.[5] Using simulation in this manner provides an opportunity to 'test' the system and the team prior to managing patients in the new system. Increasingly, tools such as the NASA Task Load Index Scale (NASA TLX) are used in association with simulation to assess perceived workload under varying conditions or with different team configurations.[5] A similar intervention is the use of *in situ* simulation. The goals of this type of simulation can include evaluation of teamwork, readiness, systems, and resources in the clinical setting.[16]

Additionally, new equipment being considered for use in the emergency department or modifications to existing processes and the introduction of new processes are also opportunities for the use of simulation. In our own institution, we have identified difficulties with a particular defibrillator monitor's design prior to its introduction in our department. In several simulations we observed that the synchronization button was not readily apparent to the user and resulted in defibrillation rather than cardioversion of a patient with supraventricular tachycardia. Working with clinical engineers, we highlighted the synchronization button to ensure it was more visible to the clinical user.

27.6 **Disaster training and mass casualty incidents**

An important aspect of emergency care in which teamwork and coordination is vital is that of multiple simultaneous patients or mass casualty situations. Traditionally, training for these types of disasters has been confined to tabletop or computer simulations supplemented by the delivery of *moulaged* patients to various hospitals and aid stations. Healthcare providers were limited to triaging *moulaged* patients and describing how the patients would be handled. While this qualifies as simulation, it occurs at a very low level and does not promote the critical decision-making nor allow for practice of the skills and behaviours necessary to handle this type of crisis. Following the events of 11 September 2001, increased funding for training resulted in the greater use of simulation for disaster preparedness and mass casualty training in the United States. The Advanced Bioterrorism Triage Course, Advanced Disaster Life Support, and other offerings are examples of courses that integrate high-fidelity simulation fully into a curriculum designed for physicians out of training.[7, 8]

As compared with traditional disaster drills, the incorporation of sophisticated mannequin simulators allows for the actual practice and performance of 'triage', resuscitation, and invasive procedures as compared with the typical *moulaged* volunteers in a disaster drill. This 'hybrid' type of simulation provides more realism related to the 'mix' of 'walking wounded' and critical patients.[8, 9] Another advantage of this type of hybrid simulation is the opportunity for ED staff to practise decontamination, as well as various technical procedures, while wearing the protective gear that is required for providers in these types of situations.[52, 53] What has been published on this topic indicates the difficulty of communication between the team members as well as the difficulty of performing medical procedures such as endotracheal intubation or intravenous line placement while wearing protective gear.

In Israel, simulation has been used to develop and assess the skills necessary for the management of multiple casualties. Skills such as endotracheal intubation and intraosseous line placement are performed on simulated patients by healthcare providers wearing full chemical protective gear.[53, 54] This training provides an element of realism that is not matched in other mass casualty exercises. It also provides regional and national planners with a more realistic assessment of the time frame and resources necessary should such an event occur.

27.7 **Continuing education and credentialing**

Continuing education (CE) opportunities in EM are numerous and diverse. As in other educational venues, high-fidelity simulation devices and task trainers may be utilized to augment standard didactic presentations or to create an immersive training experience for CE. The demand for this type of training is relatively high and, as content becomes more interactive, this is increasingly attractive to adult learners. The downside of training of this type remains its labour-intensive nature for the instructor.

Simulation is highly utilized for continuing procedural skills practice for high-acuity, low-frequency events. Difficult airway skills education, such as fibre-optic intubation, laryngeal mask airways, and other novel equipment are easily and safely performed utilizing airway task trainers or high-fidelity simulation devices. There are currently several commercial providers of CE which utilize high-fidelity simulation.

Baker and Salas have recommended that the various licensure and board certification organizations should assess and regulate the physician's knowledge of the 'components of a team' as well as requiring the physician to 'demonstrate competence in team leadership, mutual performance monitoring, back up behaviour and adaptability'.[47] In the aviation industry, simulation has been used to assess this type of competency. The Line Operational Evaluation (LOE) 'requires pilots and co-pilots to demonstrate acceptable teamwork skills during this critical certification event'. Further, this type of training and evaluation is mandated during initial certification as well as during periodic recertifications conducted in simulators. The importance of ongoing reinforcement and assessment of technical competence and teamwork behaviours is a major factor in the evolution of aviation as a high-reliability industry.[47]

In the United States, the American Board of Anesthesiology requires simulation-based recertification of all boarded anesthesiologists every ten years.[55] Individual institutions have also started to require simulation-based training as part of their requirements for maintenance of medical staff privileges and performance-based credentialing. Many institutions have based these requirements on emerging data that demonstrates a decreased risk of litigation for high-risk specialties like EM that complete periodic simulation training. The optimal length and interval between such training is not clear at this time. It does appear that this represents a trend for simulation-based training from individual specialty boards and institutions that will only increase as simulation becomes more available.

27.8 **Conclusion**

The utilization of simulation in EM is evolving. Clear applications for the use of simulation for the education of technical skills exist in EM as in other specialties. However, the use of simulation for non-technical skills, including teamwork training, is recognized as equally important. Though the field is maturing, there is a need for additional evidence that directly links simulation training to improved patient outcomes. EM is still defining the optimal ways to use simulation for education and safety. It appears that there are specific needs in

EM that may only be adequately addressed through simulation, including the evaluation of clinical environments, systems and equipment, and training for mass casualty incidents. As expertise evolves, it is likely that additional applications will be identified.

Disclaimer

The views expressed herein are those of the authors and are not to be construed as official or reflecting the views of the United States Department of Defense.

References

1 Okuda Y, Bond W, Bonfante G, McLaughlin S, Spillane L, Wang E, et al. National growth in simulation training within emergency medicine residency programs, 2003–2008. Acad Emerg Med 2008;**15**(11):1113–1116.

2 Barsuk JH, Cohen ER, Feinglass J, McGaghie WC, Wayne DB. Use of simulation-based education to reduce catheter-related bloodstream infections. Arch Intern Med 2009;**169**(15):1420–1423.

3 Patterson MD, Geis GL, Lemaster T, Wears RL. Impact of multidisciplinary simulation-based training on patient safety in a paediatric emergency department. BMJ Quality & Safety 2012.

4 Kobayashi L, Overly FL, Fairbanks RJ, et al. Advanced medical simulation applications for emergency medicine microsystems evaluation and training. Academic Emergency Medicine: Official Journal of the Society for Academic Emergency Medicine 2008;**15**(11):1058–1070.

5 Geis GL, Pio B, Pendergrass TL, et al. Simulation to assess the safety of new healthcare teams and new facilities. Simulation in Healthcare: Journal of the Society for Simulation in Healthcare 2011;**6**(3):125–133.

6 Johnson KGG, Oehler J, Houlton J, Tabangin M, Myer C, Kerrey B. High fidelity simulation to design a novel system of care for pediatric critical airway obstruction. The American Society of Pediatric Otolaryngology. San Diego, CA; April 2012.

7 Kaji AH, Bair A, Okuda Y, Kobayashi L, Khare R, Vozenilek J. Defining systems expertise: effective simulation at the organizational level—implications for patient safety, disaster surge capacity, and facilitating the systems interface. Academic Emergency Medicine: Official Journal of the Society for Academic Emergency Medicine 2008;**15**(11):1098–1103.

8 Kobayashi L, Shapiro MJ, Suner S, Williams KA. Disaster medicine: the potential role of high-fidelity medical simulation for mass casualty incident training. Med Health RI 2003;**86**(7):196–200.

9 Kobayashi L, Suner S, Shapiro MJ, Jay G, Sullivan F, Overly F, et al. Multipatient disaster scenario design using mixed modality medical simulation for the evaluation of civilian prehospital medical response: a 'dirty bomb' case study. Simulation in Healthcare: Journal of the Society for Simulation in Healthcare 2006;**1**(2):72–78.

10 Ilgen JS, Sherbino J, Cook DA. Technology-enhanced simulation in emergency medicine: a systematic review and meta-analysis. Acad Emerg Med 2013;**20**(2):117–127.

11 Falcone RAJ, Daugherty M, Schweer L, Patterson M, Brown RL, Garcia VF. Multidisciplinary pediatric trauma team training using high-fidelity trauma simulation. J Pediatr Surg 2008;**43**:1065–1071.

12 Patterson MD, Geis GL, Falcone RA, Lemaster T, Wears RL. *In situ* simulation: detection of safety threats and teamwork training in a high-risk emergency department. BMJ Quality & Safety 2012.

13 Kobayashi L, Dunbar-Viveiros JA, Devine J, Jones MS, Overly FL, Gosbee JW, et al. Pilot-phase findings from high-fidelity *in situ* medical simulation investigation of emergency department procedural sedation. Simulation in Healthcare: Journal of the Society for Simulation in Healthcare 2012.

14 Kobayashi L, Patterson MD, Overly FL, Shapiro MJ, Williams KA, Jay GD. Educational and research implications of portable human patient simulation in acute care medicine. Acad Emerg Med 2008;**15**(11):1166–1174.

15 Miller D, Crandall C, Washington C, 3rd, McLaughlin S. Improving teamwork and communication in trauma care through *in situ* simulations. Acad Emerg Med 2012;**19**(5):608–612.

16 Steinemann S, Berg B, Skinner A, DiTulio A, Anzelon K, Terada K, et al. *In situ*, multidisciplinary, simulation-based teamwork training improves early trauma care. Journal of Surgical Education 2011;**68**(6):472–477.

17 Counselman FL, Borenstein MA, Chisholm CD, Epter ML, Khandelwal S, Kraus CK, et al. The 2013 model of the clinical practice of emergency medicine. Academic Emergency Medicine: Official Journal of the Society for Academic Emergency Medicine 2014;**21**(5):574–598.

18 Harvey EM, Wright A, Taylor D, Bath J, Collier B. TeamSTEPPS((R)) simulation-based training: an evidence-based strategy to improve trauma team performance. Journal of Continuing Education in Nursing 2013;**44**(11):484–485.

19 Turner P. Implementation of TeamSTEPPS in the emergency department. Critical Care Nursing Quarterly 2012;**35**(3):208–212.

20 Risser DT, Rice MM, Salisbury ML, Simon R, Jay GD, Berns SD. The potential for improved teamwork to reduce medical errors in the emergency department. The MedTeams Research Consortium. Annals of Emergency Medicine 1999;**34**(3):373–383.

21 Rosen MA, Salas E, Wu TS, Silvestri S, Lazzara EH, Lyons R, et al. Promoting teamwork: an event-based approach to simulation-based teamwork training for emergency medicine residents. Academic Emergency Medicine: Official Journal of the Society for Academic Emergency Medicine. 2008;**15**(11):1190–1198.

22 Yule S, Flin R, Paterson-Brown Sea. Development of a rating system for surgeons' non-technical skills. Med Educ 2006;**40**(11):1098–1104.

23 Reznek M, Harter P, Krummel T. Virtual reality and simulation: training the future emergency physician. Academic Emergency Medicine: Official Journal of the Society for Academic Emergency Medicine 2002;**9**(1):78–87.

24 Graber MA, Wyatt C, Kasparek L, Xu Y. Does simulator training for medical students change patient opinions and attitudes toward medical student procedures in the emergency department? Academic Emergency Medicine: Official Journal of the Society for Academic Emergency Medicine 2005;**12**(7):635–639.

25 Kyaw Tun J, Granados A, Mavroveli S, Nuttall S, Kadiyala AN, Brown R, et al. Simulating various levels of clinical challenge in the assessment of clinical procedure competence. Annals of Emergency Medicine 2012;**60**(1):112–120e5.

26 Barsuk JH, McGaghie WC, Cohen ER, O'Leary KJ, Wayne DB. Simulation-based mastery learning reduces complications during central venous catheter insertion in a medical intensive care unit. Crit Care Med 2009;**37**(10):2697–2701.

27 McGaghie WC, Issenberg SB, Cohen ER, Barsuk JH, Wayne DB. Medical education featuring mastery learning with deliberate practice can lead to better health for individuals and populations. Acad Med 2011;**86**(11):e8–9.

28 Wayne DB, Barsuk JH, O'Leary KJ, Fudala MJ, McGaghie WC. Mastery learning of thoracentesis skills by internal medicine residents using simulation technology and deliberate practice. J Hosp Med 2008;**3**(1):48–54.

29 Grall KH, Stoneking LR, DeLuca LA, Waterbrook AL, Pritchard TG, Denninghoff KR. An innovative longitudinal curriculum to increase emergency medicine residents' exposure to rarely encountered and technically challenging procedures. Advances in Medical Education and Practice 2014;**5**:229–236.

30 American College of Emergency Physicians Policy Statement on Emergency Ultrasound Guidelines. Dallas, TX: ACEP; 2008.

31 Academy of Emergency Ultrasound: Society for Academic Emergency Medicine; [cited 2014 10 May 2014]. Available from: <http://community.saem.org/saem/groupdetails?CommunityKey=13f1ec b4-4d12-4802-a1c1-81f784318fc3>

32 Mateer J, Plummer D, Heller M, Olson D, Jehle D, Overton D, et al. Model curriculum for physician training in emergency ultrasonography. Annals of Emergency Medicine 1994;**23**(1):95–102.

33 Satish U, Streufert S. Value of a cognitive simulation in medicine: towards optimizing decision making performance of healthcare personnel. Qual Saf Health Care 2002;**11**(2):163–167.

34 Satish U, Streufert S, Marshall R, Smith JS, Powers S, Gorman P, et al. Strategic management simulations is a novel way to measure resident competencies. American Journal Of Surgery 2001;**181**(6):557–561.

35 Kovacs G, Croskerry P. Clinical decision making: an emergency medicine perspective. Academic Emergency Medicine: Official Journal of the Society for Academic Emergency Medicine 1999;**6**(9):947–952.

36 Croskerry P, Tait G. Clinical decision making: the need for meaningful research. Acad Med 2013;**88**(2):149–150.

37 Croskerry P, Singhal G, Mamede S. Cognitive debiasing 1: origins of bias and theory of debiasing. BMJ Quality & Safety 2013.

38 Croskerry P, Singhal G, Mamede S. Cognitive debiasing 2: impediments to and strategies for change. BMJ Quality & Safety 2013.

39 Croskerry P. Cognitive forcing strategies in clinical decision making. Annals of Emergency Medicine 2003;**41**(1):110–120.

40 To err is human: building a safer health system. Linda T, Kohn JMC, Donaldson MS, editors. Washington, DC: National Academy Press; 2000, 271.

41 Fletcher G, Flin R, McGeorge P, Glavin R, Maran N, Patey R. Anaesthetists' non-technical skills (ANTS): evaluation of a behavioural marker system. Br J Anaesth 2003;**90**(5):580–588.

42 Flin R, Maran N. Identifying and training non-technical skills for teams in acute medicine. Qual Saf Health Care 2004;**13**(Suppl 1):i80–84.

43 Flin RGR, Maran R, et al. Framework for observing and rating anaesthetists' non-technical skills 2004 (2 November 2004); (1 May 2006). Available from: <http://www.abdn.ac.uk/iprc/papers%20 reports/Ants/ANTS_handbook_v1.0_electronic_access_version.pdf>

44 Morey JC, Simon R, Jay GD, Wears RL, Salisbury M, Dukes KA, et al. Error reduction and performance improvement in the emergency department through formal teamwork training: evaluation results of the MedTeams project. Health Serv Res 2002;**37**(6):1553–1581.

45 Salas E, DiazGranados D, Klein C, Burke CS, Stagl KC, Goodwin GF, et al. Does team training improve team performance? A meta-analysis. Hum Factors 2008;**50**(6):903–933.

46 Stout RJ, Salas E, Fowlkes JE. Enhancing teamwork in complex environments through team training. Group Dyn 1997;**1**(2):169–182.

47 Baker DP, Salas E, King H, Battles J, Barach P. The role of teamwork in the professional education of physicians: current status and assessment recommendations. Jt Comm J Qual Patient Saf 2005;**31**(4):185–202.

48 Salas E, Wilson KA, Burke CS, Priest HA. Using simulation-based training to improve patient safety: what does it take? Jt Comm J Qual Patient Saf.2005;**31**(7):363–371.

49 Salas E, Rhodenizer L, Bowers CA. The design and delivery of crew resource management training: exploiting available resources. Hum Factors 2000;**42**(3):490–511.

50 Ebright PR, Urden L, Patterson E, Chalko B. Themes surrounding novice nurse near-miss and adverse-event situations. The Journal of Nursing Administration 2004;**34**(11):531–538.

51 Weick KE, Sutcliffe KM. Managing the unexpected: resilient performance in an age of uncertainty. Second edn. San Francisco, CA: Jossey-Bass; 2007, 194.

52 Vardi A, Levin I, Berkenstadt H, Hourvitz A, Eisenkraft A, Cohen A, et al. Simulation-based training of medical teams to manage chemical warfare casualties. IMAJ 2002;**4**(7):540–544.

53 Berkenstadt H, Ziv A, Barsuk D, Levine I, Cohen A, Vardi A. The use of advanced simulation in the training of anesthesiologists to treat chemical warfare casualties. Anesthesia and Analgesia 2003;**96**(6):1739–1742, table of contents.

54 Vardi A, Berkenstadt H, Levin I, Bentencur A, Ziv A. Intraosseous vascular access in the treatment of chemical warfare casualties assessed by advanced simulation: proposed alteration of treatment protocol. Anesthesia and Analgesia 2004;**98**(6):1753–1758, table of contents.

55 Levine AI, Schwartz AD, Bryson EO, Demaria S Jr. Role of simulation in U.S. physician licensure and certification. Mt Sinai J Med 2012;**79**(1):140–153.

Chapter 28

Simulation in paediatrics

Nicole K Yamada, Janene H Fuerch,
and Louis P Halamek

Overview

- Paediatric patients differ from adult patients in significant ways.
- These differences must be acknowledged and addressed in order to develop successful paediatric simulation-based training and research programmes.
- Close collaboration between paediatric healthcare professionals and others (risk managers, school and hospital administrators, industry leaders, etc.) is required to if paediatric simulation is ever to reach its potential to significantly enhance the safety and care of children.

28.1 Introduction

Before discussing paediatric simulation-based training and research, it is important to first define what is meant by the term 'paediatric'. The adjective paediatric applies to the period of human development from birth (0 days) to young adulthood (21 years) of both male and female patients. Paediatric patients range from those born at a gestational age of 22 to 23 weeks (a little more than halfway through a full-term, 40-week pregnancy) and a birth weight of approximately 500 g to young adults standing 2 m in height and weighing more than 100 kg. The anatomic, physiologic, developmental, and psychological differences found across this spectrum of patients are wide-ranging and present tremendous challenges for those healthcare professionals charged with their care. In addition, a large number of paediatric subspecialties have evolved over the past century to address this complexity. As with adult healthcare, the field of paediatrics includes physicians, nurses, and allied healthcare professionals with expertise in areas such as newborn intensive care (neonatology), paediatric critical care, cardiology, pulmonology, gastroenterology, nephrology, anaesthesiology, general surgery, cardiothoracic surgery, and multiple other medical and surgical domains. These differences among patients and those charged with their care also present great challenges for those involved in paediatric simulation-based training and research. Realistically, simulating the wide range of body sizes, anatomic features, vital signs, physiologic responses, etc. present in this group of very diverse patients is daunting.

Healthcare professionals caring for children are faced with a myriad of challenges in addition to treating complex paediatric diseases; these challenges include but are not limited to careful consideration of the child's psychosocial developmental stage and the necessary involvement of family as surrogate decision-makers when questions as to best course of action arise. Training professionals to provide competent, compassionate, and developmentally appropriate care has been a difficult process secondary, in part, to the limitations of the traditional training paradigm that does not provide sufficient opportunity for hands-on practice in interacting with children and their families. In addition to limitations in training, there are many questions regarding optimal methods of providing care that are difficult to study in the actual clinical domain when delivering care to real paediatric patients. It is these gaps in clinical training and research that serve as optimal targets for simulation-based methodologies.

28.2 Rationale for paediatric simulation

Why devote an entire chapter to paediatric simulation-based training? Children are not small adults and paediatric simulation is not adult simulation on a 'smaller' scale. As one can see from the preceding section, there is no 'standard' paediatric patient akin to the '70 kg adult white male' so often described in the adult literature. Thus, the focus of this chapter is to highlight those unique aspects of paediatric simulation-based training and research rather than repeat information found elsewhere in this text.

One question that must be answered early on is this: given that most children are healthy and rarely present healthcare professionals with serious management issues, why develop a programme in paediatric simulation-based training and research in the first place? Paediatric healthcare professionals work in environments just as complex, dynamic, and highly technical as any found in adult medicine. This can be confirmed by walking into a neonatal or paediatric intensive care unit and standing at the bedside of a patient with persistent pulmonary hypertension of the newborn on extracorporeal membrane oxygenation (ECMO) or a paediatric patient with multisystem organ dysfunction receiving high-frequency oscillatory ventilation (HFOV), inhaled nitric oxide (INO), dialysis, and inotropic support. Demands for succinct and accurate transfer of information while under intense time pressure and the need to interact with young overwhelmed parents acting as surrogate decision-makers for patients who are too ill to speak for themselves are also inherent in these environments. Thus, the professionals working in these environments must possess not only the content knowledge and technical skills required to understand and treat the disease process but also behavioural skills to allow them to respond appropriately while under intense pressure.

Most children **are** healthy—and that is a major reason why paediatric simulation makes sense. In many ways, serious paediatric pathology is the classic low-frequency, high-risk event that lends itself well to simulation-based training. Unless they work in emergency or intensive care settings, many paediatric healthcare professionals rarely get the opportunity to recognize and treat serious disease processes let alone a true life-threatening emergency. Even for those for whom a sufficient number of opportunities do exist, one must question whether it is acceptable to essentially practice on real living patients who are not capable of providing informed consent on their own. While parents do act as surrogate decision-makers for children below the age of consent, few want to contemplate that their child is to be someone's first spinal tap, first intubation, first thoracostomy tube placement, or intestinal resection. The same rationale can be applied to simulation-based paediatric research. Simulation is an ideal methodology for studying important issues that would otherwise require obtaining consent from parents who may already be in crisis with a sick child.

Non-paediatric healthcare professionals receive little exposure to paediatric patients during their general training. In the US, most medical students spend only one to two months on a general paediatrics rotation (involving both an inpatient and outpatient component) during four years of medical school. Nursing students typically receive even less exposure to paediatric patients, and some schools have difficulty in even finding hospitals with which to partner in order for their students to learn basic paediatric care. Despite these limitations in the traditional training model, many adult healthcare professionals will, nevertheless, encounter sick children during their careers and must be able to respond quickly and correctly until the appropriate paediatric subspecialist can arrive. This is especially true in the emergency medicine setting, where sick children present at all hours of the day and night.

Because of all of these factors, one may argue that the ethical imperative for simulation is stronger in paediatrics than in any other field of healthcare.[1]

One subspecialty of paediatrics—neonatal-perinatal medicine—is unique in that the soon-to-be paediatric patient (the foetus) exists inside of an adult patient; in addition there may be one, two, three, or more paediatric patients awaiting birth inside of that pregnant adult female patient. In this instance, the possibility of a sick mother delivering a sick newborn creates a situation where optimal training occurs only when the paediatric and adult teams train together. The multitude of events (from both the maternal and neonatal perspectives) that can complicate human birth make this an especially appealing target for simulation-based training.[2, 3]

In acknowledgement of the unique needs of children and the healthcare professionals serving them, the international paediatric simulation community has its own professional organization, the International Pediatric Simulation Society (IPSS). Founded in 2008, the IPSS was 'established to promote and support multi-disciplinary simulation-based education, training and research in all subspecialties that care for infants and children'.[4] Its goals are listed in Box 28.1. The society organizes an annual meeting—the International Paediatric Simulation Symposia and Workshops (IPSSW)—that provides a forum for the clinicians, investigators, and educators in the field of paediatric simulation. The first meeting of the society was held in 2008 in Stockholm, Sweden; since that time, meetings have been held annually at various locations around the world. The formal structure of the IPSS

Box 28.1 Goals of the IPSS

1 To grow and maintain an international paediatric simulation community.

2 To foster innovation in paediatric simulation aimed at promoting excellence in paediatric and perinatal care wherever it is delivered.

3 To support and promote patient safety through the use of simulation tailored to healthcare environments where infants, children, and their families are cared for.

4 To promote high-quality paediatric simulation research.

5 To advocate internationally for the use of simulation for paediatric education and training (technology, funding and legislation, public policy).

6 To collaborate with professional and simulation societies having common goals for the benefit of patient safety and care delivered to children.

Reproduced from the International Pediatric Simulation Society (IPSS), http://ipssglobal.org/about/what-is-ipss/, (accessed 1 March 2015).

---

consists of a board of directors and ten standing committees: advocacy, public affairs and international relations; affiliations; articles and bylaws; education; executive; membership; nominating; research, technology and standards; website, communication and marketing. In addition to its annual meeting, the society hosts monthly webinars and publishes a quarterly newsletter. All of these facets of the IPSS function to serve the unique needs of the paediatric simulation community.

28.3 Simulation-based paediatric clinical training

Quite simply, simulation is practice. It should be kept in mind that the idea of using practice to improve performance is hardly novel nor is it unique to healthcare. In fact, it is fair to state that in many ways healthcare lags behind other industries where the risk to human life is high (such as aerospace, commercial aviation, mass transit, the military, nuclear power) when it comes to allocating the human, technical, and financial resources necessary to allow its professionals to achieve and maintain proficiency. It even trails low-risk occupations such as professional sports where the amount time devoted to practice far exceeds that spent in actual athletic contests between opponents. Thus, while use of the term 'simulation' is currently in vogue in healthcare, we need to remind ourselves that we can learn a great deal from our colleagues in other industries where simulation has been used for many decades to identify strengths and weaknesses in human and technical systems and subsystems.

'Healthcare simulation' is used to describe a wide spectrum of activities ranging from the relatively simple (skills stations where trainees perform technical procedures such as intravascular access and intubation on task trainers, role-playing exercises used to facilitate training in effective communication) to the highly complex (comprehensive full-scale highly realistic re-creations of clinical scenarios incorporating multiple visual, auditory, and tactile cues). The specialty of paediatrics is not a newcomer to simulation as defined in its broadest sense. Simulation that is limited in scope has been in existence for decades in programmes such as the Neonatal Resuscitation Program (NRP) of the American Academy of Pediatrics (AAP) and the Pediatric Advanced Life Support Program (PALS) of the American Heart Association (AHA). More recently, educators and clinicians have begun to formally design and implement curricula for the learning sessions they deliver and evaluate the devices utilized during these sessions (primarily task trainers) as well as the effects of the sessions on the trainees. Much of this work is targeted at achieving an acceptable level of performance (defined in various ways) in specific technical skills in the relative novice (medical or nursing student, resident, etc.).[5–7]

More complex paediatric simulation, using realistic full-body patient simulators capable of exhibiting physiologic responses to interventions delivered with actual medical equipment and conducted in a highly authentic healthcare environment, was first described in 2000.[8] The goals of such complex simulation activities are much more comprehensive and usually involve the acquisition, refinement, and integration of cognitive, technical, and behavioural skills. The key to conducting a successful full-scale, complex simulation is to engender the same response in the trainees to the simulated clinical scenario as they would exhibit in the actual hospital, clinic, or office environment when caring for real patients. When this is achieved, trainees are able to identify their strengths and, thereby, understand what skills lead to successful human performance and, even more importantly, recognize their weaknesses and develop strategies to remediate them before they become manifest during the care of real patients. Comprehensive simulation is also being employed to prototype physical structures prior to actual construction, assess operational readiness of large-scale systems, prepare specific teams to treat specific disease states in specific patients, and address training and assessment needs in complex clinical interventions such as extracorporeal membrane oxygenation.[9–18] This type of full-scale simulation is becoming more common within paediatrics and its various subspecialties, and represents one way in which paediatric healthcare can begin to close the gap between its safety and performance efforts and those of other high-risk industries.

28.4 **Simulation-based paediatric research**

Simulation-based research focuses on two major areas: (i) direct examination of simulation itself as a learning modality; and (ii) using simulation to study issues that are difficult or impractical to study in the actual clinical environment when caring for real human patients. Each of these areas will be discussed separately in the following paragraphs.

In healthcare, the gold standard of proof has historically been the prospective, sufficiently powered, randomized, controlled, multicentre trial. Such trials have proven very difficult to conduct in the area of healthcare simulation, leading some to conclude that simulation has yet to be proven as an effective strategy for skill acquisition and maintenance in healthcare. This viewpoint cannot be supported. The fact that proficiency is achieved by practising doing the right thing, in the right way, using the right equipment and other resources, while working under highly realistic conditions is accepted at face value in virtually every aspect of human activity, and healthcare should be no different. Thus, efforts to examine whether simulation in healthcare works may be best redirected to the study of how best to optimize healthcare simulation. There are many important questions regarding optimization of paediatric simulation that require answers, including but not limited to the following:

◆ How is proficiency in the various cognitive, technical, and behavioural skills necessary to deliver effective care to paediatric patients defined?

◆ Once defined, how can proficiency in these skills be objectively measured?

◆ Once defined, how can proficiency in these skills be acquired and maintained over time?

◆ How can skill acquisition and maintenance be achieved in the most efficient manner in terms of utilization of resources (time, money, physical space, effort)?

While a few studies have attempted to answer questions such as these, much work remains to be done.[19]

Simulation is a useful tool for studying questions that are difficult or impractical to study in the actual clinical environment when caring for real human patients.[20, 21] This is especially true for emergency and intensive care fields where obtaining informed consent from parents who are focused on whether their child will survive is awkward at best and injurious at worst. A number of investigators have pursued studies examining a wide range of issues in human and system performance.[22-26] Because a well-designed simulation-based study allows for the standardization of many aspects of the environment (including but not limited to the anatomical features and physiologic reactions of the simulated patient, the responses of the human beings serving as confederates in the scenario, the ambient noise level in the room, and the function of the medical devices and instruments used in the simulation), many confounding variables can be minimized or eliminated and the performance of the human subject(s) and/or system(s) undergoing the simulation can be isolated.

In much the same way that paediatric healthcare professionals have come together on an international level within the IPSS to share lessons learned for the benefit of their patients, a similar effort has spawned the International Network for Simulation-based Pediatric Innovation, Research, and Education (INSPIRE).[27] INSPIRE was established in 2011 by integrating two research networks with complementary activities, needs, and resources. Unlike the IPSS, however, INSPIRE is a 'bottom-up, grassroots organization that has formed to meet the needs of the rapidly changing landscape of paediatric simulation research'.[28] As such, it represents another unique product of the efforts of the paediatric simulation community. It has been especially productive in the area of procedural training, a particularly challenging aspect of paediatric clinical care given that the small size of many patients leaves little margin for technical error.[29-35] The overall goals of the members of the INSPIRE network are listed in Box 28.2.

Box 28.2 Goals of INSPIRE

1 Identify consensus research priorities.

2 Facilitate single and multicentre research projects.

3 Build expertise and knowledge.

4 Provide mentorship for new/novice investigators.

5 Promote an international network for simulation-based paediatric innovation, research, and education.

Source: data from International Network for Simulation-based Pediatric Innovation, Research, and Education (INSPIRE), http://inspiresim.com/, (accessed 1 March 2015).

28.5 Challenges in paediatric simulation

28.5.1 Focusing on methodology, not technology

At its core, simulation is a learning and assessment methodology and the key to effective simulation is achieving a degree of realism in scenarios that engenders authentic responses on the part of the trainees. Unlike the didactic learning sessions that many in paediatrics are accustomed to, simulation is a methodology that:

+ focuses on learning rather than teaching;

+ gives more control over the learning environment to the trainees;

+ places much of the responsibility for learning on the trainees;

+ integrates cognitive, technical, and behavioural skills;

+ does not lend itself necessarily to tightly scripted deliveries of content knowledge defined by time (i.e. the 45-minute lecture); and

+ de-emphasizes written tests in favour of performance-based assessments of skills that are carried out while under realistic time pressure generated by changes in patient physiologic state.

In simulation, the responsibility for learning falls on the trainees as they perform scenarios and then reflect on their actions during facilitated debriefings.

Learning objectives drive everything in simulation: scenario design, equipment used, content of debriefing, evaluation tools, etc. Poorly defined learning objectives are likely to lead to substandard learning experiences and ill-prepared trainees. Identifying learning objectives makes it possible to identify measures of assessment that will demonstrate that new skills have been gained. It is helpful when determining learning objectives to consider the types of skills that learners must acquire in order to achieve those objectives. In general, these skills fall into three major categories: cognitive ('what we think' or content knowledge), technical ('what we do' or hands-on, manual interventions), and behavioural ('how we think and do' while working as a team).[36] As an example, safe and effective intubation of the newborn is a key learning objective in neonatal-perinatal medicine. In order to achieve this learning objective one must master the abbreviated list of skills found in Box 28.3. As can be seen from this list, effective and safe intubation of a neonate is a learning objective that is achieved only by integrating multiple elements of the three major skill sets.

The process of developing pertinent learning objectives includes determining whether the learners' needs are best met by training as a single discipline or as part of a multi-disciplinary team and deciding whether novices can/should be integrated with experts during training. Consideration also should be given to an estimation of the length of time required for acquisition of particular skills, their half-lives, and the timing of retraining.

Box 28.3 A partial list of skills necessary for successful intubation of the newborn

Cognitive skills

- Know the indications for intubation of the newborn.
- Know how to recognize these indications when present.
- Know what equipment (size of endotracheal tube, laryngoscope blade) to use in order to accomplish intubation.
- Know the indications of a successful intubation.

Technical skills

- Correctly assemble the laryngoscope.
- Hold the laryngoscope in the left hand.
- Use the laryngoscope to expose the trachea to view.
- Insert the endotracheal tube into the trachea.
- Assess for proper placement of the endotracheal tube in the trachea.
- Secure the endotracheal tube at the appropriate depth

Behavioural skills

- Communicate effectively with team members regarding the need for intubation, specific pieces of equipment, etc.
- Distribute the workload so that specific tasks are assigned to the team members most likely to carry them out successfully.
- Delegate responsibility and supervise appropriately.
- Call for help when necessary.

Many recommendations for the length and frequency of training experiences are not evidence-based and are arbitrary at best. These issues are especially relevant to paediatric simulation because of the wide spectrum of patient sizes, varying physiologies, and distinct disease states that are seen in the paediatric population.

While technologies have the potential to enhance the realism of scenarios, they can also serve to distract from learning if they do not facilitate acquisition of learning objectives. As mentioned previously, the technologies currently available in paediatric simulation are limited in number and utility; therefore, paediatric simulation is even more dependent on sound methodological strategies for success than its adult counterpart.

28.5.2 **Developing useful technologies**

The current state of the art in paediatric human patient simulators is inadequate to meet the needs of the diverse group of professionals that might benefit from widespread implementation of simulation-based training. The full range of patient sizes represented in the paediatric patient population is under-represented by the paediatric simulators that are commercially available. Many of these simulators are not capable of realistically indicating their state of relative health or disease. Of those that do harbour some type of internal physiologic modelling, the models are often based on adult physiology and 'adapted' in some way for the paediatric patient. This type of engineering ignores the unique anatomy and physiology of paediatric patients and results in a substandard learning experience. Areas where extrapolation of adult physiology to paediatric patients may result in significant inaccuracies include but are not limited to the following:

- Cyanotic congenital heart disease with persistent low haemoglobin oxygen saturation (SaO_2): the low SaO_2s (70–85%) commonly seen in these patients are compensated for by unusually high haematocrits that ensure adequate oxygen content and delivery and are completely compatible with survival. When SaO_2s in this range are seen in adults they usually presage ventricular fibrillation and death.

- Right-to-left shunting of unoxygenated blood through a patent ductus arteriosus (PDA): the ductus arteriosus normally closes off in the days following birth at full term; this process is delayed or never occurs in the premature neonate. Persistence of a PDA can result in cardiopulmonary failure. There is no anatomical equivalent in the adult.

- Congenital malformations such as diaphragmatic hernia (CDH): CDH, with its concomitant pulmonary parenchymal and vascular hypoplasia, may be associated with persistent pulmonary hypertension of the newborn, significant right-to-left shunting of unoxygenated blood, and severe cyanosis and acidosis. Again, there is no anatomic equivalent in the adult population.

- Cardiac death: in the neonatal and paediatric populations, death is usually preceded by bradycardia followed by asystole. In adults, dysrhythmias such as ventricular fibrillation usually constitute the terminal event.

- Events preceding death: in the neonatal patient population, respiratory failure is a far more common cause of cardiac arrest than intrinsic cardiac disease. This is true even for a large percentage of children beyond the first month of life. In the adult, cardiac disease is the usual underlying cause of cardiac arrest.

♦ Drug metabolism: drug metabolism is developmentally regulated throughout the first days, months, and years of life and thus can differ tremendously from that of the adult. In addition, metabolism of pharmaceutical agents is heavily influenced by the patient's underlying disease and state of organ (dys)function. As mentioned previously, accurate representation of both healthy and deranged paediatric physiology is extremely limited.

Development of hybrid technologies that combine materials like the plastics used for physical patient simulators with visual displays and haptic interfaces capable of generating the images and tactile sensations associated with patient care will create learning opportunities that are currently impossible to achieve in the absence of a real patient. This combination of physical and virtual reality is sorely needed in paediatrics and obstetrics for the following reasons:

♦ Paediatric patients come in many different sizes and while it is not necessary to simulate every conceivable stage of human development it is nevertheless important to simulate those stages where significant differences in anatomy and physiology dictate different approaches to care. An obvious example of this is the neonate—there are many anatomic and physiologic differences between preterm and term neonates and these mandate careful consideration when selecting pharmaceuticals, determining the size of catheter for insertion into the umbilical artery, etc.

♦ Purely mechanical devices are unlikely to ever be able to simulate vaginal birth, with enough fidelity to generate realistic responses by trainees, in a cost-effective manner. The same is true of highly invasive procedures.

Thus, combining physical simulators with virtual reality interfaces designed to compensate for the physical simulators' limitations will play a major role in paediatric and obstetric high-fidelity simulation.

Until there is better collaboration among paediatric healthcare professionals, scientists with knowledge of simulation- and virtual reality-based technologies, and industry leaders, significant inadequacies will continue to plague efforts to achieve higher levels of realism and improved training experiences.

28.5.3 Securing necessary human and technical resources

Unless one is fortunate enough to work at a children's hospital, paediatrics is often a small (<10%) component of the care delivered at community and university hospitals. Thus, it can be difficult for any single paediatric subspecialty to generate enough human and technical resources to sustain a viable simulation programme. Sharing resources with adult programmes can help to defray overall costs and create potentially powerful collaborations and interesting programmes (such as combined neonatal-obstetric team training). Every paediatric simulation programme should be one component of a comprehensive effort to enhance human performance and improve patient safety during the care of children.[37]

28.5.4 **Optimizing return on investment**

Officials responsible for managing education and training budgets may question why traditional lecture settings involving relatively large numbers of trainees and smaller numbers of instructors should be replaced by experiences demanding a much higher instructor: trainee ratio. And they would be correct in their scepticism if the learning objectives involve only cognitive skills (content knowledge). Proponents of paediatric simulation-based training must be able to explain the unique benefits their programmes offer; some of these are listed in Box 28.4. Simulation-based activities must be related to the care of patients in some manner. While much of the early work in paediatric simulation has focused on developing programmes for the relative novice, little has been done to evaluate the return on the investment (ROI) of the time, effort, money, and space that has accompanied this work. Because early career trainees usually pay for their training directly in terms of tuition or indirectly by working long hours for relatively low pay, there is no significant driving force mandating formal calculation and justification of ROI in this population. As the field devotes more resources to developing continuing learning and assessment programmes for experienced healthcare professionals and multidisciplinary team training becomes the norm, those paying for such programmes (hospitals, clinics, and the healthcare professionals themselves) will make determination of ROI a mandate.

Simulation is not the optimal methodology for all learning objectives. For example, learning objectives that consist primarily of cognitive skills or content knowledge may be best acquired by reading self-study manuals and textbooks or interacting within online learning environments. Similarly, technical skills that require many repetitions in order to achieve mastery may be optimally acquired and refined by working with task trainers at skills stations (as opposed to practice within comprehensive simulated environments). However, for learning objectives that are primarily behavioural in nature or that encompass components of all three skill sets (cognitive, technical, behavioural), simulation is an ideal learning methodology; it is reasonable to hypothesize that the majority of learning objectives in healthcare belong in this category.

Box 28.4 Some benefits of paediatric simulation-based training

- ◆ Permits training in environments (intensive care units) that are usually inaccessible to less experienced trainees.
- ◆ Creates training opportunities for rarely encountered but highly challenging/risky situations (resuscitation, delivery of difficult news).
- ◆ Allows for training opportunities in paediatric domains ranging from general paediatrics to intensive care, counselling to high-tech areas such as ECMO.
- ◆ Permits formal objective performance assessment.

Those in quality improvement and risk management can serve as useful resources in determining priorities for training and in providing objective data to assess the outcomes of any training programme. Finally, working with colleagues with expertise in healthcare finance will provide guidance in analysing the cost-benefit ratio of simulation-based training. Given the financial constraints in paediatric healthcare, these relationships are arguably more important in paediatric than adult simulation.

28.6 **Conclusions**

Simulation-based training and research has the potential to revolutionize paediatric healthcare but this potential will be reached only if it is developed and implemented in a manner that addresses the unique needs of children and those caring for them. The term 'disruptive technology' describes the rapid evolution that occurs when a technologic breakthrough allows business to capitalize on its potential; this term was coined by Clayton Christensen in 1997.[38] Christensen later changed his terminology to 'disruptive innovation' in 2003; this may be a reasonable description of the potential of the simulation-based training methodology to change education, training, and performance assessment in paediatric healthcare.[39] If not self-motivated and self-regulated by professional and hospital associations within healthcare itself, such change will likely be driven by outside forces such as industrial regulatory bodies and the government. In fact, organizations such as the Joint Commission (JC) have already made recommendations for simulation-based training in the perinatal domain.[40] Thus, the challenge to those involved in paediatric simulation is to determine how to best utilize this powerful tool to optimize paediatric training and facilitate meaningful research before other less-informed entities relieve us of our responsibility.

References

1 **Ziv A, Wolpe PR, Small SD, Glick S.** Simulation-based medical education: an ethical imperative. Simul Healthc 2006;**1**(4):252–256.

2 **Murphy AM, Halamek LP.** Simulation-based training in neonatal resuscitation. NeoReviews 2005;**6**(11):e489–492.

3 **Lipman SS, Daniels KI, Arafeh J, Halamek LP.** The case for OBLS: a simulation-based obstetric resuscitation curriculum. Sem Perinatol 2011;**35**:74–79.

4 IPSS, <http://ipssglobal.org>, accessed 01 Sep. 2014.

5 **Dumont T, Hakim J, Black A, Fleming N.** Enhancing postgraduate training in pediatric and adolescent gynecology: evaluation of an advanced pelvic simulation session. J Pediatr Adolesc Gynecol 2014 Sep 22. pii: S1083–3188(14)00110–7. doi: 10.1016/j.jpag.2014.01.105. Epub ahead of print PMID: 25256870.

6 **Gupta AO, Ramasethu J.** An innovative nonanimal simulation trainer for chest tube insertion in neonates. Pediatrics 2014;**134**(3):e798–805.

7 **Vukin E, Greenberg R, Auerbach M, et al.** Use of simulation-based education: a national survey of pediatric clerkship directors. Acad Pediatr 2014;**14**(4):369–374.

8 Halamek LP, Kaegi DM, Gaba DM, et al. Time for a new paradigm in pediatric medical education: teaching neonatal resuscitation in a simulated delivery room environment. Pediatrics 2000;**106**(4):e45–51.

9 Austin EN, Bastepe-Gray SE, Nelson HW, et al. Pediatric mass-casualty education: experiential learning through university-sponsored disaster simulation. J Emerg Nurs 2014;**40**(5):428–433.

10 Su L, Spaeder MC, Jones MB, et al. Implementation of an extracorporeal cardiopulmonary resuscitation simulation program reduces extracorporeal cardiopulmonary resuscitation times in real patients. Pediatr Crit Care Med 2014 Aug 26. Epub ahead of print PMID: 25162513.

11 Stone K, Reid J, Caglar D, et al. Increasing pediatric resident simulated resuscitation performance: a standardized simulation-based curriculum. Resuscitation 2014;**85**(8):1099–1105.

12 Tobler K, Grant E, Marczinski C. Evaluation of the impact of a simulation-enhanced breaking bad news workshop in pediatrics. Simul Healthc 2014;**9**(4):213–219.

13 Kennedy JL, Jones SM, Porter N, et al. High-fidelity hybrid simulation of allergic emergencies demonstrates improved preparedness for office emergencies in pediatric allergy clinics. J Allergy Clin Immunol Pract 2013;**1**(6):608–617.e1–14.

14 Ventre KM, Barry JS, Davis D, et al. Using *in situ* simulation to evaluate operational readiness of a children's hospital-based obstetrics unit. Simul Healthc 2014;**9**(2):102–111.

15 McMorrow A1, Davis JW, Mayes C. Planning for a rare clinical challenge—simulating a sextuplet delivery. Simul Healthc 2013;**8**(5):350.

16 Dadiz R, Weinschreider J, Schriefer J, et al. Interdisciplinary simulation-based training to improve delivery room communication. Simul Healthc 2013;**8**(5):279–291.

17 Anderson JM, Murphy AA, Boyle BB, Yaeger KA, Halamek LP. Simulating extracorporeal membrane oxygenation (ECMO) emergencies, part II: qualitative and quantitative assessment and validation. Simul Healthc 2006;**1**:228–232.

18 Anderson JM, Murphy AA, Boyle BB, Yaeger KA, Halamek LP. Simulating extracorporeal membrane oxygenation (ECMO) emergencies to improve human performance, part I: methodologic and technologic innovations. Simul Healthc 2006;**1**:220–227.

19 Cheng A, Auerbach M, Hunt EA, et al. Designing and conducting simulation-based research. Pediatrics 2014;**133**(6):1091–1101.

20 Halamek LP. Simulation as a methodology for assessing the performance of healthcare professionals working in the delivery room. Semin Fetal Neonatal Med 2013;**18**(6):369–372.

21 Halamek LP. The rationale and strategy for rigorous human performance assessment in neonatal-perinatal medicine. NeoReviews 2013;**14**:e379–e386.

22 Geurtzen R, Hogeveen M, Rajani AK, et al. Using simulation to study difficult clinical issues: prenatal counseling at the threshold of viability across American and Dutch cultures. J Simul Healthc 2014;**9**(3):167–173.

23 Chitkara R, Rajani AK, Oehlert JW, Halamek LP. Accuracy of human senses in the detection of neonatal heart rate during standardized simulated resuscitation: implications for delivery of care, training and technology design. Resuscitation 2013;**84**(3):369–372.

24 Rajani AK, Chitkara R, Oehlert J, Halamek LP. Comparison of umbilical venous and intraosseous access during simulated neonatal resuscitation. Pediatrics 2011;**128**(4):e954–958.

25 Chitkara R, Rajani AK, Lee HC, Snyder SF, Halamek LP. Comparing the utility of an ergonomic neonatal resuscitation cart with a generic code cart: a randomized, controlled, crossover trial. BMJ Qual Saf 2013;**22**(2):124–129.

26 Agarwal S, Swanson S, Yaeger KA, Murphy AA, Halamek LP. Utilizing simulation to compare the standard pediatric code cart with a pediatric code cart based on the Broselow tape. Pediatrics 2005;**116**(3):e326–e333.

27 International Network for Simulation-based Pediatric Innovation, Research and Education (INSPIRE), <http://inspiresim.com>, accessed 01 Sep. 2014.

28 International Network for Simulation-based Pediatric Innovation, Research and Education (INSPIRE), <http://inspiresim.com/about-inspire/how-did-we-become-inspire/>, accessed 01 Sep. 2014.

29 International Network for Simulation-based Pediatric Innovation, Research and Education (INSPIRE), <http://inspiresim.com/category/proced/> accessed 01 Sep. 2014.

30 **Chang TP, Kessler D, McAninch B, et al**. International Simulation in Pediatric Innovation, Research, and Education (INSPIRE) Network. Script concordance testing: assessing residents' clinical decision-making skills for infant lumbar punctures. Acad Med 2014;**89**(1):128–135.

31 **Auerbach M, Chang TP, Reid J, et al**. Are pediatric interns prepared to perform infant lumbar punctures? A multi-institutional descriptive study. Pediatr Emerg Care 2013;**29**(4):453–457.

32 **Kessler DO, Arteaga G, Ching K, et al**. Interns' success with clinical procedures in infants after simulation training. Pediatrics 2013;**131**(3):e811–820.

33 **Johnston LC, Auerbach M, Kappus L, Emerson B, Zigmont J, Sudikoff SN**. Utilization of exploration-based learning and video-assisted learning to teach GlideScope videolaryngoscopy. Teach Learn Med 2014;**26**(3):285–291.

34 **Haubner LY, Barry JS, Johnston LC, et al**. Neonatal intubation performance: room for improvement in tertiary neonatal intensive care units. Resuscitation 2013;**84**(10):1359–1364.

35 **Li S, Rehder KJ, Giuliano JS Jr, et al**. For the National Emergency Airway Registry for Children NEAR4KIDS Investigators and Pediatric Acute Lung Injury and Sepsis Investigator PALISI Network Investigators. Development of a quality improvement bundle to reduce tracheal intubation-associated events in pediatric ICUs. Am J Med Qual 2014 Aug 20. pii: 1062860614547259. Epub ahead of print PMID: 25143411.

36 **Halamek LP**. Teaching versus learning and the role of simulation-based training in pediatrics. J Pediatr 2007;**151**(4):329–330.

37 **Halamek LP**. Improving performance, reducing error, and minimizing risk in the delivery room. In: Fetal and neonatal brain injury: mechanisms, management, and the risks of practice. Stevenson DK, Benitz WE, Sunshine P, Hintz S, Druzin M, eds. Cambridge, UK: Cambridge University Press, 4th edn; 2009.

38 **Christensen CM**. The innovator's dilemma. Boston, MA: Harvard Business School Press; 1997.

39 **Christensen CM**. The innovator's solution. Boston, MA: Harvard Business School Press; 2003.

40 The Joint Commission, <http://www.jointcommission.org/assets/1/18/sea_30.pdf>, accessed 01 Sep. 2014.

Chapter 29

Obstetric simulation

Shad H Deering

Overview

◆ Practising for obstetric emergencies with simulation training has demonstrated the ability to significantly decrease maternal and foetal/infant morbidity and mortality, and is now recommended and recognized by major regulatory bodies.

◆ Emergencies in obstetrics are common and may result in significant morbidity and mortality for the mother and the foetus.

◆ A well-thought out curriculum and evaluation forms are essential to provide realistic and beneficial training.

◆ Both teamwork and technical performance are important components to evaluate during training.

◆ Training done on the actual delivery unit may be more beneficial than in a laboratory setting, as it allows for the assessment of technical skills and the opportunity to evaluate for systems issues that can be corrected.

29.1 Brief history and evidence

There are few areas of medicine where simulation training is more necessary and potentially beneficial than obstetrics. In 2012, a joint publication, endorsed by seven different national societies, titled 'Quality Patient Care in Labor and Delivery: A Call to Action' was released. It focused on areas where improvements are needed to ensure optimal care on labour and delivery and specifically recommended simulation training as part of a comprehensive strategy to improve outcomes in obstetrics. In addition, over the past several years, several studies have been published demonstrating improved outcomes in actual patients. One of the best examples of this is related to deliveries complicated by shoulder dystocia.

In the United Kingdom, Draycott et al. implemented a training programme for personnel involved in labour and delivery management. This training was mandatory and used a relatively inexpensive hybrid birthing simulator to teach and allow practice of the basic manoeuvres for management of a shoulder dystocia delivery.[1] After implementing this training, the group found that the use of McRobert's position drastically increased during actual deliveries from 29.3% to 87.4% and there was a decrease in the head-to-body delivery time from three minutes to two minutes. Neonatal outcomes also improved. The risk of neonatal injury at births complicated by shoulder dystocia decreased from 9.3% to 2.3% post-training, and the risk of brachial plexus injury fell from 7.4% to 2.3%.

These findings were replicated in the United States. In 2011, Grobman et al. implemented a similar programme that showed a decrease in the incidence of brachial plexus injury after deliveries complicated by shoulder dystocia from 10.1% to 4.0% (p < 0.001).[2]

The objectives of this chapter are to provide the reader with a good understanding of the current state of obstetric simulation and how to best construct and run effective obstetric simulation scenarios.

29.2 **Obstetric simulation training**

When planning obstetric simulation training that will make a difference, there are several factors that must be considered. Siassakos et al. reviewed programmes where delivery units demonstrated improved patient outcomes after simulation training.[3] They identified the following common elements:

- **Institution-level incentives:** these may be in form of decreased medical malpractice premiums, or held as a requirement for credentialing.

- **Relevant, in-house training for all staff**: the programmes that demonstrated improvements all trained nearly 100% of their staff. In addition, many of them conducted the training in the actual hospital rather than at outside facilities.

- **Non-threatening training environment:** ensuring that providers who attend training understand the purpose of the training, to improve patient safety and outcomes, is critical. Creating a hostile or threatening testing climate can decrease staff participation and performance.

- **Development of local solutions:** allowing the on-site providers to both identify issues and produce their own solutions can improve ownership of the changes made and help ensure they are implemented and sustained.

- **Realistic training tools:** simulators used do not have to be the most expensive or high-tech to be effective, but they should be realistic enough to allow for appropriate interventions to be undertaken. The use of patient actors, either with a hybrid simulator or as the simulator's family member, may be helpful in improving communication.

- **Multiprofessional teamwork training:** because emergencies are handled by a team and not individuals, training together is important to ensure the team works well together during obstetric emergencies.

The steps involved in creating and conducting obstetric simulation include the following:

- define what you want to teach
- decide who you will be training

- write learning objectives
- determine the training location
- choose a simulator
- design simulation scenario and evaluation/debriefing forms
- practise the simulation
- conduct simulation and debriefing
- review training and obtain feedback

While these steps can be applied to any specialty, in the following sections the chapter will discuss each of these steps in detail and specifically how they are applied to obstetric simulation.

29.2.1 **Define what you want to teach**

In obstetric simulation, there are both technical and overall management/communication skills that need to be taught. For technical skills, such as operative vaginal delivery, vaginal laceration repair or manoeuvres to relieve a shoulder dystocia, it is helpful to have specific skill stations set up that allow for deliberate teaching and practice to ensure correct performance. For overall management of obstetric cases and emergencies, such as postpartum haemorrhage, you may want to focus on both the technical skills as well as teamwork and communication, which will involve running full scenarios rather than just skills stations.

Any simulation training that uses the birthing mannequins is also an opportunity for teamwork/communication training and evaluation.[4] The challenge involved in doing this usually stems from being able to have the ancillary staff available to participate and finding a time that is not too busy on labour and delivery if that is where the training will take place.

29.2.2 **Decide who you will be training**

The level of simulation will depend on who you are planning to train. This will dictate both the skills to be taught as well as shape the specific learning objectives. As an example, for providers that actually perform operative vaginal deliveries, your learning objectives may focus on indications, counselling, and actual performance whereas if you are training labour and delivery nurses on the same topic, you would focus less on actual technique and more of the critical assistant role that they play.

29.2.3 **Write learning objectives**

Before you decide on a simulator, write down your specific learning objectives. These may be purely technical in terms of teaching skills such as laceration repair, or you may want to focus more on communication and teamwork. Regardless of what your goals are, setting out clear objectives will make your training more effective.

29.2.4 **Location of obstetric simulation training**

There is always debate about where obstetric simulation training should occur, with reasonable arguments for several different approaches. For the most part, the decision must be made between conducting training on the labour and delivery unit or at a separate dedicated location.

The benefit to conducting training at a location away from labour and delivery is that the staff involved are less likely to be pulled into other clinical duties during the simulation training time. In addition, if you can procure a permanent space, then you do not have to set up and then put away the equipment and you have a better ability to consider installing video-recording devices, which are helpful in reviewing training and assist with debriefing. On the other hand, training on the actual labour and delivery ward adds a degree of realism that cannot be completely replicated in a laboratory.

Training on the labour unit allows providers to practice technical skills as well as to incorporate multidisciplinary training, and see what unique systems problems may occur in actual cases. For example, if you simulate a shoulder dystocia and the staff asks the nurse to call for help, if you are on your own labour and delivery unit, that nurse has to find the phone, use the correct phone number, or physically go and find the appropriate person in the exact same manner as they will during a real dystocia. If the simulation is done in a lab, then the act of finding someone to help can be simulated, but it will not identify any of the systems issues. The down side to training on the actual labour and delivery unit is that scheduling may be difficult as the acuity at any given time cannot be predicted with certainty, and patient safety will always trump training. Another logistical issue is that you will have to transport the mannequin to the unit for training if it is not normally stored in that area.

Where you decide to conduct your training will depend on multiple factors, as discussed above. If you are training students, residents (registrars), and staff on procedures, this can be accomplished well away from the labour and delivery ward. If you have the ability and desire to provide a more realistic team approach, then simulation training on actual labour and delivery suites may be a better choice.

29.2.5 **Choose a simulator**

While many will begin planning for simulation by asking what simulator they should use or purchase, this should always come later in the process. There are several companies that supply a wide range of obstetric simulators, with more being made available every year. Specific features of these mannequins with regards to the individual simulations are discussed in detail in the following sections.

A list of the simulations that common birthing trainers can support can be found in Table 29.1 and Internet links for several manufacturers can be found at the end of this chapter.

What follows is a reasonable representation of some of those used most often.

29.2.5.1 Birthing mannequins

Birthing mannequins range from just the lower portion of the female torso to a complete adult female with arms and legs. Determining exactly which one is best for your needs is a balance of cost and the anticipated use. The good news about obstetric simulation is that

Table 29.1 Comparison of common obstetric simulator capabilities

Simulator	NOELLE	PROMPT	SimMom	Sophie's Mum	Fidelis	Mama Natalie
Manufacturer	Gaumard Scientific	Laerdal	Laerdal	Model-Med	CAE	Laerdal
Price Range + (< $1,000) ++ (< $10,000) +++ (> $10,000) ++++ (>$20,000)	+ to ++++	++	++++	++	++++	+
Simulations supported						
Spontaneous vaginal delivery	X	X	X	X	X	X
Forceps/Vacuum delivery	X	X	X	X	X	X
Breach vaginal delivery	X	X	X	X	X	X (inflatable foetus, not good for manoeuvres)
Umbilical cord prolapse	X	X	X	X	X	X
Shoulder Dystocia	X	X	X	X	X	X
Postpartum haemorrhage	X		X	X*	X	X
FHR monitoring	X*		X*		X*	
Internal monitor placement	X		X		X	
Caesarean Section	X*		X*		X*	
Eclampsia	X	(patient controlling the simulator can simulate seizure)	X		X	(patient controlling the simulator can simulate seizure)
Maternal cardiac arrest	X		X		X	
External cephalic version	X*					

* Note that there are several different models in these product lines. It is important to review the specific model with regards to its full capabilities as some of the capabilities require additional products from the manufacturer.

there are relatively low-cost solutions that can accomplish the majority of training object-ives. Some of the more common birthing mannequins in use are briefly described below.

29.2.5.1.1 **NOELLE® birthing mannequins** The NOELLE® mannequins are generally full-size females complete with arms and legs, though there are more simple birthing man-nequins that only include the lower torso. There are several different models of this man-nequin available, and some of them include monitors that allow the trainer to show both the foetal heart rate tracing and maternal vital signs. The full-size mannequins by Gau-mard allow for most all of the obstetric simulations included in this chapter to be run. The foetus may be delivered either by a motor that is contained within the abdomen, or pushed out by hand. Newer models have additional features that allow for measurement of force applied during delivery, external cephalic version, and caesarean section (see Figure 29.1).

29.2.5.1.2 **PROMPT® birthing simulator** The PROMPT® birthing simulator consists of the lower torso of an adult female, and includes only the top portions of the thighs. The birthing foetus that is included on some models contains a force-feedback mechanism that allows the trainer to monitor the amount of force applied during delivery. In order to control the foetus during delivery with this model, it requires someone playing the part of the patient to sit on the bed and push the foetus out. This is why it is often considered a hybrid simulator. A new version of this model that will be available soon will add the abil-ity to train for postpartum haemorrhage (see Figure 29.2).

29.2.5.1.3 **Sophie and her Mum** This model is also a hybrid simulator which is similar to the PROMPT® birthing simulator; however, the legs do not articulate. The pelvic tissue is well designed and it is one of the most realistic for practising operative vaginal delivery. There is also a module available for it that allows for practising postpartum haemorrhage (see Figure 29.3).

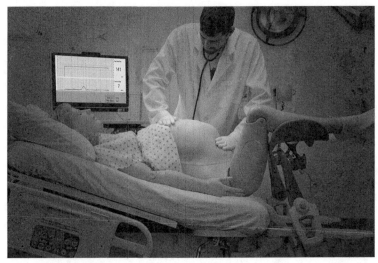

Fig. 29.1 NOELLE® birthing simulator.
Reproduced by kind permission of Gaumard Scientific. Copyright © 2015 Gaumard Scientific, FL, USA.

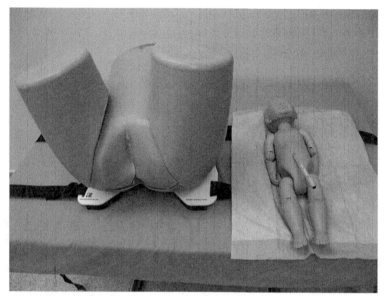

Fig. 29.2 PROMPT® birthing simulator.
Reproduced by kind permission of Laerdal Medical Ltd. Copyright © 2015 Laerdal Medical Ltd., UK.

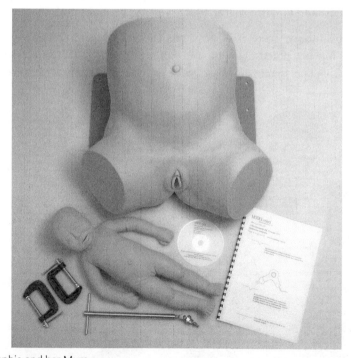

Fig. 29.3 Sophie and her Mum.
Reproduced by kind permission of Model-Med Pty Ltd. Copyright © 2015 Model-Med Pty Ltd, Melbourne, VIC, Australia.

29.2.5.1.4 **Mama Natalie** The Mama Natalie is a low-fidelity and low-cost simulator (less than $1,000) that was designed for use in developing countries. It is worn by a simulated patient who controls the foetus for delivery. The foetus is inflatable with either air or water. There is a large simulated blood reservoir included that allows for a significant postpartum haemorrhage. The entire simulator packs into an easy-to-carry backpack. Though it is designed for low-resource areas, it can be a very effective simulator for many obstetric complications (see Figure 29.4).

29.2.5.1.5 **SimMom** This is a new full-body birthing simulator that is similar in capabilities and appearance to the NOELLE® line of simulators. It allows for all of the basic obstetric simulations to be run and includes a robust maternal/foetal monitoring capability which makes practising maternal cardiac arrest scenarios possible.

29.2.5.1.6 **CAE Fidelis** This is a new full-body simulator that has been recently released. Though there is not a lot of experience with its use at this time, it is a high-fidelity full-body birthing simulator with capabilities listed in Table 29.1.

29.2.5.2 Specific task trainers

There are also a number of specific task trainers that are available for obstetrics at this time, though most all of the simulations discussed in this chapter can be accomplished on standard birthing mannequins. The most common procedures that can be taught with task trainers are episiotomy, perineal laceration repair, and amniocentesis.

29.2.5.2.1 **Episiotomy** There are several models available and described in the literature for training and practising episiotomy and third/fourth-degree laceration repairs. These range from homemade simulators, such as using a thawed beef tongue or a carwash

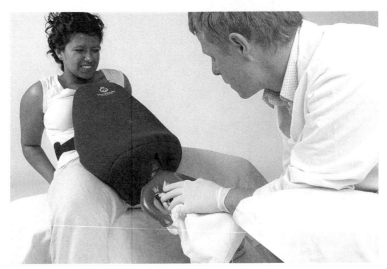

Fig. 29.4 MamaNatalie Birthing Simulator.
Reproduced by kind permission of Laerdal Medical Ltd. Copyright © 2015 Laerdal Medical Ltd, UK.

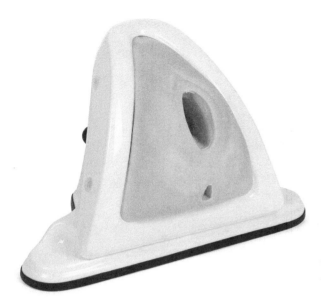

Fig. 29.5 Episiotomy model.
Reproduced by kind permission of
Limbs and Things Ltd. Copyright
© 2015 Limbs and Things Ltd.,
Bristol, UK.

sponge, to more advanced anatomical models.[5] The Limbs and Things models are some of the most realistic at this time, and have been used at different centres in validation studies.[6] A picture of an episiotomy model is seen in Figure 29.5.

29.2.5.2.2 **Amniocentesis/cordocentesis** Commercially available amniocentesis/cordocentesis trainers are available from Limbs and Things (Bristol, UK) and Blue Phantom. The first model contains two separate placentas and simulated umbilical cords that can be refilled with mock blood to practise both amniocentesis and cordocentesis. The model is relatively simple to use, and the only issue we have found in working with it is that there is no representation of subcutaneous tissue, so the procedure is significantly easier than real life. During our training, we often place the Limbs and Things model inside of an inexpensive birthing simulator to allow the provider to drape the procedure area (see Figure 29.6 and Figure 29.7). The Blue Phantom model is in a body form with an abdominal wall and a more realistic image.

29.2.5.2.3 **Design simulation scenario and evaluation/debriefing form** For each simulation, creating an instruction packet for the staff who will run the simulation will result in better and more standard training. This should include a brief overview of the simulation, and learning objectives, as well as a simple flow diagram of how to run the drill. This flow diagram should explain how the simulation begins, and define a clear point at which the simulation will end. For example, with a shoulder dystocia scenario, it can begin as the provider enters the room and the foetal head is made to deliver. At our institution, we will usually continue the simulation until the trainee delivers the posterior arm, performs a Zavenelli manoeuvre, or states that they do not know any other manoeuvres that they can do.

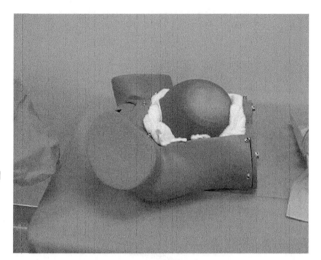

Fig. 29.6 Limbs & Things cordocentesis simulator placed inside a birthing simulator.

Reproduced by kind permission of Limbs and Things Ltd. Copyright © 2015 Limbs and Things Ltd., Bristol, UK.

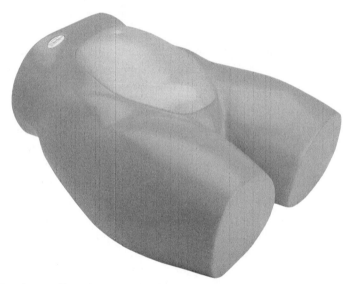

Fig. 29.7 Blue Phantom® amniocentesis simulator.
Reproduced by kind permission of CAE Healthcare. Copyright © CAE Healthcare, 2015.

Another area that should be covered in the instructions is the role of any additional personnel other than the staff running the scenario. For instance, if you are going to have someone play a nurse or family member, make sure to include their role and basic responses in the instructions so they are standardized for all the participants. We have found that if you can add a concerned and vocal 'family member' to the simulations that it adds a lot to the reality of the situation and we highly recommend doing this if you are able.

In addition, we usually include a basic troubleshooting list and common questions that the trainee may ask and what the standard response will be during the scenario for each question.

When making a grading form for your simulation, it is usually easiest to include both objective and subjective sections. For example, the objective section may have simple yes or no questions regarding the actions taken by the trainee during the simulation while the subjective section may include a standard Likert scale and is meant to assess more global issues such as, how well did the provider perform overall or how prepared was the provider for the scenario encountered. Additional sections and/or checklists may be included to evaluate how well the team counselled the patient or to focus on key documentation points.[7]

In order to make evaluation forms more relevant, it is helpful to discuss the important performance measures with your staff and local experts, because these may vary between sites. After you have designed your grading form, the best way to determine if it works well is to record someone, even yourself, going through the simulation and then have two or three people watch and grade you and comment on the evaluation forms themselves. This will allow you to see if the form is simple enough for them to understand how to fill it out, if they are relatively consistent in their assessments, and if there is anything you might want to add or delete from the forms as well.

With regards to specific format, as opposed to several years ago, there are many examples available online. The current format and an example used by the American College of Obstetrics and Gynecologists (ACOG) simulation consortium can be found in a recent article on simulation for obstetric emergencies by Deering et al.[8]

29.2.6 Practise the simulation

After you have created the simulation scenario and forms, it is important to then practise running through the simulation before implementing it. There will almost always be something that has been overlooked or, more likely, the trainees will ask for something you did not anticipate that takes the scenario away from the learning objectives you intended.

29.2.7 Conduct simulation and debriefing

Exactly how you run the training sessions will depend on how many simulation staff you have to run the simulations, how many people you have to train, and time constraints. For example, you will set things up very differently if you are trying to train 20 residents in a four-hour session versus only four. If there is a large number trainees, or you are conducting multidisciplinary training, then group teaching afterwards may be more efficient than the individual debriefing that can be accomplished with smaller numbers. It is important, however, that you allow trainees to practise physically on the mannequin after/during the scenario, and to practise the skills you are trying to teach.

One of the most significant challenges is often deciding what to do with trainees between simulations as others run through the simulation, because having them just sit around is a waste of valuable time. Some ways to decrease any down time are to either have two or three stations that they rotate between and then do additional teaching/training after they have completed all stations or have the trainee write a procedure or delivery/event note after they go through the simulation. These notes can then be used as part of the debriefing process and provide a good opportunity for instruction on documentation after emergencies/procedures.

For many of the obstetric scenarios the actual simulation part only will only require 5–10 minutes, so you can realistically have multiple people run through them and then bring them together afterwards for feedback, instruction, and additional practice on the simulator.

In general, here is how we run our multidisciplinary simulation training exercise for shoulder dystocia:

Step 1: The birthing mannequin is set up in a room on a delivery table with legs in stirrups. The staff controlling the foetus and delivery sets up for the delivery.

Step 2: The first provider is given the clinical scenario just outside the room. They take a few minutes to read it and then enter the room and the scenario begins. As they recognize the complication, the provider will call for assistance and perform manoeuvres to relieve the dystocia.

Step 3: After the simulation ends, the entire team is gathered together and a formal and standardized debriefing occurs. During this, key points and the learning objectives are reviewed.

Step 4: After the debriefing is completed, individual providers are given the opportunity to practise manoeuvres and additional instruction is given during this time.

29.2.8 Debriefing

There is a definite skill to giving feedback and debriefing after simulation, and entire courses have been developed to assist with this process. The key is to ensure that the session is productive and not punitive, as this will be counterproductive to both learning and future training. After this, allow the trainees to practise on the actual mannequin with supervision and assist them in anything they had difficulty with during the scenario.

29.2.9 Review training and obtain feedback

After you have completed training, obtaining feedback from learners about how the session went is important to ensure you achieved your learning objectives and allow for changes if needed for future training. It is helpful to have a standard feedback form for records and to make sure you ask the questions you are interested in.

29.3 Common issues and barriers to training

No matter how good the planning, or how needed the training is, there will always be barriers to implementing simulation training in any field. In obstetrics, some of the most common challenges are cost, leadership support, and space.

Though many of the simulators, especially the hybrid ones, mentioned are relatively inexpensive (< $10,000), this may still be a significant investment for many institutions. The full-body high-fidelity birthing mannequins are usually more expensive, ranging from $20,000–70,000, and require additional expertise to make full use of the technology and monitoring systems. In most cases, however, the consumable costs for obstetric simulators are minimal, with the delivery foetus being the part most often needing to be replaced.

Despite all of the evidence that is available for the benefits of obstetric simulation, without support from leadership, these programmes will not reach their full potential. To ensure this support is present, we recommend involving key personnel, including clinical, administrative, and patient-safety representatives, in the process and planning from the beginning. Showing the evidence and expected outcomes as well as a coherent plan for implementation can overcome these barriers in most cases.

Space for storage and training is always a challenge. If your institution has a simulation centre, then this may be easier. Otherwise, for truly *in situ* programmes, identifying a standard location for storage and/or training should be included in the planning from the beginning stages.

29.4 **Conclusions**

Simulation training in obstetrics has the potential to prevent a significant number of poor outcomes. It is an essential part of training today and can be accomplished with a relatively small investment of both time and funding. Evidence has been published and research continues to demonstrate how it can improve outcomes for actual patients and training resources are readily available to assist with implementation.

References

1 Draycott TJ, Crofts JF, Ash JP, et al. Improving neonatal outcome through practical shoulder dystocia training. Obstet Gynecol 2008;**112**(1):14–20.

2 Grobman WA, Miller D, Burke C, Hornbogen A, Tam K, Costello R. Outcomes associated with introduction of a shoulder dystocia protocol. Am J Obstet Gynecol 2011;**205**(6):513–517.

3 Siassakos D, Crofts JF, Winter C, Weiner CP, Draycott TJ. The active components of effective training in obstetric emergencies. BJOG 2009;**116**:1028–1032.

4 Robertson B, Schumacher L, Gosman G, Kanfer R, Kelley M, DeVita M. Simulation-based crisis team training for multidisciplinary obstetric providers. Sim Healthcare 2009;**4**:77–83.

5 Sparks RA, Beesley AD, Jones AD. The 'sponge perineum': an innovative method of teaching fourth-degree obstetric perineal laceration repair to family medicine residents. Fam Med 2006;**38**(8):542–544.

6 Nielsen PE, Foglia LM, Mandel LS, Chow GE. Objective structured assessment of technical skills for episiotomy repair. Am J Obstet Gynecol 2003;**189**:1257–1260.

7 Goffman D, Heo H, Chazotte C, Merkatz IR, Bernstein PS. Using simulation training to improve shoulder dystocia documentation. Obstet Gynecol 2008;**112**(6):1284–1287.

8 Deering SH, Rowland J. Obstetric emergency simulation. Seminars in Perinatology 2013;**37**:179–188.

Websites for obstetric simulation supplies/models

NOELLE® birthing mannequin:

<http://www.gaumard.com>

PROMPT® birthing simulator (pelvis and upper legs):

<http://www.laerdal.com/us/doc/224/PROMPT-Birthing-Simulator>

Mama Natalie:

<http://www.laerdal.com/us/mamaNatalie>

Amniocentesis models:

<http://limbsandthings.com/global/products/cordocentesis-trainer>

<http://www.bluephantom.com/product/Amniocentesis-Ultrasound-Training-Model.aspx?cid=429>

Sophie's Mum birthing simulator (pelvis and upper legs):

<http://paradigmmedicalsystems.com/sophie-and-her-mum/>

SimMom:

<http://www.laerdal.com/us/SimMom>

CAE Fidelis birthing simulator:

<http://www.caehealthcare.com/patient-simulators/maternal-fetal-childbirth-simulator>

Curriculum and simulations

ACOG Simulation Consortium:

<http://www.acog.org/About-ACOG/ACOG-Departments/Simulations-Consortium>

Chapter 30

Creating virtual reality medical simulations: a knowledge-based design and assessment approach

Dale C Alverson, Thomas P Caudell, and Timothy E Goldsmith

Overview

- Virtual reality (VR) can enhance learning by providing students as an example here.

- Our VR simulation development is based on the concept of providing a distributable simulator environment in which individual trainees and instructors can work together virtually as teams despite physical separation at different locations.

- Using a multiplayer collaborative participatory environment, enabled over advanced Internet networks, offers a platform for 'just-in-time' team training, training on demand, refreshment training, and performance assessment that can complement onsite simulation.

- As in other forms of simulation, VR also can be applied to individuals, as well as teams, and the simulator technology or user interface matched with the goals of the simulation, needs of the learners/trainees, and their best learning style.

- VR simulations provide a means for interactive, experiential, problem-based learning and integrated into simulation centres, an overall curriculum or training milieu, creating safe environments to make mistakes, a sense of presence, and engagement to enhance learning.

- VR simulation should be matched with the specific training goals and objectives; it may be designed for skill training, and cognitive assessment and decision-making, or both.

- In our initiatives, VR simulations are based on a rules-based artificial intelligence (AI) engine developed in conjunction with subject-matter experts (SMEs) and computer programmers that dynamically governs changes in physiology, physical findings, movement and events, as well as responses to the user.

Overview *(continued)*

- Important concepts can be embedded into the VR simulation scenario applying a knowledge-based design using the SME's knowledge structure as a gold standard.

- In addition, the expert knowledge structure can be used to compare the novice learner to the expert, provide a measure of the effect of the simulation in improving the learner's knowledge structure, and progression toward becoming an expert.

- VR simulation development requires a coordinated, collaborative transdisciplinary team of subject-matter experts, computer scientists, engineers, graphic and sound artists, communication network specialists, educators, cognitive psychologists, and evaluators.

- VR can include high-fidelity graphics and animation that can be changed to match the needs of the simulation scenario.

- VR can also enable reification of abstract concepts that provides a method wherein those abstractions can be perceived, rendered, and visualized as something concrete with which the users can interact.

30.1 Introduction to creating virtual reality medical simulations

This chapter describes a method for creating a virtual reality (VR) simulation for medical education and training along with assessing student's knowledge and skill. An example of how the tools and methods can be applied is provided. VR simulations can be used on site as part of a simulation centre or independently off site, by individual learners or teams of learners, as well as used interactively by teams over distance at different sites in distributed VR environments. VR allows students and trainees to be uniquely immersed and engaged in lifelike situations where they can learn without suffering the consequences that may occur due to lack of experience.[1]

VR developers can create environments through a process called **reification** that helps students comprehend abstract concepts by making them appear concrete.[2] In these simulations, students are allowed to interact with objects and processes that are not normally accessible, but because of their explicit nature learners can grasp concepts that are ordinarily difficult to comprehend. In this manner, individuals can utilize their senses to perceive better the relevance of important concepts, entering virtual worlds outside normal experience, interacting through 'perceptualization': a combination of visualization, sound, touch, and perhaps even taste and smell. These principles have been applied in developing a 'fantastic voyage' into the human kidney, in which the 'voyager' can interact and manipulate the important elements in the virtual world, and thus begin to grasp the important abstract concepts that are often difficult to learn, understand and teach.

The creation of a VR simulation requires that a development team have skills in computer science and engineering, visualization, computer graphics, artificial intelligence

(AI), three-dimensional (3D) modelling, and knowledge-based design. Subject-matter experts (SMEs) pertinent to the content material being taught and learning goals and objectives in the simulation are also key participants.

This chapter captures these concepts and sets out a process for developing VR simulation, including describing specific steps, methods, and tools. It also briefly provides a method for evaluating the impact of VR stimulation on learning and performance. Finally, it gives a specific example of VR simulation and suggests future approaches to research and development.

30.2 **Knowledge-structure approach**

Underlying much of our work in designing and evaluating VR simulations is the idea of an explicit representation of knowledge, and in particular the representation of knowledge by a human expert.[4] Several decades of research in cognitive science show that experts acquire a vast amount of domain-specific knowledge but equally important is how they represent this knowledge in long-term memory.[3-5] Indeed, it is the structure of this knowledge that differentiates an expert from more novice learners. Experts share a common structural organization of concepts and, as a consequence, are more likely to see certain relevant, abstract relationships and connections the same way. Further, there have been various attempts to empirically elicit individuals' knowledge structures with much of this work occurring in an educational setting.[6-8]

We use a three-phase method for eliciting and evaluating an individual's knowledge structure: (i) elicit some behavioural index of an individual's organization of domain concepts; (ii) represent these elicited data as a formal representation (e.g. network) that captures the important structural properties of the knowledge; and (iii) evaluate the goodness or level of expertise of this derived representation.

The elicitation phase first identifies a master set of terms and concepts from textbooks, manuals, reports, and SMEs. The experts then rate the centrality of these terms to the knowledge domain and from the averaged ratings we select a smaller subset of terms. The SMEs then rate the relatedness of each pair of central terms, and the average of these pairwise relatedness ratings serves as the basis for deriving a single expert knowledge structure.

We apply the Pathfinder algorithm[9] to these ratings to derive a formal network model of the concepts and their semantic relationships. Pathfinder generates a connected graph, or knowledge network, that depicts local concept relationships as directly linked nodes in the graph. Pathfinder knowledge networks were found to predict well students' classroom performance.[10-12]

Finally, in the evaluation phase, a person's knowledge structure (i.e. Pathfinder knowledge network) is evaluated to assess its level of competence. We use a referent-based evaluation to compare a student's knowledge structure with a corresponding expert knowledge structure. Using this measure we find that experts have more similar knowledge structures to one another than do less experienced people, and the degree of similarity between a student's knowledge structure and an expert's is an index of how much the student knows about the domain.

The resulting expert knowledge structure is used for two purposes: to guide the development of the VR simulation and to serve as a gold standard against which to assess students' learning of the domain.

30.2.1 Assessing student learning in VR

A principal goal in creating a VR simulation is to foster student learning of the domain. Ultimately, the knowledge students acquire from VR training would be evaluated by having them apply the acquired skills in a realistic context. However, such assessments are difficult to carry out immediately after learning; to gauge the effectiveness of VR training we use the structural assessment of knowledge method.

We obtain knowledge structures from students for the same set of concepts used in the expert structure. We do this before the student experiences the VR simulation and then immediately after VR training. The change in pre-/post-training similarities to the expert network is viewed as an index of learning. Knowledge structures are particularly appropriate for assessing complex, conceptual understanding[13]—exactly the type of knowledge that is the focus of our VR simulations.

Undoubtedly, there are other and perhaps more valid measures of student learning, such as how well knowledge transfers to other courses of study or how well it transfers to a clinical setting.[14] In future work, we plan to examine how acquired conceptual knowledge transfers to novel tasks. We hypothesize that participants receiving simulation training will not only develop improved conceptual understanding of the domain, but also that their understanding will transfer to tasks requiring novel applications of the knowledge.

30.3 Creating the VR simulations and processes for development

30.3.1 Knowledge-based design

Although others have taken a cognitive approach to building medical simulators and trainers[15] we believe that our approach to designing VR simulations from a structural knowledge approach is unique. The essence of the approach is to use the core concepts and relationships of an expert knowledge structure to guide the design of the simulated environment. As part of this process, the VR development team brainstorms with SMEs to identify multiple approaches for representing conceptual relationships; from this process storyboards emerge. The development team creates prototypes in a visualization tool or game engine, initially using coarse models, animations, and sounds. SMEs then help refine elements of the simulation that best represent their conceptual understanding of the structure and process being simulated. A concept audit is conducted for each potential simulated environment to ensure that critical associations in the expert knowledge structure occur within the simulation. An initial rule-based AI, which controls the simulation, is also created to capture the general interactions of conceptual elements using SME-validated rules.

Once an initial VR training environment is created, we can then use student learning to refine the VR simulation. The change in students' knowledge structures as a result of VR training serves as an immediate and objective index of training effectiveness. We examine what aspects of the students' knowledge structures change over the course of training, or more importantly what aspects do not change. For example, assume that domain experts have concepts A, B, and C tightly linked together as a meaningful substructure in the expert knowledge network. Assume further that these links are absent from the students' knowledge structures after VR training. We would then want to examine how these concepts and their relationships are represented in the simulation and how this representation might be altered to make more salient the concept associations. Hence, achieving agreement between students' and experts' knowledge structures serves as an objective goal for guiding and refining the simulation.

The VR simulation design team iteratively refines game content and rules to arrive at the validity level required to begin learning experiments. Human subjects' knowledge structures are measured before and after system exposure and statistically compared with those of the SMEs. Changes are correlated with representational elements from the audit matrix to determine how they potentially contributed to the changes. Designers use the analysis to evolve or redesign the representation and possibly re-evaluate which key concepts are included. The process is repeated until post-exposure subject performance best matches that of the experts.

30.3.2 Validation of the VR simulations

Each VR simulation should be subjected to various levels of validation: face, content, construct, concurrent, and predictive.

30.3.2.1 Establishing face validity

SMEs review the VR simulation to determine whether the representation of the material and concepts matches their expected appearance of the content. Through an iterative process with the SMEs, the VR representation is refined.

30.3.2.2 Establishing content validity

The VR scenario and treatment algorithms are assessed for content accuracy to ensure that the curriculum goals have been incorporated, as well as for degree of fidelity and detail. Each scenario is evaluated in depth to determine if it is appropriate and situation specific. The scenario, simulation algorithm, and content are then revised as needed.

30.3.2.3 Establishing concurrent validity

Each simulation scenario's outcomes related to measures of student learning are compared with an established 'gold standard' teaching method to assess whether learning goals have been met, with the ultimate objective to assure comparable outcomes or favourable enhancement of the teaching programme when using the VR simulations.

30.3.2.4 Establishing construct validity

Scenarios are evaluated to ensure that performance in the VR simulation discriminates among novice, intermediate, and expert users based on prior assessment of the participant as to their level of knowledge or skills before the simulation experience. Performance criteria that differentiates those skill or knowledge levels should be demonstrable and measurable within the VR simulation and not based on competency in using the VR simulation tools alone.

30.3.2.5 Determining predictive validity

Scenarios can also be evaluated according to how well they predict subsequent performance or knowledge transfer to other real or simulated scenarios. The effects of pre-training and didactic information given to subjects prior to VR training can be evaluated by examining performance, stress level, and knowledge retention. Retention will be assessed at specified intervals, evaluating the effect of mastery on the ability to transfer knowledge in a manner that is retained over time.

30.3.3 **VR simulations tools**

30.3.3.1 Flatland: a computer software platform for VR simulation

Flatland served as the VR application development environment.[16] Flatland allows software authors to construct, and users to interact with, arbitrarily complex graphical and aural representations of data and systems. It is written in C/C + + and uses the standard OpenGL graphics language to produce all graphics. In addition, Flatland uses the standard libraries for window, mouse, joystick, and keyboard management. It is object-oriented, multi-threaded, and uses dynamically loaded libraries to build user applications in the virtual environment (VE). As an open-source code, Flatland can be run on a variety of operating systems, including IRIX, Linux, Unix, Mac OSX, and Windows. The end result is a VR immersive environment with sight and sound, in which the operator uses joy wands and virtual controls to interact with computer-generated learning scenarios that respond logically to user interaction. Virtual patients can be simulated in any of several circumstances, with any type of disease or injury.

Flatland is designed to make use of any position-tracking technology. A tracker is a multiple degree of freedom measurement device that can, in real time, monitor the position and/or orientation of multiple receiver devices in space, relative to a transmitter device. In the standard Flatland configuration, trackers are used to locate handheld wands and to track the position of the user's head. Head position and orientation are needed in cases that involve the use of head-mounted displays or stereo shutter glasses.

User interaction is a central component of Flatland, and as such, each object is controllable in arbitrary ways defined by the designer. Currently, there are four possible methods for the control of objects: (i) pop-up menus in the main viewer window; (ii) the keyboard; (iii) 2D control panels either in the environment or separate windows; and (iv) external systems or simulations. In the future there will also be available 3D menus and controls in the virtual environment, as well as possible voice recognition.

The immersed user or avatar interacts with the virtual patient or other virtual objects using a joy wand equipped with a six degree of freedom tracking system, buttons, and a trigger. The wand's representation in the environment is a virtual human hand. The user may pick up and place objects by moving the virtual hand and pulling the wand's trigger. Multiple user avatars can participate in the virtual environment simultaneously and

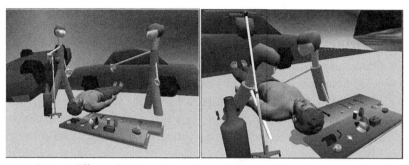

Fig. 30.1 Students at different locations interacting together as full body avatars in the virtual environment as they perform diagnostic evaluation and management of a virtual patient.

interact with each other independently of location or distance.[17–19] The avatars can also interact verbally while in the VR environment (see Figure 30.1).

Fully immersed users are represented within the virtual environment as avatars and can be observed by others from outside the virtual world via computer monitor or on a projection screen. They wear a head-mounted display associated with the trackers, allowing them a sense of presence and interaction within the virtual environment. For cases where total immersion is not required, users may use see-through Augmented Reality displays that allow the superposition of virtual and real-world scenes.[20] Team members within the virtual environment will be able to see each other as full human figures and interact as if they were physically present, even when those students are separated by significant distances. Immersed students can examine the virtual patient by independently controlling their viewpoint and motion within the virtual world. The ratio between real time and virtual time can be varied to allow events to progress slower or faster. The immersed users can work with others in a learning group to gather information and initiate interventions. During the simulation process, the students and tutor can discuss the case as it unfolds, pause the scenario as appropriate in order to talk about their observations, hypothesize, and generate learning issues (see Figure 30.2).

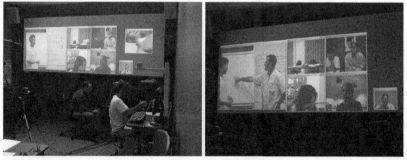

Fig. 30.2 Using the Access Grid the students and a tutor at different locations can observe the simulation, discuss the case as it unfolds, and pause the scenario as appropriate in order to talk about their observations, hypothesize, and generate learning issues.

30.4 **Studies of VR simulations**

30.4.1 **The virtual patient: a case of head trauma—'Mr Toma'**

In the Mr Toma case, a student arrives at an accident scene where paramedics have removed a victim from a car and prepared him for treatment.[19] The task is to diagnose the patient's injury and stabilize him for transport. The player can apply a range of instruments, bandages, and drugs at will. The rule-based AI system controls the behaviour of every internal patient element, including the patient's physiology, treatment responses, and drug effects. Knowledge from SMEs populates the AI system, which mirrors the way the experts cognitively structure this knowledge. Using our knowledge structure assessment methods, we have demonstrated that trainee VR immersion effectively increases students' understanding level[9] (see Figure 30.3).

30.4.2 **Reified models: Nephron Project**

The virtual nephron model was an interactive puzzle that included the glomerulus, proximal tubule, descending and ascending loop of Henle, distal tubule, and collecting duct[21, 22] (see Figure 30.4). The simulation showed solute paths demonstrating secretion and reabsorption between the nephron and peritubular capillary, ATP-ase sodium/

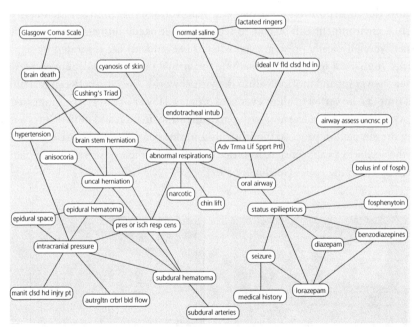

Fig. 30.3 An expert knowledge network can be used as the standard against which the novice learner can be compared.

Reproduced from: Stevens S M, et al. 'Virtual reality training improves students' knowledge of medical concepts'. Medicine Meets Virtual Reality 2005;13:519–525. Reproduced with permission from IOS Press. Copyright © 2015 the authors.

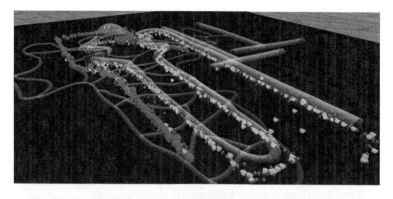

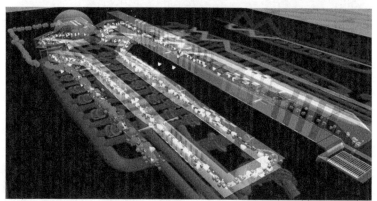

Fig. 30.4 The reified nephron represented in the virtual environment with which participants can interact and explore to better understand physiological concepts.

Reproduced from Alverson D C, et al. 'Reification of abstract concepts to improve comprehension using interactive virtual environments and a knowledge-based design'. Medicine Meets Reality 2006;14:13–18. Reproduced with permission from IOS Press. Copyright © 2015 the authors.

potassium exchange, medulla urea concentration, and urea recirculation between the collecting duct and loop of Henle. A rule-based AI system developed in collaboration with kidney experts controlled all of the nephron physiology, component functionality, and their reaction to various drugs.

30.4.2.1 Knowledge-structure approach with the Nephron Project

To derive an expert knowledge structure of normal nephron functioning we first identified a master list of terms and concepts from six SMEs who teach in a first-year medical student class. We then asked these experts to rate the centrality or relevance of these terms to the topic of renal functioning. We pared down the list to 29 terms by selecting those terms with the highest averaged relevance values. These same experts rated the semantic relatedness of each pair of these terms, and then we used these averaged ratings across the experts to derive the final expert knowledge structure. We applied Pathfinder[9] to create a network from the relatedness ratings. Figure 30.5 shows the resulting network of core terms and their

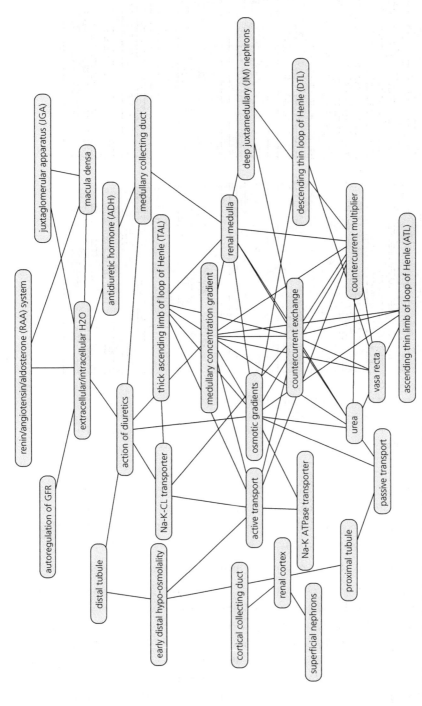

Fig. 30.5 An empirically derived expert knowledge network for virtual nephron.

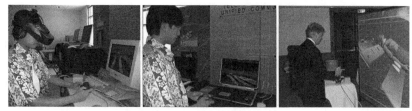

Fig. 30.6 A variety of user interfaces can be incorporated for interaction in the virtual reality environment with or without a head-mounted display, rendered on a monitor or projection screen, and using different gaming-type devices.

Reproduced from Gutiérrez F, et al. 'The effect of degree of immersion upon learning performance in virtual reality simulations for medical education'. Medicine Meets Reality 2007;15:155–160. Reproduced with permission from IOS Press. Copyright © 2015 the authors.

relationships. Terms that are closely connected by either a direct link or a close path are more semantically related to one another than terms that have more distant connections.

30.4.3 Discussion

The results showed an enhanced positive impact on improving knowledge structure related to nephron function when the virtual nephron simulation was employed. Overall, the data suggested that training in a 3D VR simulation was beneficial to student learning as assessed by traditional classroom exams.

30.5 Future VR simulation developments and next steps

Future VR simulations are likely to offer users a variety of interfaces to enhance usability and functionality, such as systems projected on standard monitors or screens without head-mounted displays, as well as VR gloves or other types of user interfaces found in standard gaming devices. The acceptance and familiarity of these types of systems, their ease of use, decreased complexity, and affordability should help to advance the adoption of VR simulation (see Figure 30.6).

Integration of other sensory modalities, such as sound,[16, 21] touch, and even smell can enhance the sense of presence for the participants and the feeling of being there as opposed to being there in the real world. In addition, the degree of immersion and the level of fidelity necessary to provide for adequate user engagement and sense of presence could be studied in the development of the most effective forms of simulation that are also cost-effective.

30.6 Conclusions

This chapter described a step-by-step approach for creating a VR simulation for medical education, training, and performance assessment, as well as a discussion of the tools and methods needed to create VR simulations.

A simulation-based approach offers the opportunity to learn in a relatively realistic problem-solving environment, to practise skills without danger, to explore real and artificial situations, to modify the time scale of events, and to interact with simplified versions of the process or system being simulated.

Combining the elements of high-performance computing, AI, human–computer interface, perceptualization, high-fidelity graphics, 3D models, and knowledge-based design distributed over the next generation of the Internet creates the rubric of VR simulation that can enhance human understanding and learning. These efforts, which complement the development of advanced computing, digital media, and gaming expertise, are converging to develop new models for interdisciplinary research and education that can provide tools for improving human understanding in a complex virtual world—a truly 'fantastic voyage'.

Acknowledgements

The project described was supported partially by grant 2 D1B TM 00003–02 from the Office for the Advancement of Telehealth, Health Resources and Services Administration, Department of Health and Human Services. Its contents are solely the responsibility of the authors and do not necessarily represent the official views of the Health Resources and Services Administration.

The project was also partially made possible by grant number W81XWH-04-1-0875 from the USAMRAA. Its contents are solely the responsibility of the authors and do not necessarily represent the official views of USUHS, the US Department of Defense, or the Henry M. Jackson Foundation for the Advancement of Military Medicine, Inc.

We wish to acknowledge the contributions of Holly Phillips, Kathryn Ann Caudell, Panaiotis, Victor Vergara, Deb LaPointe, Leslie Danielson, Jennifer Spisla, and Geoff Alexander to the development and testing of the Nephron Project.

References

1 Alverson DC, Saiki SM, Jr, Caudell TP, Summers K, Panaiotis, Sherstyuk A, et al. Distributed immersive virtual reality simulation development for medical education. J of Int Assoc of Med Sci Educ 2005;**15**:19–30.

2 Alverson DC, Saiki SM, Jr, Caudell TP, Goldsmith T, Stevens S, Saland L, et al. Reification of abstract concepts to improve comprehension using interactive virtual environments and a knowledge-based design: a renal physiology model. In: Westwood JD, Haluck RS, Hoffman HM, Mogel GT, Phillips R, Rob RA et al., eds. MMVR 14: Accelerating change in health care: next medical toolkit, Vol. IV Studies in health technology and informatics Amsterdam, the Netherlands: IOS Press; 2006, 13–18.

3 Chi MTH, Glaser R, Farr MJ. The nature of expertise. Taylor and Francis; 1988.

4 Anders Ericsson KA, Charness N, Hoffman RR, Feltovich PJ, eds.. The Cambridge handbook of expertise and expert performance. Cambridge: Cambridge University Press; 2006.

5 Chase WG, Simon HA. The mind's eye in chess. In: Chase WG, ed. Visual information processing. New York, NY: Academic Press; 1973.

6 Geeslin WE, Shavelson RJ. Comparison of content structure and cognitive structure in high school students learning of probability. J Res Mat Educ 1975;**6**:109–120.

7 Shavelson RJ, Staton GC. Construct validation: methodology and application to three measures of cognitive structure. J Educ Meas 1975;**12**:67–85.

8 Jonassen DH, Beissner K, Yacci M. Structural knowledge: techniques of representing and acquiring structural knowledge. Hillsdale, NJ: Lawrence Erlbaum; 1993.

9 Schvaneveldt RW, ed. Pathfinder associative networks: studies in knowledge organization. Norwood, NJ: Ablex Publishing Corporation; 1990.

10 Johnson PJ, Goldsmith TE, Teague KW. Structural knowledge assessment: locus of the predictive advantage in Pathfinder-based structures. J Educ Psychol 1994;**86**:617–626.

11 Trumpower DL, Goldsmith TE. Structural enhancement of learning. Contemp Educ Psychol 2004;**29**:426–446.

12 Goldsmith TE, Johnson PJ, Acton, WH. Assessing structural knowledge. J Educ Psychol 1991;**83**:88–96.

13 Bransford J, Brown AL, Cocking RR. How people learn: brain, mind, experience and school. Washington, DC: National Academy Press; 2000.

14 Ilic D, Nordin RB, Glasziou P, Tilson JK Villanueva E. Development and validation of the ACE tool: assessing medical trainees' competency in evidence based medicine. BMC Med. Ed. 2014;**14**:114.

15 Cannon-Bowers J, Bowers C, Stout R, Ricci K, Hildabrand A. Using cognitive task analysis to develop simulation-based training for medical tasks. Mil Med 2013;**178**:15–21.

16 Caudell T, Summers KL, Holten IV J, Hakamata T, Mowafi M, Jacobs J, et al. Virtual patient simulator for distributed collaborative medical education. New Anat. 2003;**270B**:23–29.

17 Mowafi M, Summers KL, Holten J, Greenfield JA, Sherstyuk A, Nickles D, et al. Distributed interactive virtual environments for collaborative medical education and training: design and characterization. In: Westwood JD, Haluck RS, Amsterdam H, eds. MMRV 12: Building a better you: the next tools for medical education, diagnosis, and care, Vol. 98. Studies in health technology and informatics. Amsterdam, the Netherlands: IOS Press; 2004;**98**:259–261.

18 Alverson DC, Saiki SM, Jacobs J, Saland L, Keep MF, Norenberg J, et al. Distributed interactive virtual environments for collaborative experiential learning and training independent of distance over Internet2. (abs) MMVR 12. Newport Beach, CA; 2004.

19 Jacobs J, Caudell T, Wilks D, Keep MF, Mitchell S, Buchanan H, et al. Integration of advanced technologies to enhance problem-based learning over distance: Project TOUCH. New Anat 2003;**270B**:16–22, 64–80.

20 Caudell TP, Mizell DM. 'Augmented reality, an application of heads-up display technology to manual manufacturing processes', Proceedings of the 25th HICSS. Milutinovic and Shriver, eds, Vol. II, 659–669 (January 1992).

21 Panaiotis, Vergara V, Sherstyuk A, Kihmm K, Saiki SM, Jr, Alverson DC, et al. Algorithmically generated music enhances VR nephron simulation. In: Westwood JD, Haluck RS, Hoffman HM, Mogel GT, Phillips R, Rob RA, et al., eds. MMVR 14: Accelerating change in health care: next medical toolkit, Vol. IV Studies in health technology and informatics Amsterdam, the Netherlands: IOS Press; 2006, 422–427.

22 Dawson-Saunders B, Feltovich PJ, Coulson RL, Steward DE. A survey of medical school teachers to identify basic biomedical concepts medical students should understand. Acad Med 1990;**65**(7):448–454.

Chapter 31

Role of cognitive simulation in healthcare

Usha Satish, Satish Krishnamurthy, and Mantosh Dewan

Overview

◆ Simulations allow healthcare providers to hone their skills and enhance patient safety without endangering the patient or hurting their self-confidence.

◆ Cognitive simulations provide a realistic replication of complex and demanding healthcare professional's workday. Cognitive simulations help assess and train the underlying process variables of medical decision-making, including planning, strategy, multitasking, critical thinking, and overall perspective.

◆ Healthcare providers are often challenged by VUCAD (volatility, uncertainty, complexity, ambiguity, and by problems with delayed feedback such as test results) when decisions have to be made. Healthcare providers need to have the ability to respond to complex challenges by processing information optimally in addition to factual content knowledge necessary. Strategic management simulations (SMSs) provide an optimal opportunity to acquire both.

◆ SMS assesses and trains 'how' we think.

◆ Standard testing of cognitive parameters are usually performed individually and the interaction of various parameters are extrapolated to real life subsequently. SMS simultaneously evaluates multiple cognitive parameters simultaneously in a 'real life' like situation. This real-world atmosphere allows for a more realistic (ecologically relevant) assessment of competency.

◆ In addition, SMS can help in retraining individuals in areas of their suboptimal performance. SMS can be used for individual or team evaluation or training.

◆ SMS successfully identifies superior performance among normal subjects (superior functioning managers, medical residents, and nursing students). SMS is effective in evaluating a change in functioning due to medications or environmental chemicals or due to disordered brain function

◆ SMS technology provides a strong complement to existing simulator technologies which greatly enhance specific procedural or algorithmic skills.

31.1 **Introduction to the role of cognitive simulation in healthcare**

> High-quality learning is impossible in the absence of high-quality patient care; likewise, high-quality patient care is impossible without high-quality learning. Attention to both is needed.
>
> Leach and Philibret, 2006.

Healthcare delivery in the twenty-first century is extremely complex. This complexity arises in part from the many technologies, physical infrastructure, cognitive challenges, unpredictable patient needs, and diverse workforce requirements that characterize modern care.[1] While the information to be learned on an ongoing basis is exploding, so are the expectations of better and a more exact delivery of care by the consumer. A number of constituencies are becoming increasingly interested in measuring the performance of physicians in their day-to-day clinical practices, especially since the Institute of Medicine's report suggested that the quality of care may often be less than optimal.[2]

Purchasers of healthcare services are concerned about the effects of suboptimal care on workforce productivity, and seek to maximize the quality of care provided. Consumers of care want to be able to identify high-quality physicians and institutions but lack the effective means to do so. Although some groups have measured and reported quality of care for individual medical groups and physicians, these efforts have been limited.[3] The combination of changes in healthcare delivery, shortened hospital stays, more home and ambulatory care, variations in care not explained by science, declining reimbursements, and, above all, the inexorable and visible failure of the current system to deliver safe care, has been described as the 'perfect storm'.[4] Safer and more predictable care is needed. Paul O'Neill has said that he knows of no other industry that accepts a 38% reimbursement on amounts billed.[4] McGlynn has said that we deliver care known to be best only 54% of the time.[5] These numbers may be related.[4]

In addition to delivering healthcare, the healthcare system also needs to focus on training new generations of physicians, nurses, and others who can meet these challenges better. The time to train an intern through residency into a specialty physician is short. 'As dramatic as the transformation from medical school matriculant to graduate is, the growth from beginning intern to residency (registrar) graduate is even more remarkable. Four weeks after graduating from medical school, interns begin residency training; often in a new hospital in a new city (or country), neophytes in their chosen specialty, unfamiliar with their peers and supervisors as well as their new medical centre's physical environment, protocols and systems. Three to six years later, they depart, ready for sub-specialty training or for independent practice of their discipline.'[6] This challenge is only compounded by the fact that academic medicine is in crisis around the world according to International Campaign to Revitalize Academic Medicine report 'Future of Academic Medicine: Five Scenarios to 2025'.[7] The report states that medical education does not prepare graduates for careers in modern medicine.[7] In addition, the great pressures on health services and the introduction of healthcare reform mean that academic medicine is squeezed.[7] In order to tailor the medical education to these new demands, the Royal

College of Physicians and Surgeons in Canada has redefined the meaning of physician competence to encompass seven different roles instead of defining competence just by the medical content that they know.[8]

One of the key determinants of a competent healthcare provider is how they make the decision. In a recent report brief from the Institute of Medicine to address the wide variation of healthcare practices and, therefore, spending, the recommendation to the Center for Medicare and Medicaid Services (CMS) was to focus on decision-making by the healthcare provider.[9] This chapter summarizes the utility of cognitive simulations which focus on how to improve decision-making skills in healthcare providers and reviews the work that has been done using strategic management simulations (SMSs).

31.2 **Definition**

The Society for Simulation in Healthcare[10] defines simulation in healthcare as a technique—not a technology—to replace or amplify real patient experiences with guided experiences that evoke or replicate substantial aspects of the real world in a fully interactive manner.[11] Artificial environments such as flight simulators for the training of airline pilots, the USS Enterprise's Holodeck, movie set-like towns and alleys for military to train within, computer models of weather prediction using 'what if' scenarios, and hospital drills all fall within this definition.[10] All of these techniques for learning and training have been successful in improving pattern recognition thought process, specific skills, outcomes, and post-encounter evaluations.

Despite being a relative newcomer to simulation, medicine has moved simulation from the vanguard to the cutting edge of validated practice in medical education and the professional development of practising physicians.[12] Widespread use of computers has enabled simulating real environments and its application to the field of healthcare possible. Healthcare simulations provide the means to educate healthcare workers how to provide better care for patients. Maintenance of certification that includes lifelong learning is a requirement for physicians from all specialties. Various tasks involved in taking care of a patient, namely clinical skills, algorithmic management of emergent conditions, surgical procedures, thinking skills, and teamwork have all been successfully simulated with good results.

The recipient of care, subjects covered, skills learnt, time required, and the cost of simulation vary widely. A variety of institutions have a centre for simulation, and several societies and journals devoted to simulation exist, reflecting an explosive interest in this area. The prime goal for all these simulations is improved patient safety by honing clinical skills without endangering the patient or denting the practitioner's self-confidence. Simulation has the potential for the evolution of a new teaching paradigm for the new millennium.[13] These simulations can be rerun, stopped, or otherwise altered to enhance educational value. Thereby, creating a non-threatening learning environment where multiple options could potentially be tested, worked through, and mastered. 'Every patient deserves a competent physician every time. Every resident deserves competent teachers and an excellent learning environment. Simulation serves both of these core principles.'[4]

31.3 **Underlying principles: the need for simulations**

In 'To Err Is Human: Building a Safer Health System', the Institute of Medicine encouraged the medical community to reach out to other domains for insight and inspiration for different models of performance and teaching.[2] Effective use of simulation technology is a substantial contributor to making commercial air transportation the safest available mode of travel. Human error is routinely blamed for disasters in the air, on the railways, in complex surgery, and in healthcare generally.[14] While one action or omission may be the immediate cause of an incident, closer analysis usually reveals a series of events and departures from safe practice; each influenced by the working environment and the wider organizational context. Understanding the characteristics of a safe and high-performing system, therefore, requires research of the context, the development and maintenance of individual skills, the role of high technology, the impact of working conditions on team performance, and the nature of high-performance teams. Simulation is an essential tool in the learning and understanding of high-performing systems. Safety in these high-reliability organizations (HROs) is ultimately understood as a characteristic of the system—the sum total of all the parts and their interactions.[15] This cultural evolution required the creation of a continuous improvement process. This process includes, first, an event-reporting system that processes data into meaningful knowledge, creating opportunity for meaningful change within an organization. Second, it required simulations to study systems and to implement changes within an organization. The importance of effective teamwork in aviation is critical to safety.

Human beings make mistakes. Contemporary airline safety is a significant measure of the product of this loop of operational reporting, analysis in simulation, and training in simulation. State-of-the-art airline crew training—the Advanced Qualification Program (AQP)—emerged out of simulation studies during which reported actual events were recreated in simulation. The AQP identified specific team skills that enhance safety through effective use of all available resources—human, hardware, and information. The process achieved a greater degree of integration of the team skills in part because AQP team training and practice increases awareness of human and system error, and provides techniques and skills that will minimize their effects. This is accomplished through awareness of crew member attitudes and behaviour, and the use of practical management skills.[15]

An important variant of simulators are cognitive simulations. Simulations replicate several aspects of a learner's environment simultaneously. This provides a realistic replication of a healthcare professional's workday that involves several complex demands that have to be processed simultaneously. In other words, cognitive simulation technologies help assess and train the underlying process variables of medical decision-making, including but not limited to planning, strategy, multitasking, critical thinking, and overall perspective.

This technology provides a strong compliment to existing simulator technologies, which greatly enhance specific procedural or algorithmic skills.

31.4 **Requirements for effective medical decision-making**

Competency in professional endeavours may require much more than finding a single 'correct' response to some particular situation.[16, 17] There are task situations where a single correct action or where multiple correct actions will solve the problems at hand, but not all challenges fit that pattern. Complex tasks—including medical decision-making tasks—can generate unpredictable dynamics that defy treatment with standard content knowledge approaches.[18, 19] When a task is highly challenging and does not fit a memorized or documented pattern, an additional set of skills is necessary; adequate competency in information-processing is essential.[20]

Just as factual knowledge, information-processing skills must be learned and this form of training cannot be transmitted through books or lectures.[21] In fact, modern learning theorists clearly distinguish the processes involved in the acquisition and use of specific content knowledge and the acquisition and use of intellectual processing skills that are free of specific knowledge content.[22] The latter skills represent cognitive strategies that an effective decision-maker uses to regulate his or her own processes of attending, learning, remembering, and thinking,[23] involving external (incoming) information as well as internal or remembered information and concepts.[24] These 'information-processing strategies' are not fixed; they must adjust to changes in task challenges—for example, different patients with different sets of morbidities and conditions—and they must adjust to gains in knowledge over time.[25] Learning to apply such processing strategies requires guided personal experience.

We respond to an environmental stimulus based on our interpretation of 'normal' for the situation we are in. Our sense of normal depends on extent of exposure to that particular situation, our knowledge, and our ability to learn. Response to a stimulus depends on our alertness, ability to focus (without distractions akin to sterile areas in the cockpit where no one is allowed to distract the pilot and the co-pilot during take-off or landing), knowledge of the context, accurate interpretation of the stimulus, and threshold level for a response. Last but not the least, the execution of the response needs to be error-free. The results need to be monitored for desired outcome and the response is modified if the outcome is deviating from the optimum (see section 31.5.2.1).

In addition, the physician or medical team is often challenged by VUCAD (volatility, uncertainty, complexity, ambiguity, and by problems with delayed feedback such as test results)[20] when decisions have to be made. How can we make sure that physicians will effectively manage a network of interrelated problems that involve ambiguity, inconsistency, novelty, and surprise?[26] We have known for some time that learning, transfer of knowledge, and ability are impacted by both **task structure and task complexity**, and by the **structural information-processing competence** of the individual (physician) involved.[27] We need to ensure that medical personnel have the factual content knowledge needed to respond to the task at hand, but we also need to make sure that they can respond to complex challenges by processing information optimally. Simulations, if used as part of an appropriate training system, provide an optimal opportunity to acquire both.

31.5 **Fundamental concepts of SMSs and its relevance to healthcare and HROs**

Cognitive simulations have the intrinsic capability of replicating several aspects of a learner's environment simultaneously. This provides a realistic replication of a healthcare professional's workday that involves several complex demands that have to be processed simultaneously. This technology provides a strong complement to existing simulator technologies which greatly enhance specific procedural or algorithmic skills.

Standard testing of cognitive parameters are usually performed individually and the interaction of various parameters are extrapolated to real life subsequently. The true impact of a mild memory loss and a decreased attention span in a head-injured patient might mean that she/he will not be employable. SMSs simultaneously evaluate multiple cognitive parameters simultaneously in a 'real life' like situation. This 'real life' like situation means that the subject experiences VUCAD, which are part of everyday decision-making. SMSs can demonstrate milder deficits in head-injured patients in the relative absence of standard neuropsychological deficits.[28] The real-world atmosphere of the task and setting, involving multiple potentially interactive components of task demands as well as multiple and interactive options to engage in various aspects of behaviour allows for a more realistic (ecologically relevant) assessment of competency. SMS is unique in the absence of requirements to engage in specific actions or to make decisions at specific points in time, the absence of stated demands to respond to specific information, the freedom to develop initiative, and freedom for strategy development and decision implementation allows each participant to utilize his/her own preferred or typical action, planning, and strategic styles.

Most of the simulations are interactive and directly responsive to the actions taken by the subject. SMS records the responses of the subject in relation to the evolution of the scenario but does not alter the course of the simulation. This feature is known as quasi-experimental simulation and allows comparison of performance of different subjects using the same scenario. This property has allowed determination of norms for different levels of functioning in normal subjects. Comparison of a subject with or without a drug or medication can be evaluated. Reported studies include effects of caffeine,[29] alcohol,[30] etc.

SMSs described below go beyond simply recreating the learner's complex environment and allowing the learner to practise or be evaluated. In addition, SMSs can also help both the learners and teachers to understand performance in the simulation in relation to a number of well-validated factors as well as help in retraining.[31] SMS has been used to evaluate generic thinking in a wide variety of subjects. SMS successfully differentiates performance among normal subjects (superior-functioning managers versus average-functioning managers;[32] better medical residents versus average- or poorly functioning residents[33]). SMS is effective in evaluating a change in functioning due to medications[34] or environmental chemicals, or due to disordered brain function.[28] It is commonly known in the managerial world that a CEO who is successful in selling cars can be successful in selling any other widget. This implies that successful managers think differently and this 'how of thinking' is important in addition to specific knowledge of cars or the specific widget.

Whereas team task analysis as detailed by Burke et al.[35] focuses on designing a simulation for a specific situation, SMS evaluates generic thinking processes. As mentioned previously, both content-specific knowledge as well as generic decision-making competencies are essential for optimal functioning. Further, SMS uses several different scenarios, all of which evaluate the same generic-thinking processes such that effect of learning from repetition is eliminated. Effectiveness of focused training of areas of deficiencies in a subject can be objectively evaluated using SMS.

31.5.1 Description of the SMS

SMSs assess both basic cognitive and behavioural responses to task demands as well as cognitive and behavioural components that are commonly subsumed under the rubric of executive functions. High levels of predictive validity, reliability, and applicability of the SMS to real-world settings have been repeatedly demonstrated in both North America and Europe.[31, 36] The method provides more than 80 computer-gathered and calculated measures of functioning, loading on 12 reliable factors (based on factor analytic varimax rotation for more than 2,000 prior subjects). Among others, simulation data predict success on indicators such as 'job level at age', 'income at age', 'number of persons supervised', and 'number of job promotions during the past 10 years' (corrected for industry, location, etc.).[31] These simulations can be administered to both individual participants as well as teams. While individual simulation runs offer feedback to a participant on their individual decision-making pattern, group performances yield rich data on how teams function together. Further, team evaluations also provide detailed information on each of the individual team participants, thereby enhancing the feedback and improvement potential. These are particularly important to the performance of teams of physicians and other healthcare providers. Potential applications for team performance include handling of mass casualties and disaster situations. During a simulation, participants make decisions during a one half-hour task period. The absence of requirements to engage in specific actions or to make decisions at specific points in time, the absence of stated demands to respond to specific information, the freedom to develop initiative, and freedom for strategy development and decision implementation allows each participant to use his/her own preferred or typical action, planning, and strategic styles. The real-world atmosphere of the task and setting, involving multiple potentially interactive components of task demands as well as multiple and interactive options to engage in various aspects of behaviour allows for a more realistic (ecologically relevant) assessment of competency.

31.5.2 SMS measurement outputs

Data in response to the factors listed in Table 31.1 are captured and provided via computer-generated scores and represented in two primary output modalities. These outputs are used for feedback and potential training as required.

Table 31.1 Definition of SMS measures

Measures	Definitions
i) Activity level	ii) Overall level of activity (measures both focused activity that is directed to a specific context and activity that is directed toward overall goals)
iii) Response speed	iv) Speed of responses in both terms of emergent and non-emergent situations
v) Task orientation	vi) Ability to focus on a task at hand and also focus on 'larger' goals
vii) Initiative	viii) Ability to generate activity without an overt external stimulus that would aid in successful task completion. Elements pertaining to initiative in context and strategy are also measured)
ix) Information management	x) Ability to seek and use information efficaciously
xi) Strategy	xii) Ability to form systematic plans and actions that are optimally sequenced and goal-directed in the long term
xiii) Breadth of approach	xiv) Ability to think along multiple dimensions and find different solutions to problems
xv) Planning	xvi) Ability to make task-oriented plans in the short and long term
xvii) Emergency responses	xviii) Ability to think critically and strategically under conditions of emergency and stress

31.5.2.1 Time-event matrix

Figure 31.1 shows direct graphic representations of performance, and are captured during the performance period. A good analogy to describe this complex output is like a magnetic resonance imaging scan of decision-making. These graphs are represented with various combinations of lines and symbols that represent different aspects of decision-making. Based on appropriate interpretation these graphs accurately predict the 'underlying process' of thinking in a participant.

In general, richer performance by the subject during the simulation is indicated by a more complex graph. Time during the simulation is plotted on the horizontal axis and the vertical axis represents the variety of decisions made by the participant. Individual actions are represented by a point that is placed vertically above the time when the action occurred and horizontally in line with the particular decision code. Information provided or incoming information is denoted with a star. If an action corresponds to incoming information, one or more stars (depending on the number of pieces of information) are placed on the same horizontal level where the action is located, with stars placed at the point when each item of information was received. The action is circled to indicate that it was responsive to an event or a message.

If the participant thinks and acts strategically, these actions are connected with diagonal lines. If these actions are strategy based on use of opportunity and information that is already provided these lines are coloured red. If the strategies represent visionary thinking

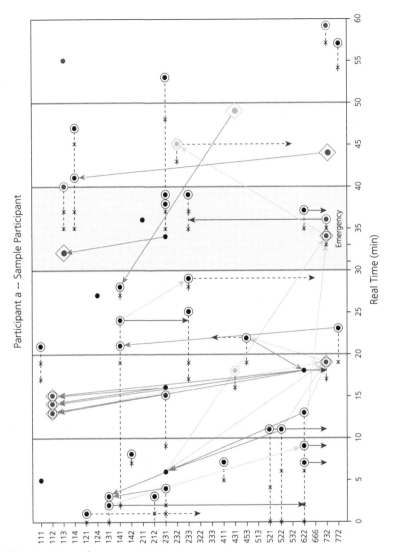

Fig. 31.1 Time-event matrix.

and are not necessarily cued, they are represented by green lines. Blue lines also an integral part of this output represents the ability to create plans. In addition, there are several other symbols and line formations that represent elements of critical thinking such as initiative, multitasking, and sustained planning, among others.

A serious emergency is introduced at some point in all the SMS scenarios. The emergency requires rapid and decisive action. Performance patterns during this time point can be compared with other time points in the simulation to judge both the effectiveness of crisis handling as well as preparation for a crisis and recovery patterns after crisis.

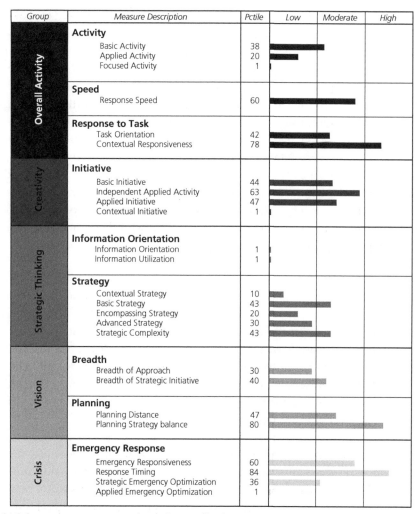

Group	Measure Description	Pctile	Low	Moderate	High
Overall Activity	**Activity**				
	Basic Activity	38			
	Applied Activity	20			
	Focused Activity	1			
	Speed				
	Response Speed	60			
	Response to Task				
	Task Orientation	42			
	Contextual Responsiveness	78			
Creativity	**Initiative**				
	Basic Initiative	44			
	Independent Applied Activity	63			
	Applied Initiative	47			
	Contextual Initiative	1			
Strategic Thinking	**Information Orientation**				
	Information Orientation	1			
	Information Utilization	1			
	Strategy				
	Contextual Strategy	10			
	Basic Strategy	43			
	Encompassing Strategy	20			
	Advanced Strategy	30			
	Strategic Complexity	43			
Vision	**Breadth**				
	Breadth of Approach	30			
	Breadth of Strategic Initiative	40			
	Planning				
	Planning Distance	47			
	Planning Strategy balance	80			
Crisis	**Emergency Response**				
	Emergency Responsiveness	60			
	Response Timing	84			
	Strategic Emergency Optimization	36			
	Applied Emergency Optimization	1			

Fig. 31.2 Strategic management simulation profile chart.

This profile shown in Figure 31.2 represents the 12 factors listed above in terms of percentile scores. The scores reflect low, moderate, and high levels of performance based on normative data. These profiles are used to ascertain the performance pattern of a participant in the various parameters of decision-making. Further, since these measures are fine-tuned in terms of the definition of a given parameter and its implications in the real world, it helps make the training more focused and thereby time-effective.

31.6 **SMS and healthcare**

31.6.1 **Healthcare applications**

David Leach outlines several reasons why simulations should be used for medical education.[4] To ensure patient safety, clinical skills have to be learnt as far away from the patient as possible. Simulations allow actions to be planned, studied, and debriefed to allow safer patient care. Simulation is a great tool for educating residents. Simulations can be used as a formative tool for resident development. Simulation can be used to expose mastery of both rules and values. Familiarity with protocols becomes clear during simulations. At the same time, it is also possible to require improvisation as the learner manages emerging situations. Rules are either demonstrated or not; improvisation calls forth adaptive expertise. Improvisation exposes values. It is an efficient and safe way to explore competence. Residents can intentionally make mistakes and learn about their consequences during simulations. Simulation can determine how residents respond in different contexts. Simulation can be used to populate a portfolio of assessed experiences that enable residents to demonstrate their abilities. Simulation offers a controlled way to learn systems-based practice. Simulations can be constructed that involve multiple interdependent variables. Simulation can document how residents think, as well as what they think. Every resident deserves competent teachers and an excellent learning environment.[4]

31.6.2 Improving medical education

The use of SMS for recruitment and training in healthcare education has the potential to markedly improve the quality of physician and nursing graduates.[33, 37] How specifically does SMS help produce a better health professional? What novel technology does it add to our regular methods? How do we determine who is a good physician? It is well accepted that there are many important attributes of a good physician such as knowledge, skills, and a caring, professional demeanour. However, there is increasing acceptance that the single most meaningful outcome of medical education is to produce physicians whose clinical care results in good clinical outcomes for their patients.[38, 39]

To produce good physicians, traditional healthcare education is focused on knowledge. Standardized examinations test the depth of this knowledge and its application to the clinical situation. However, studies have consistently found that scores on examinations are not correlated with, or predictive of, a good doctor (Carnegie Report 2010).[40] More importantly, there is a lack of data correlating any aspect of a physician's medical education and the clinical outcome of their patients.

Subject knowledge (i.e. 'what' of thinking) alone does not correlate with functioning at the level of a good doctor. SMS adds the process or the 'how' of thinking, which is more sophisticated than the concept of 'critical thinking'.[37] How a person thinks (or how the content knowledge is used) as assessed by SMS has been shown in numerous studies to be highly correlated with level of functioning in a number of non-medical professions under 'real world' conditions marked by VUCAD, as described earlier. In the healthcare arena, there are several studies with findings that are instructive to producing better physicians and nurses.

31.6.3 Application of SMS to physician education and training

In a seminal study, graduating residents in psychiatry were rated on a number of key parameters. The traditional measures included their performance on a national in-training

examination (a test of knowledge and its clinical application) and a national psychotherapy examination (a computerized test of principles of psychotherapy and their clinical
application that estimates an essential skill). Non-traditional ratings included faculty
ranking (a global ranking based on 'who would you send you send your mother to?')
and measures on the SMS. Faculty ranking—the measure that is the best surrogate for
the best physician—was not correlated to either of the traditional scores; they did correlate strongly with measures on the SMS.[41] Similar findings have been reported in surgical
residents. The SMS profile correlated more robustly with their performance than did their
scores on the in-training national examination.[33, 42]

Moving forward, the goal is to build on these findings and use SMS to recruit more
suitable students and to train them to excellence. For instance, it would be ideal to recruit
bright students who are gifted in the 'how' of thinking. Soon we will have SMS measures
on more than 500 students at one medical school and ratings on their performances.[43] This
will allow us to set the minimum standard required to be a good physician and answer the
age-old question: 'How tall is the shortest giant?" If every medical student met this minimum standard, it would markedly diminish or eliminate dropouts (currently 3% of all US
students and much higher in Caribbean medical schools), diminish the need for remediation (which is expensive for both the system and student; currently 20% of US students
take five or more years to graduate), and potentially improve the patient outcomes of the
patients of these medical graduates.

More recently, programmes are beginning to use the SMS as one of the key variables
to select residents. They recognized that some residents struggle despite coming in with
outstanding examination scores and excellent letters. Remediation through their six-
year programme is taxing. They aim to select highly functional—in addition to highly
credentialed—trainees.[43]

Training with SMS is particularly effective and efficient because it has training modules
that are focused on separate parameters—e.g. initiative or information management, rather than generic global training. For now, given an unfiltered class of students, a number
of institutions are using SMS to train students. Their goal is not merely to produce physicians but to graduate physicians who excel in the real world.[44] Similarly, several residency
programmes have used the SMS-based training as part of their curriculum.[41, 42] The goal
is to help residents maximize their potential for excellent clinical care, teamwork, and
leadership.

31.6.4 Application of SMS to nursing education

Discerning that cognitive simulation would be a natural partner to manikin-based simulation, nursing programmes have also begun to use the SMS for evaluation and training
of process measures. There are several important findings from this study. First, faculty
rank at graduation did not correlate with the rank at admission, calling into question the
traditional way we select students based on tests of knowledge and letters. Second, students who received SMS training showed marked improvement in important measures
that predict better functioning in the real world. Third, the SMS-trained group had higher

SMS scores on graduation compared with Group B, which was the training-naïve group, on graduation.[37]

There are clear data that SMS can be a powerful tool to help us select the most suitable students to nursing school, medical school, and residencies. Further, SMS-based feedback and training results in a significant improvement on SMS parameters; importantly, these parameters have been shown to reflect real-world functioning. Simulation technologies that improve knowledge and skills help make better doctors and nurses; adding cognitive simulation technology such as the SMS takes a step closer to consistently producing excellent physicians and nurses.

31.7 **Conclusion**

Clearly, simulations have the distinct advantage of providing 'real world' experiences to the learner without causing harm to patients or learners. Simulations can be designed to replicate virtually all complex realities and offer training and retraining using well-standardized paradigms. Simulations are increasingly used for training in and evaluation of procedural skills in surgery and anaesthesia, for example. We believe that simulation can also be a highly effective way to evaluate decision-making and leadership skills in medicine, providing students and residents with insights into their own abilities and needs, and assisting faculty in reliably assessing competence in these areas.

The complexity of teaching the art and science of medicine is a quest that will be a continued challenge to healthcare professionals. However, it would be wise to bear in mind the virtue of constant learning and improvement as noted by Mahatma Gandhi's words of wisdom, 'Live as if you were to die tomorrow, learn as if you were to live forever'.

References

1 **Karlsberg DW, Pierce RG.** Anonymity: an impediment to performance in healthcare. Health Serv Insights 2014;7:19–23. DOI: 10.4137/HSI.S14869

2 **Kohn L, Corrigan J, Donaldson M, eds.** To err is human: building a safer health system. Washington, DC: National Academy Press; 2000, 146.

3 **Landon BE, Normand ST, Blumenthal D, Daley J.** Physician clinical performance assessment: prospects and barriers. JAMA 2003;**290**:1183–1189.

4 **Leach D.** Simulation: it's about respect. ACGME Bulletin December 2005.

5 **McGlynn EA, Asch SM, Adams J, et al.** The quality of healthcare delivered to adults in the United States. N Engl J Med 2003;**348**(26):2635–2645.

6 **Cooke M, Irby DM, O'Brien BC, eds:** Educating physicians: a call for reform of medical school and residency. Stanford, CA: Jossey Bass; 2010, 113.

7 Milbank Memorial Fund, *The Future of Academic Medicine: Five scenarios to 2025*, <http://www.milbank.org/uploads/documents/0507FiveFutures/0507FiveFutures.pdf>, accessed 01 Sep. 2014.

8 The CanMEDS 2005 physician competency framework. Better standards. Better physicians. Better care. (Frank JR, ed.). Better standards. Better physicians. Better care. The CanMEDS 2005 physician competency framework. Ottawa: The Royal College of Physicians and Surgeons of Canada; 2005.

9 Variation in healthcare spending. Target decision making and not geography. Available at <http://www.iom.edu/geovariation>

10 Society for Simulation in Healthcare (SSH), *About Simulation*, <http://www.ssih.org/About-Simulation>, accessed 01 Sep. 2014.

11 **Gaba DM.** The future vision of simulation in healthcare. Qual Saf Health Care 2004;**13**(Suppl. 1): i2–i10.

12 **Leach D.** Editor's Introduction. ACGME Bulletin December 2005.

13 **Dunn WF.** Simulators in critical care education and beyond. Society of Critical Care Medicine: Introduction; 2004.

14 **Reason J.** Human error. New York, NY: Cambridge University Press; 1990.

15 **Hamman W, Rutherford W.** The language of aviation simulation training: relevance for medical education. ACGME Bulletin 2005; 5–7.

16 **Breuer K, Streufert D.** Authoring of complex learning environments: design considerations for dynamic simulations. J Struct Learn 1996;**12**:315–321.

17 **Scandura JM, Stone DC, Scandura AB.** An intelligent role tutor CBI system for diagnostic testing and instruction. J Sruct Learn 1986;**9**:15–61.

18 **Streufert S.** Complexity and complex decision-making: convergences between differentiation and integration approaches to the prediction of task performance. J Exp Soc Psychol 1970;**6**:494–509.

19 **Hall N.** Explaining chaos: a guide to the new science of disorder. New York, NY: WW Norton; 1993.

20 **Streufert SC.** Behavior in the complex environment. New York, NY: John Wiley; 1978.

21 **Streufert S, Swezey R.** Complexity, managers and organizations. New York, NY: Academic Press; 1985.

22 **Gagné RM.** The conditions of learning and theory of instruction. New York, NY: Holt Rinehart and Winston; 1985.

23 **Breuer K.** Cognitive development based on process-learning environments. In: Dijstra S, Krammer HPM, van Merrienboer JJG, eds. Instructional models in computer-based learning environments. Berlin: Springer Verlag; 1992.

24 **Tennyson RD, Thurlow K, Breuer K.** Problem oriented simulations to develop and improve higher order thinking strategies. Comput Hum Behav 1987;**3**:151–165.

25 **Toffler D.** Zukunftschance. Munich: Deutscher Taschenbuch Verlag;1980.

26 **Isenberg DJ.** How senior managers think. Harvard Bus Rev 1984:**84608**.

27 **Buss AR.** Learning, transfer and changes inability factor: a multivariate model. Psychol Bull 1972;**80**:106–112.

28 **Satish U, Streufert S, Eslinger PJ.** Complex decision-making after orbitofrontal damage. Neurocase 1999;**5**:355–364.

29 **Streufert S, Satish U, Pogash R, et al.** Excess coffee consumption in simulated complex work settings: detriment or facilitation of performance? J Appl Psychol 1997;**82**(5):774–782.

30 **Streufert S, Pogash RM, Roache J, et al.** Effects of alcohol intoxication on risk taking, strategy, and error rate in visuomotor performance. J Appl Psychol 1992;**77**(4):515–524.

31 **Streufert S, Nogami G, Swezey RW, et al.** Computer assisted training of complex managerial performance. Computers Hum Behav 1988;**4**:77–88.

32 **Streufert S, Pogash R, Piasecki M.** Simulation-based assessment of managerial competence: reliability and validity. Personnel Psychol 1988;**41**:537–557.

33 **Satish U, Streufert S, Marshall R, et al.** Strategic management simulation is a novel way to measure resident competencies. Am J Surg 2001;**181**:557–561.

34 **Streufert S, DePadova A, McGlynn T, Pogash R, Piasecki M.** Impact of beta blockade on complex cognitive functioning. Am Heart J 1988;**116**(1 Pt 2):311–315.

35 **Burke CS, Salas E, Wilson-Donnelly K, Priest H.** How to turn a team of experts into an expert medical team: guidance from the aviation and military communities. Qual Saf Health Care 2004;**13**(Suppl. 1):i96–i104.

36 Breuer K, Satish U. Emergency management simulations: an approach to the assessment of decision-making processes in complex dynamic crisis environments. In: From modeling to managing security. Norway: Norwegian Academic Press; 2003, 145–155.

37 LaMartina K, Ward-Smith P. Developing critical thinking skills in undergraduate nursing students: the potential for strategic management simulations. JNEP 2014;**4**(9):155–162. DOI: 10.5430/jnep.v4n9p155

38 Dewan M, Manring J, Satish U. The new milestones: do we need to take a step back to go a mile forward? Acad Psychiatry 2014.

39 Nasca T, Weiss K, Bagian J, Brigham T. The accreditation system after the 'next accreditation system'. Acad Medicine 2014;**89**:24–26.

40 Cooke M, Irby DM, O'Brien BC, eds. Educating physicians: a call for reform of medical school and residency. San Francisco, CA: Jossey-Bass; 2010.

41 Satish U, Manring J, Gregory R, Krishnamurthy S, Streufert S, Dewan M. Novel assessment of psychiatry residents: SMS simulations. ACGME Bulletin January 2009; 18–23.

42 Krishnamurthy S, Satish U, Foster T, Streufert S, Dewan M, Krummel T. Components of critical decision making and ABSITE assessment: toward a more comprehensive evaluation. Journal of Graduate Medical Education December 2009; 273–277.

43 Korentager R. Components of critical decision making in plastic surgery residents: selecting the best. Annual symposium on simulation in healthcare. Kansas; December 2014.

44 Chumley H, Satish U, Dewan M. Simulation-based learning to improve higher cognitive functions. Presented at the 20th anniversary meeting of the Society in Europe for Simulation Applied to Medicine, Poznan, Poland June 12–14, 2014. Published abstract on p. 78 available at <http://sesampoznan.eu/uploads/files/sesam2014_abstracts.pdf>

Glossary of medical and simulation terms, acronyms, and abbreviations

AAMC Association of American Medical Colleges

AAP American Academy of Pediatrics

A&E Accident & Emergency (Department)

AB Antibiotic

ABA American Board of Anesthesiologists; a medical specialty organization responsible for accrediting specialist anaesthetists (anesthesiologists)

ACCME The Accreditation Council for Continuing Medical Education (US)

ADPIE-C The steps of the nursing process typically include: Assessment, Diagnosis, Planning/Outcomes, Implementation, Evaluation then Communication

ABG Arterial Blood Gas

ACARS Aircraft Communications Addressing and Reporting System

ACCESS Anaesthesia Computer-controlled Emergency Situation Simulator

ACEP American College of Emergency Physicians

ACES Advancing Care Excellence for Seniors (US)

ACGME Accreditation Council for Graduate Medical Education (US)

ACF Ante-cubital Fossa

ACLS/ALS Advanced (Cardiac) Life Support course

ACRM Anaesthesia Crisis Resource Management

ACS American College of Surgeons

ACT Acute Care Team

ADMS Advanced Disaster Management Simulator

ADO Anaesthesia Department Orderly (anaesthesia technician): a trained anaesthesia assistant

adrenaline A vasopressor drug used in resuscitation and treatment of anaphylaxis and cardiac arrest

AEEC Airline Electronics Engineering Committee

AHA American Heart Association

AHCP Allied Healthcare Providers

AI Artificial Intelligence: the study and design of intelligent agents where an intelligent agent is a system that perceives its environment and takes actions

AICD Automatic Implantable Cardioverter-Defibrillator; also known as ICD

ALS See ACLS

albuterol Salbutamol, a common bronchodilator drug (US)

ambulance officer Emergency Medical Technician/Paramedic; a trained professional who delivers emergency pre-hospital care

AMPLE Trauma history mnemonic acronym to remember key questions in trauma assessment: Allergies, Medications (anticoagulants, insulin, and cardiovascular medications especially), Previous medical/surgical history, Last meal (time), Events/Environment surrounding the injury (exactly what happened). See also SAMPLE history.

ANA American Nurses Association

anaesthesia The practice and science of anaesthesia

anaesthetist A physician who administers anaesthesia

andragogy The method and practice of teaching adult learners; adult education

anesthesia The practice and science of anaesthesia (US) or the state of anaesthesia

anesthesiologist A physician who practises anaesthesia (US)

anesthesiology The practice and science of anaesthesia (US)

ANTS Anaesthetists' Non-technical Skills

ANTS-AP Anaesthetic Non-technical Skills for Anaesthetic Practitioners

ANZCA Australian and New Zealand College of Anaesthetists

APSF Anesthesia Patient Safety Foundation (US)

AQP Advanced Qualification Programme

ARINC Aeronautical Radio Incorporated

AROM Artificial Rupture of Membranes (obstetrics)

ASA American Society of Anesthesiologists

ASA PS (1–6) American Society of Anesthesiologists Physical Status; a patient classification system

ASIASIM Federation of Asian Simulation Societies

ASPE Association of Standardized Patient Educators

ASPiH Association for Simulated Practice in Healthcare (UK)

ASPIRIN A tool for successful communication: Acknowledge the problem; Situational analysis; Provide some solutions; Implement; Review the outcome; Inform stakeholders; Next steps

ASRS Aviation Safety Reporting System

ASSH Australian Society for Simulation in Healthcare

ATLS Advanced Trauma Life Support course (similar to EMST)

attending A medical practitioner who has undergone training in a specialty and is practising in that specialty (US)

AV Audiovisual (equipment or system)

avatar A graphical representation of a person participating in a virtual environment whether in the form of a three-dimensional model as used in cyberspace or virtual reality environments

AVPU Alert, Voice, Pain, Unresponsive; an acronym for a patient's responsiveness

Below 10 Below 10,000 ft communication; limiting unnecessary communication during a critical procedure; 'Sterile Cockpit Rule'

BEME Best Evidence Medical Education

BICEPS A military debriefing tool; Brevity, Immediacy, Centrality, Expectancy, Proximity, Simplicity

BiPAP Bi-level Positive Airway Pressure

BKAT Basic Critical Care Knowledge Assessment Test

BLS Basic Life Support course

boot camp A rigorous course for participants that are new to the field

bougie an airway catheter designed to assist tracheal intubation

BP Blood pressure or British Pharmacopoeia

briefing A meeting for giving information or instructions to participants in a course. Similar to pre-briefing.

BURP Backwards, Upwards, Rightwards Pressure; a manoeuvre to improve laryngeal view during tracheal intubation

BVM Bag Valve Mask (ventilation)

call-back and read-back The practice of repeating orders or instructions to enhance communication

call-out Members of a medical team state their actions, observation, and concerns out loud

CanMEDS An educational framework identifying and describing seven roles that lead to optimal health and healthcare outcomes: medical expert (central role), communicator, collaborator, manager, health advocate, scholar and professional (Royal College of Physicians and Surgeons of Canada)

CASE Comprehensive Anesthesia Simulation Environment (Stanford University)

CBC Complete Blood Count; Full Blood Count

CbD Case-based Discussion

CCO Critical Care Outreach

CCrISP Care of the Critically Ill Surgical Patient (course)

CCTV Closed-circuit Television

CCU Coronary Care Unit; in some regions Critical Care Unit

cell Cellphone or cellular phone (US); a mobile phone

CGI Computer-generated Image

CHSE Certified Healthcare Simulation Educator; an educational programme from the Society for Simulation in Healthcare

CHSOS Certified Healthcare Simulation Operations Specialist; an educational programme for the simulation operations specialist from the Society for Simulation in Healthcare

CISD Critical Incident Stress Debriefing

CLC Closed Loop Communication

CME Continuing Medical Education: a formal system of further education in a medical, nursing, or paramedical field (also known as MOPS and CPD)

CMS Content Management System (of a website) or Centers for Medicare and Medicaid Services (US)

CMV Controlled Mechanical Ventilation

code A cardiac arrest (slang)

composite video An analogue video transmission standard

consultant A medical practitioner who has undergone training in a specialty and is practising in that specialty; an attending (US) or faculty

COTS Commercial off-the-shelf (product)

CPAP Continuous Positive Airway Pressure

CPB Cardio-Pulmonary Bypass

CPD Continuing Professional Development: a formal system of further education in a medical, nursing, or paramedical field

CPR Cardiopulmonary Resuscitation

CQI Continuous Quality Improvement

Crit Haematocrit (slang)

CRM Crisis Resource Management; also Cockpit Resource Management; Crew Resource Management

CRMIE CRM Instructor/Examiner

CRNA Certified Registered Nurse Anaesthetist

CSL Compound Sodium Lactate (Hartmann's solution, BP); a balanced salt solution for intravenous use

CTA Cognitive Task Analysis

CTT Crisis Team Training

CVC Central Venous Catheter

CVP Central Venous Pressure

CXR Chest X-ray

D5W 5% dextrose in water (IV solution)

DAC Data Acquisition and Control system

DAM Difficult Airway Management

debriefing The period following a simulation activity or real-world experience where participants have the opportunity to discuss, analyse, and reflect on the event and its meaning

DESC Describe, Express, Specify, Consequences; an assertive training tool

DISC An acronym for:
Dominance: relating to control, power and assertiveness
Influence: relating to social situations and communication
Steadiness: relating to patience, persistence, and thoughtfulness
Compliance

DLP Digital Light Processing

DNR Do Not Resuscitate

DOPS Direct Observation of Procedural Skills

DP Diagnostic Peritoneal Lavage

DVI Digital Visual Interface (video display)

D/W Discussed with

EAR Expired Air Resuscitation

ECFMG Educational Commission for Foreign Medical Graduates (US)

ECG Electrocardiogram

ECMO Extra-corporeal Membrane Oxygenation

ECS Emergency Care Simulator (a CAE Healthcare product)

ED Emergency Department (see A&E)

EHA European Heart Association

EJ External Jugular (vein or catheter)

EKG Electrocardiogram (US)

ELT Experiential Learning Theory

EM Emergency Medicine

EMAC Effective Management of Anaesthetic Crises course (ANZCA course)

EMD Electro-mechanical Dissociation; now known as Pulseless Electrical Activity

EMS Emergency Medical Service or System

EMST Emergency Management of Severe Trauma course (similar to ATLS)

EMT Emergency Medical Technician/paramedic; a trained professional who delivers emergency pre-hospital care

EN Enrolled Nurse

epinephrine A vasopressor drug used in resuscitation and treatment of anaphylaxis (US); 'Epi' or adrenaline

ER Emergency Room (US); a dedicated area in a hospital for the treatment of emergencies

ETCO$_2$ End-tidal carbon dioxide

ETI Endotracheal Intubation

ETT Endotracheal Tube

EUROSIM Federation of European Simulation Societies

FAA Federal Aviation Authority (US)

FAST Focused Assessment with Sonography for Trauma

FBC/FBP Full Blood Count/Picture

FDA Food and Drug Administration (US)

flipped classroom A reversal of traditional teaching where students gain first exposure to new material outside of class, usually via reading or lecture videos, and then class time is used for assimilating knowledge through strategies such as problem-solving, discussion, or debates

FLS Fundamentals of Laparoscopic Surgery course

FOI Fibre-optic Intubation; Freedom of Information

FRC Functional Residual Capacity

FSEMC Flight Simulator Engineering Maintenance Committee

FSTC Flight Simulator Technical Committee

FTE Full-time Equivalent; workload of an employed person

gamification Using gaming concepts outside the gaming industry

GAS Gainesville Anesthesia Simulator; anaesthesia (slang)

GMC General Medical Council (UK)

GME Graduate Medical Education

GP General (Family) Practitioner

graded assertiveness A communication system expressing increasing levels of concern during a crisis, using a tool such 'PACE(R)'

H&P History and Physical examination

handoff Transfer of care from one person to another (US)

handover Transfer of care from one person to another (UK)

haptics Relating to devices or systems which provide a user force feedback; a sense of touching or feeling an object represented in a virtual environment, in particular relating to the perception and manipulation of objects

HBD Here Be Dragons (dangerous or unexplored territories in a game or activity)

HDMI A proprietary audio/video interface

HEADSS/HEEADSSS An acronym for the topics that a physician wants to be sure to cover: home, education, (eating), activities/employment, drugs, suicidality, sex, (safety)

HLM Heart–Lung Machine

HMD Head-mounted Display

house officer A first-, second-, or third-year medical graduate (resident) who has not commenced specialty training

HPS Human Patient Simulator (a CAE Healthcare product)

HRO High-reliability Organization

HTA Hierarchical Task Analysis

HTN Hypertension

HR Human Resources

IABP Intra-aortic Balloon Pump

IAFSTA International Airline Flight Simulator Technical Association

IATA International Air Transport Association

IBM International Business Machines

IC Integrated Circuit

ICC Intercostal Catheter (a chest drainage tube)

ICAO International Civil Aviation Organization

ICD Implantable Cardioverter-Defibrillator (AICD)

ICP Intra-cranial Pressure

ICU Intensive Care Unit; a dedicated ward for the care of critically ill patients

IFCS Intelligent Flight Control Systems

IJ Internal Jugular (vein or catheter)

ILCOR International Liaison Committee on Resuscitation

ILS Immediate Life Support (course)

I'M SAFE Illness, Medication, Stress, Alcohol, Fatigue, Eating. From the FAA checklist for pilots prior to flying. Also used in healthcare.

IMSH International Meeting on Simulation in Healthcare

INASCL International Nursing Association for Simulation and Clinical Learning

intensive care physician Intensivist; a medical specialist in intensive care medicine

intern Intern, or first-year resident; a first-year medical graduate

internist Internal medicine physician (US)

IPE Interprofessional Education

IPL Interprofessional Learning

IPP Interprofessional Practice

IPPB/IPPV Intermittent Positive Pressure Breathing/Ventilation

IPPI Integrated Procedural Performance Instrument

IRAS Interactive Real-time Audio System

IRB Institutional Review Board

ISBAR/ISOBAR a handover tool:
      Identify who you are
      Situation—describe the problem
      Observations (vital signs)
      Background—clinical context
      Assessment—what you think is going on
      Recommendation/requirement—what you think needs to be done, what you need the other person to do

ISS In-situ Simulation; simulation activities done at the workplace

IT Information Technology

ITU Intensive Therapy Unit (UK); dedicated ward for the care of critically ill patients

IV Intravenous (line, catheter, cannula)

JCAHO Joint Commission on Accreditation of Healthcare Organizations (US); now known as Joint Commission

JiTT Just-in-Time Teaching

JSST Japan Society for Simulation Technology

knobology Familiarity with controls on an instrument or device

KSB Knowledge, Skills, Behaviour

KSS(H) Korea Society for Simulation (in Healthcare)

L&D Labour and Delivery

LA Local Anaesthetic or Left Atrium

LCD Liquid Crystal Display

LCME Liaison Committee on Medical Education; an accrediting body for educational programmes at schools of medicine in the US & Canada

LED Light Emitting Diodes

LGBTQIA Lesbian, Gay, Bisexual, Transsexual, Queer, Intersex, Asexual

lidocaine A local anaesthetic drug, also used in treatment of arrhythmias (US)

lignocaine A local anaesthetic drug, also used in treatment of arrhythmias

LIPSERVICE An acronym for successful communication: Language; Introduction; Privacy dignity and cultural issues; Subjective questioning; Examination; Review; Verdict; Information; Check understanding; End or exit

LMA Laryngeal Mask Airway; 'Larry' (slang)

LOE Line Operational Evaluation (aviation)

LOFT Line Oriented Flight Training

LPN Licensed Practical Nurse (US)

LR Lactated Ringers intravenous solution

lux The SI unit of illuminance

LVAD Left Ventricular Assist Device

lytes Electrolytes (slang)

MCC Medical Council of Canada

MCQ Multiple Choice Question (or Examination)

MEPA Managing Emergencies in Paediatric Anaesthesia (course)

meperidine Pethidine, an opioid drug (US), Demerol®

MET/MERT Medical Emergency Team; Medical Emergency Response Team

MFM Maternal Foetal Medicine

MICU Mobile Intensive Care Unit; a specialized ambulance

Mini-CEX Mini Clinical Exercise

Mini-PAT Mini Peer-assessment Tool

MMVR Medicine Meets Virtual Reality conference

MOCA Maintenance of Certification in Anesthesiology (American Board of Anesthesiology®)

MOPS Maintenance of Professional Standards; a formal system of further education in a medical, nursing, or paramedical field

MRI Magnetic Resonance Imaging

MSF Multi-source Feedback

MSR Israel Centre for Medical Simulation

MUVE Multi-user Virtual Environments

NASA National Aeronautics and Space Administration

NASCAR National Association of Stock Car Auto Racing

NBOME National Board of Osteopathic Medical Examiners (US)

NCSBN National Council of State Boards of Nursing (US)

NHS National Health Service (UK)

NICE National Institute for Clinical Excellence (UK)

NLN National League of Nursing

NMB Neuromuscular Blockade or Blocker (paralysing drug)

nor-adrenaline A vasopressor drug used in resuscitation and treatment of cardiovascular emergencies

nor-epinephrine A vasopressor drug used in resuscitation and treatment of cardiovascular emergencies (US)

NOTSS Non-technical Skills for Surgeons

NPA Naso-pharyngeal Airway

NPC A non-playable character (gaming)

NS Normal Saline (IV solution)

NTS Non-technical Skills

nurse anaesthetist A nurse who has undergone training in the field of anaesthesia; a CRNA (often shortened to anesthetist in the US)

NZSSH New Zealand Society for Simulation in Healthcare

OB/GYN Obstetrics & Gynaecology; 'O&G'

observations or 'obs' A set of clinical measurements of a patient: temperature, pulse, respirations (rate), blood pressure ± pain score; vital signs

ODA Operating Department Assistant: an anaesthesia assistant (UK)

ODD Oesophageal Detector Device

OR Operating Room (US); a dedicated area where surgery is performed

OSATS Objective Structured Assessment of Technical Skills

OSCE Objective Structured Clinical Examination

OOW Out of Warranty

OT Operating Theatre; a dedicated area where surgery is performed; also Occupational Therapy

OPQRST-AAA Mnemonic used for assessment of a patient's symptoms of an acute illness; Onset of the event; Provocation or palliation; Quality of the pain; Region and radiation; Severity; Time (history). AAA adds Aggravating/alleviating factors, Associated symptoms, Attributions/adaptations.

PA Physician Assistant; also Personal Assistant

PACE(R) A graded assertiveness tool for speaking up: Probe, Alert, Challenge, Emergency, (React)

PACU Post-anaesthesia Care Unit; a Recovery Room

PALS Paediatric Advanced Life Support

PBL(D) Problem-based Learning (Discussion)

PC Personal Computer or Politically Correct

PEA Pulseless Electrical Activity; formerly EMD (Electro-mechanical Dissociation)

PEARLS Promoting Excellence and Reflective Learning in Simulation

pedagogy The method and practice of teaching

pethidine An opioid drug; meperidine (Demerol®, US)

PFS Patient-focused Simulation

PHTLS Pre-hospital Trauma Life Support (course)

PICU Paediatric Intensive Care Unit

PPE Personal Protection Equipment

PPH Post-partum Haemorrhage

PRP Performance Review Panel

Pre-briefing The practice of releasing relevant information to participants in an immersive course to enhance their preparation. Similar to briefing

PSS Patient-specific Simulation

PT Physiotherapist; Physical Therapist (US); a person trained in physiotherapy

PTZ Pan Tilt Zoom (camera movement)

QI Quality Improvement

QSEN Quality and Safety Education for Nurses

RA Right Atrial or Room Air

RACE Acronym for fire emergencies: Rescue, Alert, Confine, Extinguish

R&D Research and Development

radiographer A person trained to safely operate X-ray apparatus; an X-ray technician (US)

RCA Root Cause Analysis

read-back The practice of repeating instructions to enhance communication

Red Blanket Protocol Rapid transfer of a trauma patient from the Emergency Department to the Operating Suite

registrar A trainee in a medical specialty

reification Making an abstract concept appear as something concrete with which a person can interact or creating a data model for a previously abstract concept

resident A junior doctor; a house officer

residency A medical specialty training programme (US)

RN Registered Nurse

ROI Return on Investment

ROSC Return of Spontaneous Circulation

Royal College of Anaesthetists A medical specialty organization responsible for accrediting specialist anaesthetists (UK)

RR Recovery Room; a dedicated ward that receives patients following anaesthesia and/or surgery; PACU

RRC Residency Review Committee

RRS Rapid Response System

RRT Rapid Response Team

RSI Rapid-sequence Induction (also known as Crash Induction)

RS232 An electrical engineering communication standard ('Recommend Standard number 232')

RT Respiratory Technician (UK) or Respiratory Therapist (US); a person trained in respiratory and ventilator care

SAD Supraglottic Airway Device

SAED Semi-automatic External Defibrillator

SAEM Society for Academic Emergency Medicine

salbutamol A common bronchodilator drug; albuterol (US)

SAMPLE History mnemonic acronym to remember key questions for a person's assessment: Signs and Symptoms; Allergies; Medications; Pertinent medical history, injuries, illnesses; Last meal/intake; Events leading up to the injury and/or illness. See also AMPLE history.

SBAR A handover tool; see ISBAR

SBE Simulation-based Education

SBT Simulation-based training

SCOAP Surgical Care and Outcomes Assessment Programme

SD Shoulder Dystocia

serious game A game or entertaining activity with a purpose other than strict entertainment

SESAM Society in Europe for Simulation Applied to Medicine

SETGO What the student Saw
What Else the group saw
What the student Thinks
What Goal do we want to achieve
Any Offers of how we get there?

SIG Special Interest Group

SimCentre Simulation Centre

SimHealth Annual Conference of Australian Society of Simulation in Healthcare

SimOps A Simulation Operations Specialist

SimTecT Annual Simulation Technology and Training Conference held by Simulation Australia

simulationist A professional involved in providing simulation activities, products, and services

SimWars A competition, in which interprofessional teams demonstrate communication, teamwork, and clinical management skills in a simulated environment

SIRC Simulation Innovation Resource Center (US)

Six Sigma A set of techniques and tools for process improvement

SME Subject-matter Expert

SMS Strategic Management Simulations or Short Message Service (a mobile phone text message)

SNAPPI A call-out tool for review during an emergency:
Stand back and get the attention of the team
Notify the team of patient status (vital signs, etc.)
Assessment of the situation (what you think is going on)
Proposed plan for treatment
Priorities (what needs to be done first, etc.)
Invite ideas and suggestions

SNAPPS An acronym; where the trainee:
Summarizes the case
Narrows the differential diagnosis
Analyses the differential diagnosis
Probes (the learner asks the teacher about areas they don't understand)
Plans management
Selects an issue for self-directed learning

SOM School of Medicine

SOP Standard Operating Procedure

SP Standardized Patient

SPLINTS Scrub Practitioners' List of Intraoperative Non-technical Skills

SpO$_2$ Oxygen saturation—measured by a pulse oximeter

SPOT Student Perception of Teaching

SPRAT Sheffield Peer-review Assessment Tool

SSH The Society for Simulation in Healthcare

SSI Surgical Site Infection

STA Society for Technology in Anesthesia

Sterile Cockpit Rule Avoiding unnecessary communication during a critical procedure

succinylcholine A short-acting muscle relaxant (US); often called 'sux'

suxamethonium A short-acting muscle relaxant (UK); often called 'sux'

S-video A signalling standard for standard-definition video

TATRC Telemedicine and Advanced Technology Research Center (US Army)

TBT Team-building Training

TCP/IP Transmission Control Protocol/Internet Protocol: a suite of communications protocols used to connect computers on the Internet

TeamSTEPPS An evidence-based teamwork system to improve communication and teamwork skills among healthcare professionals

TEE Trans-esophageal Echocardiography (US)

TLX Task Load Index

TOE Trans-oesophageal Echocardiography

TTO Team Time Out (World Health Organization Surgical Safety Checklist)

TTV/TTJV Trans-tracheal Ventilation; Trans-tracheal Jet Ventilation

Two-challenge Rule One team member may assume the duties of another team member who fails to respond to two consecutive challenges (from aviation)

U&E Urea and Electrolytes

UCLA University of California at Los Angeles

UPS Universal Patient Simulator (a Laerdal product)

USB Universal Serial Bus; an interface standard to allow peripheral devices to be connected to computers

USMLE United States Medical Licensing Examination

USP United States Pharmacopeia

VE Virtual Environment

VGA Video Graphics Array (display standard)

vital signs A set of clinical measurements of a patient: temperature, pulse, respirations (rate), blood pressure ± pain score

viva (or viva voce) An oral examination

VOP Volume of Practice; the number of each type of clinical procedure undertaken during training period

VR Virtual Reality; a computer-simulated environment that gives a sense of being present in a virtual environment and within which a participant can interact in a seemingly real or physical way

Index